Infant Nutrition and Feeding

Edited by R. Mauricio Barría

Published in London, United Kingdom

Infant Nutrition and Feeding
http://dx.doi.org/10.5772/intechopen.104345
Edited by R. Mauricio Barría

Contributors
Alejandra Itzel Contreras Rivas, Alex Kojo Anderson, Alex Luiz Pozzobon Pereira, Alex Tumusiime, Aryal Laxmi, Bernal Galicia Claudia, Brenda Nabawanuka, Carolina Roldão, Christyann Lima Campos Batista, Clement Munguiko, Dhaliwal Dolly, Edgar M. Vasquez Garibay, Emmanuel Kimera, Enos Mirembe Masereka, Erkihun Tadesse Amsalu, Francisco Hernández Fragoso, Gabriela Padilla Mendoza, Gaston Eduardo Estudillo Jimenez, Gill Rubina, Haseeb Yumna B, Haythem Bachrouche, Imtihanatun Najahah, Isai Natan Yescas Osorio, Jan Sorensen, Julian Aryampa, Kathy Whyte, Kenyonyozi Rubagumya, Linda Grace Alanyo, Lucas Amanda, M. Carmen Vidal-Carou, M. Luz Latorre-Moratalla, M. Teresa Veciana-Nogués, Md. Jannatul Ferdaus, Monika Jain, Nega Degefa Degefa, Nelly C. Muñoz-Esparza, Oriol Comas-Basté, Patricia Triviño Vargas, Prince Kwabena Osei, Priya R. Hegde, Ramya Koneru, Rekha Lakashetti, Roberta Claro Silva, Shambel Aychew Tsegaw, Sinead M. M Hurley, Vandana, Vinutha U. Muktamath, Yeshimebet Ali Dawed

First published in London, United Kingdom, 2024 by IntechOpen
IntechOpen is the global imprint of INTECHOPEN LIMITED, registered in England and Wales, registration number: 11086078, 167-169 Great Portland Street, London, W1W 5PF, United Kingdom

British Library Cataloguing-in-Publication Data
A catalogue record for this book is available from the British Library

Additional hard and PDF copies can be obtained from orders@intechopen.com

Infant Nutrition and Feeding
Edited by R. Mauricio Barría
p. cm.
Print ISBN 978-1-83768-553-0
Online ISBN 978-1-83768-554-7
eBook (PDF) ISBN 978-1-83768-555-4

For EU product safety concerns:
IN TECH d.o.o., Prolaz Marije Krucifikse Kozulić 3, 51000 Rijeka, Croatia,
info@intechopen.com or visit our website at intechopen.com.

Meet the editor

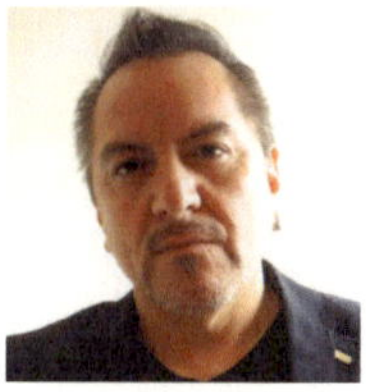

Dr. Mauricio Barría is a nurse, master of science in clinical epidemiology (MSc), and doctor in public health (DrPH). He is an associate professor at the Faculty of Medicine of the Universidad Austral de Chile, where he has been the creator and director of the Evidence-Based Health Office (2010–2017) and is currently director of the Institute of Nursing (since 2017). His areas of undergraduate and graduate teaching and research include maternal-child health, neonatal care, and evidence-based practice. He has conducted numerous research projects and has already published over 70 articles. Additionally, Dr. Barría serves on the editorial board and acts as a peer reviewer for journals in the fields of nursing, pediatrics, and public health.

Contents

Preface

Infant nutrition, particularly during the first years of life, is a crucial aspect of child-care, given its implications for future health. Despite ongoing concerns about this issue and the implementation of various public policies aimed at recommending and promoting optimal infant feeding practices, which should result in the best nutritional and health outcomes, there are still gaps and difficulties in different contexts and among the most vulnerable groups.

In this context, this book compiles experiences and thematic reviews on diverse domains of child nutrition and feeding, particularly during the initial two years. Through 16 chapters distributed across four sections, it presents an updated overview of the subject matter.

In the initial section, "Lactation, Human Milk and Formula Milk: Components and Effects" Chapter 1 presents a comprehensive analysis of the fundamental elements pertaining to the composition, characteristics, and stages of human milk. Furthermore, it offers a detailed account of the effects of breastfeeding on child growth and development, cognitive and socioemotional development, nutritional status, and childhood morbidity and mortality. Chapter 2 provides an overview of the fundamental elements of exclusive breastfeeding, including a description of the composition and functioning of breast milk, the factors associated with the initiation and maintenance of exclusive breastfeeding, and the benefits of its maintenance. Additionally, it outlines the actions that health professionals can take to promote and support EBF. In Chapter 3, the influence of breast milk on the modulation of epigenetic factors in the early stages of life, which have a protective effect on later development, is analyzed based on the developmental origins of health and disease (DOHaD) theory. It is then explained that, given that not all children are breastfed and according to the differential composition of breast milk and milk formula, it is necessary to study which components are necessary to incorporate into milk formulas in order to reduce the gap between children who receive breast milk and artificial formula. Chapter 4 then reviews the impact of polyamines on infant growth and health, the polyamine content in human milk, and how it is influenced by mother-infant interaction. The polyamine contents and profiles of human milk and infant formulas are compared. Finally, the section concludes with Chapter 5, which examines the composition of baby formula made from soy, rice, goat milk, and cow's milk and discusses nutrient bioaccessibility and protein functioning characteristics that are relevant to infant formula. Additionally, the necessity of studying whether the biochemical properties of infant formulas affect their composition is highlighted.

The second section, entitled "Infant Feeding Overview and Perspectives", commences with Chapter 6, which analyzes the recommendations for infant feeding during the first two years of life. The contents of this chapter include an examination of prelacteal nutrition, the composition and benefits of human milk, the practice of exclusive breastfeeding, the types of milk formulas and complementary feeding, and the essential elements required to meet the nutritional needs of infants. Chapter 7 provides a comprehensive overview of the landscape of current infant feeding patterns and cultural practices in different regions of the world. It also highlights the multiple drivers and barriers to exclusive breastfeeding in various regions. Chapter 8 shares the results of a study carried out in a rural area of India, Saharanpur. Among its findings, the study highlighted that the feeding practices of children and infants in this area are not satisfactory and that exclusive breastfeeding at the sixth month is not fully complied with. It is argued that an approach focused on generating awareness and efforts to improve infant feeding practices is required to eradicate malnutrition among rural children. Poverty alleviation programs, adult education programs, and a communication approach more focused on behavioral change on the part of workers are therefore proposed. The section ends with Chapter 9, which provides comprehensive information on suboptimal infant feeding practices and the factors that contribute to them. The chapter concludes that a multifaceted approach is necessary to address the socioeconomic, maternal, familial, and environmental factors that contribute to suboptimal infant feeding practices.

The third section, entitled "Infant Nutrition and Feeding for Infants with Special Problems" is devoted to the presentation of various contexts and special situations in which children must engage in the process of feeding. Chapter 10 addresses the care and feeding of premature infants during their hospital stay and then at home, with a particular focus on feeding difficulties and monitoring the growth and development of premature infants. Chapter 11 provides an overview of the use of human milk in the context of the neonatal intensive care unit (NICU), including a description of the differences between term and premature milk, milk collection, labeling, and storage techniques. Furthermore, the chapter examines the impact of breast milk intake on neurodevelopment in these at-risk children. Chapter 12 analyzes the initial diet of small-for-gestational-age children and presents a discussion based on available evidence regarding the optimal diet for these children to reduce the risk of developing diseases and disorders in the future. This section concludes with Chapter 13, which presents the findings of a prospective cohort study involving more than 200 mother–newborn dyads. The study evaluated the outcomes of children with ankyloglossia and the potential influence of this condition on exclusive breastfeeding and growth.

Finally, the fourth section, entitled "Breastfeeding Interventions" describes the various aspects and interventions that are necessary to promote successful breastfeeding. Chapter 14 discusses the cost-effectiveness and equity of breastfeeding interventions, highlighting the influence of social differences on the maintenance of breastfeeding practices. This chapter illustrates the application of the distributional cost-effectiveness (DCEA) framework to these interventions and how some interventions may be more effective in changing the behavior and outcomes of mothers with different socioeconomic statuses. This can be used to change inequality in effectiveness and improve equity in health. Chapter 15 analyzes and provides recommendations on evidence-based infant feeding intervention strategies for mothers, students, and health professionals. The promotion of breastfeeding is a notable example of an intervention that must be implemented at the individual, community, and political levels to improve the optimal general practice of this type of feeding. The section and the book conclude with Chapter 16, which emphasizes the importance of health education in the context of neonatal hospitalization and highlights the need to implement programs to promote breastfeeding as a vital support to develop parenting skills in mothers and fathers in neonatal units to sustain breastfeeding and obtain its multiple benefits. This chapter examines the applicability of the Ramona Mercer model as a comprehensive support for the mother's acquisition of knowledge.

As previously stated, this book addresses various aspects of infant nutrition and feeding, thereby encompassing a number of topics of interest to health professionals engaged in childcare. Its objective is to facilitate the experience and understanding of this phenomenon, thereby enabling the implementation of optimal practices in the context of nutrition.

I would like to express my gratitude to all the authors who, through their contributions based on their experience and intellectual dedication, have enabled the development of this thought-provoking book, which should prove useful for professionals involved in children's food and nutrition.

R. Mauricio Barría
Faculty of Medicine,
Institute of Nursing,
Universidad Austral de Chile,
Valdivia, Chile

Section 1

Lactation, Human Milk and Formula Milk: Components and Effects

Chapter 1

Breastfeeding Practices and Infant Development Outcomes

Vinutha U. Muktamath, Priya R. Hegde, Ramya Koneru and Rekha Lakkashetti

Abstract

The biochemistry of human milk contains a vast amount of knowledge and information that was previously un-recognised and unknown. The neonate and infant receive both nutritive and non-nutritive signals from milk, according to evidence. There is strong evidence that early, continuous breast feeding for 23 months significantly lowers neonatal and child mortality on a global scale. Breast feeding is the gold standard for an infant's survival, health, and development, according to scientific research. Due to its nutritional, immunological, and psychological advantages, it is thought to be the best start for infant life. To achieve the best possible growth, development, and health, the World Health Organisation advises mothers to exclusively breastfeed their infants for the first six months of their lives, then continue to do so while supplementing with the right foods until they are two years old or older. Infant developmental milestones and outcomes like cognitive development, socio- emotional development, psychomotor development, and language development have been linked to both the components of breast milk and the act of breast feeding.

Keywords: human milk, nutritive signals, survival, exclusively breast fed, developmental outcomes

1. Introduction

Infant health studies conducted around the world have primarily centered on and focused to understand the complex factors, both positive and negative affecting the infant's health. Given that childhood under nutrition is one of the most significant public health issues, breastfeeding is one of the most important issues for research on infant mortality and morbidity. It is estimated that 35% of deaths in children under the age of five in the world can be attributed to malnutrition. Early breastfeeding initiation, exclusive breastfeeding for the first six months of life, adequate, timely, and appropriate complementary feeding from six to 24 months of age, continued breastfeeding following the introduction of complementary foods, adequate dietary diversity in complementary foods, and adequate frequency of meals are all aspects of infant and young child feeding (IYCF) that are crucial in the first two years of life.

Breastfeeding is considered as the gold standard for an infant's survival, health, and development due to its nutritional, immunological, and psychological advantages, it is thought to be the best start for infant life. To achieve the best possible growth, development, and health, the World Health Organisation advises mothers to exclusively breastfeed their infants for the first six months of their lives, then continue to do so while supplementing with the right foods until they are two years old or older. According to WHO fact files from 2015, the first 28 days of life account for 44% of deaths in children under five [1]. Globally, the rates of exclusive breastfeeding up to 6 months of age is slightly better in South Asia (44%) as compared to dismal figures of 20% for Central and European nations [https://www.unicef.org/ info by country/ India statistics.html].

Breastfeeding (BF) is the act of transferring human milk from a mother to her infant, in which case the baby takes the milk directly from the mother's breast. Additionally, Exclusive Breastfeeding (EBF) means that the infant receives no other type of milk or liquid including water, infant formula and other pre-lacteal feeds for the first six months except vitamins and medicines. Breastfeeding is the best way to give babies the ideal nutrition they need for healthy growth and development. It is also an essential part of the reproductive process with significant health benefits for mothers. As long as they have access to accurate information and have the support of their family, the healthcare system, and society at large, almost all mothers can successfully breastfeed. The WHO advises using colostrum, the yellowish, sticky breast milk produced at the end of pregnancy, as the ideal food for the newborn, and that feeding should begin within the first hour of delivery. For the baby, human milk is regarded as being "hand crafted" or "well-suited" because of its benefits to the infant's nutritional needs, immune system, and psychological development; hence it is thought to be the best start to life [2–4].

Improvements in breastfeeding rates are critical to the attainment of the Millennium Development Goals and Post-2015 Sustainable Development Goals, especially to reduce the child mortality and improving maternal health. Adequate breastfeeding counselling and support are essential for mothers and families to initiate and maintain optimal breastfeeding practices. Because of its nutritional, anti-infective, and biological qualities, human milk has been referred to as the best food for human growth and development. It is also known to provide a lot of advantages to the growing infant. Infant developmental milestones and outcomes have been linked to both the components of breast milk and nursing as a primary factor. The achievement of the Millennium Development Goals and Post-2015 Sustainable Development Goals, particularly to reduce child mortality and improve maternal health, depends on improving successful breastfeeding practice rates. For mothers and families to start and continue optimal breastfeeding practices, adequate breastfeeding counselling and support are crucial. Because of its nutritional, anti-infective, and biological qualities, human milk has been referred to as the best food for human growth and development. It is also known to provide a number of advantages to the growing child. Breastfeeding practices and its components have both been linked to significant influences on the developmental milestones and outcomes of infants [5–7].

2. Human milk composition and the empirical evidence

A consistent and substantial evidence extensively indicates that early, exclusive, and continuous breastfeeding for 23 months significantly lowers neonatal and child mortality. According to an estimate, initiating breastfeeding within the first hour of birth could prevent 20% of neonatal deaths, according to a technical brief on the effect of early breastfeeding initiation on newborn deaths. Additionally, it was discovered that starting breastfeeding within 24 hours of birth is linked to a 44–45% lower relative risk (RR) of neonatal mortality from all causes and infection-related mortality. Suboptimal breastfeeding is linked to increased incidence of pneumonia, diarrhoea, morbidity and mortality among infants in the age range of 0–5 months and never breastfed children in 6–23 months of age. Every year about 800,000 child deaths occurs due to inadequate breastfeeding practices [8].

There is a vast body of knowledge and research on the biochemistry of human milk. The analysis of milk composition is now more sensitive, fast, and resolving thanks to improvements in analytical techniques. Compounds that had not previously been discovered or recognised have been found. We now know that milk gives a newborn both nutritionally important and non-nutritional signals. The milk is more nutrient-dense when the offspring develops quickly, and more nutrient-deficient when it does so slowly. All milks contain minerals, vitamins, proteins, and other nutrients in addition to fat, carbohydrates, and proteins. Lipids are organised in milk composition as emulsified globules coated with a membrane, proteins are dispersed colloidally as micelles, and the remaining components are a true solution. A single meal is insufficient at all other times in life.

Human milk is a mammary gland secretion which changes the composition and is not a uniform body fluid. Hind milk and foremilk are completely distinct with each other and compared to them, colostrum is different. Milk varies by the time of day. Physical properties like osmolarity and pH change as protein, fat, carbohydrate, mineral, and cell concentrations vary. It is becoming clearer how compositional changes affect the infant gut's physiology. Many constituents serve multiple purposes, including nutrition and immunity or a variety of other effects.

2.1 Stages of human milk

Colostrum, transitional milk, and mature milk are the three stages in the continuum of human milk according to traditional nomenclature, and their respective contents are important for newborns physiologic adjustment to extra-uterine life (**Table 1**).

2.1.1 Colostrum

During the first few days, colostrums, a thick, yellowish fluid, makes up the mammary secretion. Colostrums are formed when the residual mixture of substances in the mammary glands and ducts at delivery and immediately after gradually combines with freshly secreted milk. It is well known that the nature and relative proportions of the components of human colostrum differ from those of mature milk. Colostrum's yellow colour is due to –carotene; and it high ash content as well higher concentrations of sodium, potassium, and chloride than in mature milk. Compared to transitional or mature milk, more protein, fat-soluble vitamins, and minerals are present. The concentrations of Lactoferrin and secretary immunoglobulin A (SIgA) rise. At this point, the oligosaccharides, which are complex sugars, also increase and contribute to the infection protection properties in infants.

The development of Lactobacillus bifidus flora in the digestive tract and meconium passage are both made easier by colostrum. Antibodies found in human colostrum may offer defence against bacteria and viruses found in the birth canal and

Milk elements	Colostrum	Transitional	Mature	Cow milk
Lactose (g)	—	—	72.0 ± 2.5 (7%)	4.8%
Protein (g)	—	—	10.5 ± 2 (0.9%)	3.5%
Fat (g)	—	—	39.0 ± 4.0 (3.8%)	3.7%
Vitamin A (μg)	151.0	88.0	75.0	41.0
Vitamin B_1 (μg)	1.9	5.9	14.0	43.0
Vitamin B_2 (μg)	30.0	37.0	40.0	145.0
Nicotinic acid (μg)	75.0	175.0	160.0	82.0
Vitamin B_6 (μg)	—	—	12.0–15.0	64.0
Pantothenic acid (μg)	183.0	288.0	246.0	340.0
Biotin (μg)	0.06	0.35	0.6	2.8
Folic acid (μg)	0.05	0.02	0.14	0.13
Vitamin B_{12} (μg)	0.05	0.04	0.1	0.6
Vitamin C (mg)	5.9	7.1	5.0	1.1
Vitamin D (μg)	—	—	0.04	0.02
Vitamin E (mg)	1.5	0.9	0.25	0.07
Vitamin K (μg)	—	—	1.5	6.0
Ash (g)	0.3	0.3	0.2	0.7
Calories (kcal)	57.0	63.0	65.0	65.0
Specific gravity	1050.0	1035.0	1031.0	1032.0
Milk (pH)	—	—	7.0	6.8

Source: Food and Nutrition Board, National Research Council, National Academy of Sciences: Recommended Dietary Allowances, ed 10 [9].

Table 1.
Vitamin and other constituents of human milk and cow milk (per Deciliter).

those brought on by other human contact. The newborn's requirements and reserves at birth are met by the colostrum's high protein and low-fat content. The development of Lactobacillus bifidus flora in the digestive tract and meconium passage are both made easier by colostrum. The abundance of antibodies in human colostrum may offer defence against the germs and viruses found in the birth canal and those brought on by contact with other people. The newborn's needs and reserves at birth are met by the high protein and low-fat content of colostrum. Uric acid and an antioxidant that resembles ascorbate are both present in colostrum and these anti-oxidants may act in the colostrum as filters for reactive oxygen metabolites produced by neutrophils. The enzymatic processes of polymorphonuclear leukocytes and oxygen metabolism are interfered with by the aqueous human colostrum providing evidence to the theory that human milk is anti-inflammatory.

2.1.2 Transitional milk

Transitional milk is the milk produced between the colostrum and mature milk stages; its composition gradually changes and the period lasts roughly from 7 to 10 days after delivery to 2 weeks after delivery. While lactose, fat, and total calorie content rise, immunoglobulin concentration and total protein content fall. The levels of fat-soluble vitamins fall to those of mature milk while the water-soluble vitamin levels rise.

2.1.3 Mature milk

With the exception of some arctic and aquatic species that produce milks with high fat content (for example, the northern fur seal produces milk with 54% fat and 65% total solids), water makes up the majority of almost all mammalian milks. Water dissolves, disperses, or suspends all other components and due to the evaporation of water from the lungs and skin it accounts for 25% of heat loss and thus helps the newborn's body to regulate its temperature.

2.2 Benefits of human milk to infants growth and development

It provides optimum fluidity and warmth; and is very economical and convenient. Physiologically it has high lactose content and is the sweetest milk. The protein is simple to digest. Long chain polyunsaturated fats (LCP), phospholipids, and precursors to prostaglandins are all abundant and provides enzymes like amylase, lipoprotein lipase, bile salt stimulated lipases (BSSL), oxidases, lactoperoxidases, leucocyte myeloperoxidases, etc. These enzymes aid in digestion and serve as a barrier against microbes. Additionally, it contains growth modulators, growth promoters, and growth regulators. LCPs, docosahexaenoic acid (DHA) and aracidonic acid (ARA)) reduce hyperactivity and promote brain growth.

Breast milk is biochemically superior. Whey protein makes up the majority of the protein (80%), and casein makes up 20%. Whey protein is high in lactoferrin and lactalbumin. Tryptophan, the building block of serotonin, a crucial neurotransmitter, is abundant in lactalbumin. Lactoferrin is bacteriostatic and ensures iron and zinc absorption and binds iron and prevents the bacteria from accessing it. Human milk does not contain the allergens Alph-casein and Lactoglobulin. Despite the lower protein content, non-protein nitrogens are more abundant in breast milk. The infant's growth and development are significantly influenced by the non-protein nitrogen in breast milk. It also contains a lot of proteins that bind substances like vitamin D, B12, and thyroxin. Calcium absorption is guaranteed because the calcium-phosphorous ratio is greater than two; and absorption of calcium and magnesium is aided by lactose. The lack of certain minerals in whey protein lowers solute load guarantees a mild load on an infant's developing kidney. The best vitamins and minerals, including calcium, iron, and zinc, are also provided at the same time in order to meet the needs of infant growth [10–14].

3. Breastfeeding and cognitive development

Cognitive development is the intellectual equivalent of a person's biological adaptation to their environment. It describes the progressive and ongoing growth of perception, memory, imagination, conception, judgement, and reason. Additionally, cognition includes the mental processes involved in understanding information as well as the process of acquiring, organising, retaining, and applying knowledge. Following that, this knowledge is applied to problem-solving and generalisation to new situations.

From conception to age five, a variety of processes are included in early child development. It occurs concurrently with growth and describes the maturation of the function of picking up skills, behaviours, and values, as well as environmental adaptation. The complex process of a child's cognitive development is influenced by both genetic and environmental factors. The child's capacity for cognitive development is genetically determined. The child's cognitive development, however, may also be positively impacted by environmental factors, such as adequate nutrition and the parents' capacity to create a pleasant and stimulating home environment [15, 16]. Numerous studies have found a link between breastfeeding and children's cognitive development. Science has been studying the impact of breastfeeding on infant health and development for many years. Extensive research has looked at how breastfeeding affects the development of the brain, particularly two aspects of brain development: cognitive development and the development of visual acuity. There is a significant correlation between the length of exclusive breastfeeding and test results in the vocabulary and similarity tests as well as cognitive IQ [8, 17]. Among the benefits attributed to feeding children with human milk in comparison with substitutes such as infant formula, breastfeeding is also associated with advanced language development, high scores on vocabulary tests and very sensitive to speech stimuli [17–20]. Evidence is emerging that DHA is important in neural and visual development of preterm as well as term infants, especially for retinal and brain development [21, 22].

3.1 Essential fatty acids and brain development

The final trimester of pregnancy and the first six months of life are when the human brain grows more rapidly. The major building blocks of neural tissues are adequate long chain polyunsaturated fatty acids (LCPUFAs), such as docosahexaenoic acid (DHA; 22:6n-3) and arachidonic acid (AA; 20:4n-6). DHA is crucial for the development of the central nervous system during this growth spurt because it makes up up to 50% of the phospholipids in the retina and cerebral cortex. The main source of DHA and AA is breast milk. Because LCPUFA precursors have a low capacity for elongation and de-saturation, infants can only synthesise a small amount of LCPUFAs. There is mounting evidence that DHA plays a critical role in the neural and visual development of both term and preterm infants [23]. There is evidence that breastfeeding promotes increased white matter development in the later maturing frontal and association brain regions of children. In several brain regions, there are also positive relationships between breastfeeding duration and white matter microstructure that are anatomically in line with the observed enhancements in cognitive and behavioural performance measures [21, 22, 24].

3.2 Lactose as a source of galactose

As a readily available source of galactose, lactose is necessary for the synthesis of galactolipids, including cerebroside, which is crucial for the growth of the CNS (Central Nervous System). The relationship between amount of lactose content in a species' milk and its brain's relative size varies; with human milk having the highest levels of both and this is found to influence early language expression and comprehension measures in term infants and toddlers. When compared to breastfed infants, formula-fed infants with DHA supplements are found to score lower on receptive and expressive vocabulary tests at 14 months of age [25].

3.3 Immunoglobulins, hormone and growth factor content

Additionally, breast milk contains immunoglobulins, growth factors, and hormones like neurotensin, nerve growth factor, sialylated oligosaccharides, and thyroid stimulating hormone that are not present in formula milk but are essential for the functional development of the brain during the foetal and neonatal periods. T4 is the main form of hormonal iodine found in breast milk, whereas iodide is the only maternally derived component found in infant formulae (the inorganic form of iodine). Iodine deficiency has long-lasting effects on development because it prevents the production of thyroid hormone.

Hormonal iodine in breast milk is found as T_4, while infant formulae are devoid of such maternally-derived factors but contain iodide which is the inorganic form of iodine. Iodine deficiency has long-lasting effects on development because it prevents the production of thyroid hormone [12].

3.4 Cholesterol

The plasma membrane and myelin, a fatty sheath that surrounds the axons of neurons in both the central and peripheral nervous systems have cholesterol as an integral component. Breast milk contains significant amount of cholesterol (90–150 mg/L) whereas formula lacks cholesterol. It permits effective transmission of nerve impulses and synaptogenesis, which is crucial for neurodevelopment [26].

3.5 Psychological and psychobiological effect

In addition to the obvious nutritional advantages of breastfeeding for brain development, the nurturing and interaction with the mother that occurs during breastfeeding also has a positive impact on cognitive growth [3]. Maternal–infant touch and contact in the neonatal period, such as skin-to-skin contact are found to promote interactive behaviour in terms of increased maternal touch, adaptation and higher infant visual alertness; and this further predicts better cognitive outcomes among the infants [27].

4. Breast feeding and psycho-motor development

Between birth and age 3, young children experience rapid growth, development, and achievement of significant milestones, laying the groundwork for future development. Physical development is one aspect of newborn and toddler development. It relates to the growth, change, and development of the body, including the expansion of the muscles and the senses. The psychomotor domain pertains to physical bodily changes and involves motor skill use, coordination, and movement. It happens in a comparatively steady, predicable order. Changes in bone thickness, vision, hearing and muscle are all included [28]. The development of the body's size and weight is also a part of physical growth. Appropriate nutrition, which includes a balance of the right foods and enough water to drink, is essential for both growth and development. The developing brain and nervous system, growing bones and muscles, exercise, and physical activity help to increase control and coordination. Motor development refers to changes in children's ability to control their body's movements, from infants' first spontaneous waving and kicking movements to the adaptive control of reaching, locomotion and complex sport skills [29]. All bodily movements, including eye movements (as in the gaze) and an infant's developing control over their head, are referred to as motor behaviour. Large limbs or the entire body can be moved in gross motor actions, such as when walking. The use of fingers to grasp and manipulate objects is a fine motor behaviour. Exploratory behaviour includes motor actions like reaching, touching, and grasping [30].

The intrinsic qualities of the child and the mother's skill in child care form a complex interaction that affects the child's growth and nutritional outcomes. The most recent estimates of the global burden of malnutrition in children under five are that 178 million (one-third of all children) are stunted, 112 million are underweight, 55 million are wasted (19 million having severe acute malnutrition) and 13 million children are born each year with intrauterine growth retardation. Together they account for 21% of all under-5 deaths [11].

Studies have consistently shown a positive relationship between breastfeeding and motor development. Vestergaard et al. observed a positive relationship between breastfeeding duration and an earlier ability to crawl and perform the "pincer grip" and babies who were exclusively breastfed for six months were significantly more likely to be walking by one year compared with those who were exclusively breastfed for four months (60 vs. 39%) [31]. children breastfed for only 3 months show lower psychometric scores compared to the ones with 6 or more months of breastfeeding. A significant association between early initiation of breastfeeding, EBF and long duration of breast feeding is found to reduce the risk of underweight and have progressively more odds to high levels of psychomotor development when compared to those not breast fed successfully. The most affected psychometric domains by shortness of breastfeeding are communication and gross motor skills [2, 32–34].

There is consensus about the benefits of breastfeeding for infant growth and health, particularly in developing countries where it may be the only means to avoid malnutrition and a high risk of morbidity and mortality in the first year of life.

5. Breastfeeding and obesity/overweight

Adiposity refers to state of being fat or excessive accumulation of fat (Merriam-Webster, 2006). The Latin term adiposity means severe or morbid overweight an increase in overweight is linked to an increase in the risk of diseases that are linked to obesity. The body-mass-index is a general indicator of obesity (BMI). Adiposity and obesity rates have recently increased among children and adults, signalling a serious public health crisis in both developed and developing countries [24]. Children who are overweight run a high risk of continuing to be overweight as adults, putting them at risk for the related health issues like hypertension and coronary heart disease. According to a meta-analysis, breastfeeding is linked to a lower risk of being overweight than formula feeding [35].

Leptin, a hormone that is thought to regulate adult obesity, has a similar effect on infant obesity. First, individuals who were breastfed have a leptin profile that may support effective appetite control and less fat deposition. With regards to appetite regulation, According to Pérez-Escamilla et al. [36], Honduran infants changed the volume of milk they consumed in inverse relation to the energy density of their mother's breast milk. It has also been suggested that the milk fat content (hind milk), which is higher than the milk at the beginning of the feeding episode (fore-milk), indicates to the baby that the feeding episode is about to end. Babies who are fed formula are obviously not subject to such "physiological signalling," as the amount of fat in the formula does not change during the feeding episode. This implies that in babies who are fed formula, it is the carer, not the child, who sets the child's calorie intake. Second, during the first year of life, breastfed infants gain less weight than infants who are fed formula. Third, because infant formula contains more protein than breast milk, formula-fed babies have bloodstream insulin levels that are higher. This may encourage the body to store more fat. Fourth, it's possible that breast milk influences how a person's taste receptors develop, which may lead to a preference for lower-energy diets in later life [36, 37].

The higher human milk oligosaccharides (HMOs) diversity and evenness are associated with lower total and percentage fat mass in infants; breastfeeding reduced the risk of obesity in childhood significantly [6, 35]. The risk of obesity is found higher among children who are not exclusively breast fed, breast fed for short duration and formula fed infants [8, 38, 39].

6. Breastfeeding and socio-emotional development

Social-emotional development includes the child's experience, expression and management of emotions and the ability to establish positive and rewarding relationships with others. It encompasses both intra- and interpersonal processes [40].

The behavioural research indicates that in the first few minutes after birth, infants and mothers appear ready to interact. These discoveries include the newborn infant's capacity to crawl toward the breast in order to begin sucking as well as mother-infant thermoregulation. Encouragement of attachment through early contact, suckling, and rooming-in has been shown to reduce abandonment. Oxytocin plays a role in the biological regulation of the attachment felt between a mother and her infant [41]. Even though it's well agreed that EBF encourages greater cognitive growth, nothing is known about how it might affect socio-emotional development [42]. Yet, research indicates that longer breastfeeding periods are connected to a happy bias, whereas shorter breastfeeding periods were linked to a fear bias, indicating that breastfeeding experience can influence how newborns respond to emotional cues. Additionally, they perform better in the areas of adaptability and communication. Breastfeeding has also been linked to improved maternal-infant bonding and empathy during the early postpartum period, as well as a greater sensitivity to infant cues [42–44].

7. Breastfeeding and infant morbidity/mortality

There is strong evidence that early, continuous breastfeeding for 23 months significantly lowers neonatal and child mortality on a global scale. According to a technical brief on the effect of early breastfeeding on newborn deaths, starting breastfeeding within the first hour of birth could prevent 20% of neonatal deaths and lower the risk of infection-related neonatal mortality by 45%. According to epidemiological data, breast feeding would save about 800,000 lives annually, if they were breastfed within an hour of birth, exclusively fed breast milk for the first six months of life, and then continued breastfeeding until age two [45]. It was also reaffirmed in The Lancet Nutrition Series, 2016 on how important optimal IYCF (Infant and Young Child Feeding) is to a child's survival. According to estimates, optimal IYCF, particularly exclusive breastfeeding, could avert 1.4 million under-five deaths annually (out of the approximately 10 million annual deaths) [46, 47].

It is sterile and has the least chance of being contaminated microbiologically. Bacteriostatic lactoferrin prevents the growth of *Escherichia coli* and binds iron and prevents *E. coli* from accessing it. Lipases and peroxidases eliminate bacteria. Amoeba and giardia are destroyed by bile salt stimulated lipase (BSSL). PABA is crucial for malaria prevention and relatively low levels of PABA in human milk suppresses parasites to subclinical levels and provides an adequate antigenic stimulus for an immune response.

Infants are born with immature immune systems and organs that may take some time to develop into their ideal functioning states and breast milk is extremely safe and non-allergenic immunologically. Prebiotics, free fatty acids (FFA), mono glycerides, oligosaccharides, antimicrobial peptides, human milk glycans, lysozyme, lacto peroxidase, lacto ferrin, lipoprotein lipase, and epidermal growth factors, which stimulate the gastrointestinal epithelium as a barrier, are all present in breast milk which contributes to the development and enhancement of an infant's innate immune system. When compared to milk from other species, human milk is exceptional due to its high concentration of complex oligosaccharides. Oligosaccharides also have an impact on the development of the intestinal flora because they feed the beneficial Lactobacillus bifidus bacteria while inhibiting the growth of potentially pathogenic bacteria. It includes secretory elements, secretary IgA, and immunoglobulin (SIgA) which plays a crucial role in preventing microbial pathogen adhesion to the surface of the intestinal epithelium and binding their toxins thus providing the GI and respiratory tracts with surface protection. T and B lymphocytes, as well as anti-inflammatory nutrients like vitamins A, C, and E, enzymes, E prostaglandins, enzyme inhibitors, protease inhibitors, and growth factors, are also provided by breast milk. These work against rotavirus, the most common cause of diarrhoea in infants. Now, researchers in the United States and Mexico have discovered that complex carbohydrate in breast milk affords babies even more protection than the antibody specifically made to fight against fatal diseases like diarrhoea, viral infections and other diseases [48, 49]. Thus, we can say infant's first immunisation is mother's milk as these antimicrobial, anti-inflammatory, and immunologic-stimulating substances guard the infant against diarrhoea and other infectious diseases like food allergies, respiratory (asthma), urinary, otitis media, botulism, necrotizing enterocolitis, bacterial meningitis, and bacteremia. Additionally, there is proof that breastfeeding guards against less common diseases like Urinary tract infection, sudden infant death syndrome, celiac disease, Crohn's disease, ulcerative colitis, Type I diabetes, and childhood lymphoma [50–52]. Due to the low pH of the bowels, breastfed babies experience fewer diaper rashes. As babies who are breastfed for longer periods of time accept different tastes more readily than those who are not, it may also prevent picky eating syndrome, which may develop later in life [11, 53, 54].

8. Conclusion

Breastfeeding is considered as best start for an infant's survival, health, and development due to its nutritional, immunological, and psychological advantages. To achieve the best possible growth, development, and health, the World Health Organisation advocates mothers to initiate breast feeding within one hour of birth, feed colostrum, exclusively breastfeed their infants for the first six months of their lives, then continue to do so while supplementing with the right foods until they are two years old or older. Improvements in breastfeeding rates are critical to the attainment of the sustainable development goals, especially to reduce the child morbidity, mortality and improving maternal health. Both the constituents of breast milk and the act of breastfeeding have been implicated in the process playing a major role on infant developmental milestones/outcomes. It provides optimum fluidity and warmth; and is very economical and convenient. Breast milk has high lactose content and is the sweetest milk. The protein is simple to digest. Long chain polyunsaturated fats (LCP), phospholipids, and precursors to prostaglandins are all abundant and provides enzymes like amylase, lipoprotein lipase, bile salt stimulated lipases (BSSL), oxidases, lactoperoxidases, leucocyte myeloperoxidases, etc. A significant association was found between exclusive breastfeeding and long duration of breast on infant developmental outcomes *viz.* cognition, language, psycho motor and socio-emotional development. The mechanism/s underlying these effects are likely to be linked to the high nutritional sensitivity of physical, motor and brain development in the critical early period of life. The higher human milk oligosaccharides (HMOs) diversity in breast milk are associated with lower percentage fat mass in infants and reduces the risk of obesity in childhood significantly. Prebiotics, free fatty acids (FFA), mono glycerides, oligosaccharides, antimicrobial peptides, human milk lysozyme, lacto peroxidase, lacto ferrin, lipoprotein lipase, and epidermal growth in breast milk enhances infant's innate immune system thus reduces the risk of infant mortality and morbidity due to malnutrition.

Hence, adequate breastfeeding counselling and support are essential for mothers and families to initiate and maintain optimal breastfeeding practices. Training of health workers and volunteers should focus on counselling rather than just giving messages. Also, there is a need to regulate commercial brands of prelacteal feeds like herbal syrups, gripe water, etc., that display the advice that they can be given from birth. It is vital to establish breast milk bank to feed the babies whose mothers are ill or in distress and who have lost mothers.

Author details

Vinutha U. Muktamath[1*], Priya R. Hegde[2], Ramya Koneru[1] and Rekha Lakkashetti[2]

1 University of Agricultural Sciences, Dharwad, Karnataka, India

2 Centre for Multidisciplinary Development Research, Dharwad, Karnataka, India

*Address all correspondence to: vinumuktamath@gmail.com

References

[1] Elizabeth KE. Nutrition & Child Development. Hyderabad, India: Paras Medical Publisher; 2015. pp. 5-86

[2] Marriott BP, White A, Hadden L, Davies JC, Wallingford JC. World Health Organization (WHO) infant and young child feeding indicators: Associations with growth measures in 14 low-income countries. Maternal Child Nutrition. 2012;**8**:354-370

[3] Petryk A, Harris SR, Jongbloed L. Breastfeeding and neurodevelopment: A literature review. Infants Young Child. 2007;**20**(2):120-134

[4] Ramil A. Role of breastfeeding in promoting maternal & child health and policy implications in New Zealand. Health. 2016;**08**(01):75-82

[5] Ahmed A, Chaudhry AC, Riaz A, Batool A, Farooq H. Breastfeeding knowledge and practices: An anthropological study of lactating mothers of Noor pur shahan, Islamabad. Scientific International (Lahore). 2014;**26**(1):453-457

[6] Alderete TL, Autran C, Brekke BE, Knight R, Bode L, Goran MI, et al. Associations between human milk oligosaccharides and infant body composition in the first six months of life. The American Journal of Clinical Nutrition. 2015;**102**:1381-1388

[7] Anonymous. Baby-Friendly Hospital Initiative Revised Updated and Expanded for Integrated Care. Geneva, Switzerland: World Health Organisation and UNICEF; 2009

[8] Oddy WH, Mori TA, Huang R, Marsh JA, Pennell CE, Chivers P, et al. Early infant feeding and adiposity risk: From infancy to adulthood. Annals of Nutrition Metabolism. 2014;**64**(3-4):262-270

[9] National Research Council (US). Subcommittee on the tenth edition of the recommended dietary allowances. In: Recommended Dietary Allowances. 10th ed. Washington (DC): National Academies Press (US); 1989. Available from: https://www.ncbi.nlm.nih.gov/books/NBK234932/. DOI: 10.17226/1349

[10] Anonymous. Guidelines for Antenatal Care and Skilled Attendance at Birth by anms/lhvs/sns. Published by Maternal Health Division, Ministry of Health and Family Welfare, Government of India; 2010. pp. 5-84

[11] Black ER, Allen H, Lindsay B, Bhutta ZA, Caulfield LE, Onis M, et al. Maternal and child under nutrition: Global and regional exposures and health consequences. The Lancet. 2008;**371**(9608):243-260

[12] Lawrence AR, Lawrence MR. Breast Feeding-a Guide for Medical Profession. USA: Mosby; 2005. pp. 14-28

[13] Muktamath VU, Itagi SK, Hegde PR. Human Milk Composition: Potential Role in Infant Health and Disease. India: INSC International Publishers; 2021

[14] Rollins CN, Bhandari N, Hajeebhoy N, Horton S, Lutter KS, Martines JC, et al. Breastfeeding in the 21st century: Epidemiology, mechanisms, and lifelong effect. The Lancet. 2016;**387**(10017):475-490

[15] Bacharach VR, Baumeister AA. Direct and indirect effects of maternal intelligence, maternal age, income and home environment on intelligence of preterm, low-birth-weight children.

Journal of Applied Development and Psychology. 1998a;**19**:349-363

[16] Bacharach VR, Baumeister AA. Effects of maternal intelligence, marital status, income and home environment on cognitive development of low birth weight infants. Journal of Pediatric Psychology. 1998b;**23**(3):197-205

[17] Tozzi AE, Bisiacchi P, Tarantino V, Chiarotti F, D'elia L, De Mei B, et al. Effect of duration of breastfeeding on neuropsychological development at 10 to 12 years of age in a cohort of healthy children. Developmental Medicine Child Neuroscience. 2012;**54**:843-848

[18] Andres A, Cleves AM, Bellando JB, Pivik PT, Casey and Badger MT. Developmental status of 1-year-old infants fed breast milk, cow's milk formula, or soy formula. Pediatrics. 2012;**129**(6):1134-1140

[19] Belfort MB, Sheryl L, Rifas S, Kleinman KP, Guthrie LB, Bellinger DC, et al. Infant feeding and childhood cognition at ages 3 and 7 years: Effects of breastfeeding duration and exclusivity. JAMA Pediatrics. 2013;**167**(9):836-844

[20] Ferguson M, Molfese PJ. Breast-fed infants process speech differently from bottle-fed infants: Evidence from neuro electrophysiology. Developmental Neuropsychology. 2007;**31**(3):337-343

[21] Simopoulos AP. Omega-3 fatty acids in health and disease and in growth and development. American Journal of Clinical Nutrition. 1991;**54**(3):438-463

[22] Uauy R, Peirano P, Hoffman D, Mena P, Birch D, Birch E. Role of essential fatty acids in the function of the developing nervous system. Lipids. 1996;**31**(1):167-176

[23] Uauy R, Mena P, Rojas C. Essential fatty acids in early life: Structural and functional role. The Proceedings of the Nutrition Society. 2000;**59**(1):3-15

[24] Deoni SCL, Dean DC, Piryatinsky I, O'Muircheartaigh J, Waskiewicz N, Lehman K, et al. Breastfeeding and early white matter development: A cross-sectional study. Neuro Image. 2013;**82**:77-86

[25] Scott DT, Janowsky JS, Carroll RE, Taylor JA, Auestad N, Montalto MB. Formula supplementation with long-chain polyunsaturated fatty acids: Are there developmental benefits? Pediatrics. 1998;**102**(5):2101-2209

[26] Muktamath VU, Itagi SK. Breast feeding practices: Effect on infant morbidity. International Journal of Chemical Studies. 2019;**7**(6):1028-1033

[27] Feldman FR, Eidelman AI. Direct and indirect effects of breast milk on neurobehavioral and cognitive development of premature infants. Developmental Psychobiology. 2003;**43**:109-119

[28] Simpson EJ. The Classification of Educational Objectives in the Psychomotor Domain. Washington, DC: Gryphon House; 1972. pp. 18-23

[29] Adolph KE, Weise I, Marin L. Motor development. In: Nadel L, editor. Encyclopedia of Cognitive Science. London: Macmillan; 2006. p. 96

[30] Adolph KE. Learning in the development of infant locomotion. Monographs of the Society for Research in Child Development. 1997;**62**(3):251

[31] Vestergaard M, Obel C, Henriksen TB, Sorensen HT, Skajaa E, Ostergaard J. Duration of breastfeeding and developmental milestones during the latter half of infancy. Acta Paediatric. 1999;**88**(12):1327-1332

[32] Kamudoni P, Maleta K, Shi Z, Holmboe-Ottesen G. Exclusive breastfeeding duration during the first 6 months of life is positively associated with length-for-age among infants 6-12 months old, in Mangochi district, Malawi. European Journal of Clinical Nutrition. 2015;**69**:96-101

[33] Marques RS, Taddei JA, Konstantyner T, Loez FA, Marques AF, Oliveira C, et al. Anthropometric indices and exclusive breastfeeding in the first six months of life: A comparison with reference standards NCHS, 1977 and WHO, 2006. International Breastfeeding Journal. 2015;**10**(20):2-7

[34] Saliaj A, Zahaj M, Pura B. Long-term effect of breastfeeding in preschooler's psychomotor development. International Journal of Medical, Health, Biomedical, Bioengineering, Pharmaceuticals Engineering. 2015;**9**(12):823-826

[35] Arenz S, Rucheri R, Koletzko B, Kries RV. Breastfeeding and child hood obesity – A systematic review. International Journal of Obesity. 2004;**28**:1247-1256

[36] Pérez-Escamilla RL, Lutter C, Segall AM, Rivera A, Treviño-Siller S, Sanghvi T. Exclusive breastfeeding duration is associated with attitudinal, socio-economic and biocultural determinants in three Latin American countries. The Journal of Nutrition. 1995;**125**(12):2972-2984

[37] Parveen S, Sareen IB, Dahiya BR. Breastfeeding practices in post IMNCI era in rural community of Haryana. Indian Journal of Public Health Research and Development. 2012;**3**(4):205-209

[38] Gale C, Logan KM, Santhakumaran S, Parkinson JRC, Hyde MJ, Modi N. Effect of breastfeeding compared with formula feeding on infant body composition: A systematic review and meta-analysis. American Journal of Clinical Nutrition. 2012;**10**:1-14

[39] Sachwani S, Karmaliani R, Hirani SA, Khowaja AR, Lalwani E. Association between breastfeeding and childhood obesity among school- going children, 5-16 years of age in Karachi, Pakistan. International Journal of Nursing Education. 2015;**7**(2):244-248

[40] Cohen J. Helping young children succeed: Strategies to promote early childhood social and emotional development research and policy report. In: National Conference of State Legislatures and Zero to Three. Washington D.C; 2005. pp. 1-19

[41] Klaus M. Mother and infant: Early emotional ties. Pediatrics. 1998;**102**(5):1244-1246

[42] Krol MK, Rajhans P, Missana M, Grossmann T. Duration of exclusive breastfeeding is associated with differences in infants' brain responses to emotional body expressions. Frontiers in Behavior Neuro Science. 2015;**8**:1-11

[43] Kim P, Feldman F, Mayes LC, Eicher V, Thompson N, Leckman JF, et al. Breastfeeding, brain activation to own infant cry and maternal sensitivity. Journal of Child Psychology and Psychiatry. 2011;**52**(8):907-915

[44] Tasnim S. Effect of breastfeeding on child development: At birth and beyond. South East Asia Journal of Public Health. 2014;**4**(1):4-8

[45] Oot LA, Sommerfelt E, Sethuraman K, Rossimize J. Estimating the effect of suboptimal breastfeeding practices on child mortality: A model in profiles for country-level advocacy. Technical brief, Food and Nutrition Technical Assistance III Project; 2015. pp. 1-9

[46] Chandhiok N, Singh L, Singh KJ, Sahu D, Pandey A. Does breastfeeding have an effect on infant mortality in

India? An analysis of national family health survey data. Open Journal of Preventive Medicine. 2015;5:359-369

[47] Victora CG, Bahl R, Barros AJ, Franca GV, Krasevec J, Murch S, et al. Breastfeeding in the 21st century: Epidemiology, mechanisms and lifelong effect. The Lancet. 2016;**387**(10017):475-490

[48] Hajeebhoy N, Mannava P, Nguyen PH, Mai LT. Suboptimal breastfeeding practices are associated with infant illness in Vietnam. International Breastfeeding Journal. 2014;**9**(12):1-7

[49] Orivuori L, Loss G, Roduit C, et al. Soluble immunoglobulin a in breast milk is inversely associated with atopic dermatitis at early age: The pasture cohort study. Clinical Experimental Allergy. 2013;**44**:102-112

[50] Colen CG, Ramey DM. Is breast truly best? Estimating the effect of breastfeeding on long-term child wellbeing in the United States using sibling comparisons. Social Science & Medicine. 2014;**109**:55-65

[51] Eidelman AI, Schanler RJ. Breastfeeding and the use of human milk. Pediatrics. 2012;**129**(3):827-847

[52] Kramer MS, Guo T, Platt RW, Sevkovskaya Z, Dzikovich I, Collet J, et al. Infant growth and health outcomes associated with 3 compared with 6 mo of exclusive breastfeeding. American Journal of Clinical Nutrition. 2003;**78**:291-295

[53] Biesbroek G, Bosch ATM, Wang X, Keijser BJF, Veenhoven RH, Sanders EAM, et al. The impact of breastfeeding on nasopharyngeal microbial communities in infants. American Journal of Respiratory Critical Care Medicine. 2014;**190**(3):298-308

[54] Pabst HF. Immunomodulation by breast-feeding. The Pediatric Infectious Disease Journal. 1997;**16**(10):991-995

Chapter 2

Exclusive Breastfeeding

Imtihanatun Najahah

Abstract

For infants, breast milk is the best food. It is clean and safe, and has antibodies that protect against a variety of common childhood diseases. Breast milk meets all of an infant's nutrient and energy needs during the first few months of life, and it continues to meet up to one third and up to half of a child's nutritional requirements during the second half of the first year. Breast milk, here in after abbreviated as breastfeeding, is the liquid produced by the secretion of the mother's breast glands. Exclusive breastfeeding, is breast milk given to babies from birth for 6 (six) months, without adding and/or replacing it with other food or drinks. Exclusive breastfeeding is that babies are only given breast milk, without additional liquids such as formula milk, orange juice, honey, tea, water and without additional solid foods such as bananas, papaya, milk porridge, biscuits, rice porridge and team, for 6 months. There are many factors to get success exclusive breastfeeding.

Keywords: infant, exclusive breastfeeding, support, benefit, success

1. Introduction

For infants, breast milk is the best food. It is clean and safe, and has antibodies that protect against a variety of common childhood diseases. Breast milk meets all of an infant's nutrient and energy needs during the first few months of life, and it continues to meet up to one third and up to half of a child's nutritional requirements during the second half of the first year [1]. In 1990, WHO-UNICEF made a declaration known as the Innocenti Declaration. The declaration, which was born in Innocenti, Italy, aims to protect, promote, and provide support for breastfeeding. In this declaration which was also signed by Indonesia, it was explained that in order to optimally improve the health and quality of baby food, all mothers are advised to give exclusive breastfeeding from birth to 4 months of age. After the age of 4 months, babies begin to be given complementary foods/solids that are correct and appropriate, while breastfeeding is continued until the age of 2 years or more. In 1999, evidence was found that feeding too early has a negative effect on infants. Since then, UNICEF has provided clarification regarding the recommended period for exclusive breastfeeding. UNICEF's latest recommendation with the World Health Assembly (WHA) and many other countries is to set a period of exclusive breastfeeding for 6 months [2].

Breastfeeding, is the liquid produced by the secretion of the mother's breast glands. Exclusive breastfeeding, is breast milk given to babies from birth for 6 (six) months, without adding and/or replacing it with other food or drinks. Exclusive breastfeeding is that babies are only given breast milk, without additional liquids such as formula milk, orange juice, honey, tea, water and without additional solid foods such as bananas, papaya, milk porridge, biscuits, rice porridge and team, for 6 months [3].

Exclusive breastfeeding is beneficial for both mother and baby. Exclusive breastfeeding for 6 months is the optimal method of infant feeding. Breastfeeding provides the baby with nutrients for growth and development, and boosting the immune system. There is some evidence to prove that exclusive breastfeeding for 6 months provides protection against gastrointestinal infections and iron deficiency anemia. Exclusive breastfeeding also makes women amenorrhea for 6 months postpartum and helps them avoid unplanned pregnancies that end in abortion. In addition, research evidence shows that breastfeeding improves sensory and cognitive development while protecting babies against chronic illnesses and respiratory infections (common cold, cough, or pneumonia). Exclusive breastfeeding arrangements aim to

a. ensure the fulfillment of the baby's right to receive exclusive breastfeeding from birth to the age of 6 (six) months by taking into account their growth and development,

b. provide protection to mothers in giving exclusive breastfeeding to their babies and increasing the role and support of the family, community, local government, and the government for exclusive breastfeeding [4].

2. Exclusive breastfeeding

2.1 The composition of breast milk

The composition of breast milk consists of colostrum, foremilk, and hindmilk. From the beginning to the end of a feed, the composition of breast milk varies depending on the baby's age. It may also differ at various times of the day and between feeds. The thick, yellowish, or clear milk that women produce in the first few days after giving birth is called colostrum. The special properties of colostrum are antibody-rich, many white cells, purgative, growth factors, and vitamin A rich so why it is important because it protects against infection and allergy, protects against infection, clears meconium, helps to prevent jaundice, helps intestine to mature, prevents allergy, intolerance, reduces severity of infection, and prevents eye disease. Therefore, it is critical for infants to consume colostrum during their initial feedings. When a baby is born, the colostrum is ready in the breasts. Before the mature milk arrives, it is all the majority of babies require. Drinks and foods should not be given to babies before they start breastfeeding. Particularly risky are artificial feeds given before a baby has colostrum [5].

The milk that is produced after a few days is called mature milk. The breasts feel full, hard, and heavy because there is more milk. Some refer to this as the "coming in" of milk. The bluish milk that is produced early in a feed is called foremilk. The whiter milk that is produced later in a feed is known as hindmilk. Colostrum has more protein than later milk, and hindmilk has more fat than foremilk. There are two distinct types of breast milk. Hindmilk appears whiter because it contains more fat. Because this fat provides much of the energy needed to breastfeed, it is important not to take a baby off the breast before he has had everything he needs. Larger quantities of foremilk are produced, and they contain a lot of protein, lactose, water, and other nutrients. Mothers sometimes worry that their milk is "too thin" because it looks watery. Milk never appears "too thin." For a baby to have a complete "meal," they must have both foremilk and hindmilk. The transition from "fore" milk to "hind" milk is gradual. From the beginning to the end of a feed, the fat content gradually rises [5].

2.2 How the breast works

The small amount of milk that accumulates between feedings is extracted from the milk ducts under the alveoli when the baby latches onto the breast. Two hormones are released as a result of this suckling: oxytocin and prolactin. Oxytocin causes the alveoli, the cells that produce milk, to squeeze the milk out of the ducts and toward the nipple, while prolactin instructs the alveoli to produce more milk.

The system of breastfeeding is based on the law of supply and demand. The quantity of milk produced is determined by the amount of milk taken from the breast. Milk production takes place both between and during feedings. The quantity of milk produced will be influenced by the baby's breastfeeding frequency, duration, and quality. The breast produces foremilk at the beginning of a feeding. This has more fluid and lactose. The baby gets more fat and calories from the hind milk it gets later in the feeding process. To ensure that the baby receives the hind milk required to feel satisfied and gain sufficient weight, it is essential to allow the baby to finish the first side completely. Learning to breastfeed is a skill that may require some time [5].

2.3 Exclusive breastfeeding

Kramer & Kakuma (2004) repeated evidence of the effect of exclusive breastfeeding on the health and growth of infants, revealing that infants who were exclusively breastfed for up to six months showed a lower morbidity rate of digestive diseases and allergies. Provision of breast milk (breastfeeding) for premature babies greatly affects the level of their intelligence as adults, It's conclusion of the experiment for 16 years there were 424 babies conducted by Prof. Alan Lucas and colleagues at the Institute for Child Care at Great Ormond Street Hospital, London. This research shows that food management immediately after birth has a similar effect on all babies, not just premature babies. In 1982 when research began, hospitals generally gave standard infant formula to premature babies. Since the late 1980s, most UK hospitals have switched from standard infant formula to formula fortified with breast milk [6].

In developing countries, WHO recommends exclusive breastfeeding until the age of 4–6 months and continued breastfeeding accompanied by adequate and complete food intake until the baby is 2 years old, even though the baby has growth delays [7]. Gibney et al. 2009 wrote that obstacles hindering the success of breastfeeding are the many unwarranted beliefs and attitudes toward the meaning of breastfeeding, which makes mothers not practice exclusive breastfeeding for their babies in the first 6 months period. The World Health Organization (WHO) and the United Nations Children's Fund (UNICEF) both recommend that infants begin breastfeeding within the first hour of their birth and consume only breast milk for the first six months of their lives—no other foods or liquids, including water, are provided. Infants should be breastfed whenever they want to, throughout the day and night. Pacifiers, teats, and bottles should not be used. Children should begin eating safe and adequate complementary foods at the age of six months, and they should continue to breastfeed for up to two years and beyond. Common reasons why they do not exclusively breastfeed include the following:

a. An unfounded fear that the milk they produce is not enough and/or of poor quality

b. Delay in starting breastfeeding and the practice of throwing away colostrum

c. Incorrect breastfeeding technique

d. The mistaken belief that their baby is thirsty and needs extra fluids

e. Lack of support from health services

f. Marketing of breast milk substitute formula [8].

Exclusive breastfeeding can prevent nutritional problems in infants, from several research results showing that there is an effect of exclusive breastfeeding on the incidence of stunting as in a study conducted in Siaya which is the western part of Kenya with a cross-sectional study design. The results showed that 47% of toddlers there were stunted, the highest age group experiencing stunting is at the age of 13–24 months and 60% of toddlers experience stunting at the age of 2 years of life. It's showed during the 3 months of life 67% of babies who suckle within 10 times a day. From the results of the study, it was also found that infants who breastfed less than 10 times in 24 hours were 48.1% of stunted toddlers [9].

Research Yovita Ananta et al. 2016 found significantly more babies in the formula-fed group had abnormal head circumferences than in the group that were exclusively breastfed. A previous study also found that babies who were exclusively breastfed had greater head circumference values for age compared to those who were fed formula or mixtures. WHO and UNICEF recommend exclusive breastfeeding until the baby is 6 months old. Despite the many benefits of breastfeeding, the rate of exclusive breastfeeding at 6 months remains unsatisfactory. The results of a study by Yovita Ananta et al. in 2016 are as follows: The rate of exclusive breastfeeding varied from 10.5% in East Java to 66.9% in Jambi Province, with a total rate of 46.3%. In developed countries, exclusive breastfeeding at 6 months is found to be low: 16.3% in the United States, 13.8% in Canada, 13.4% in Hong Kong, 10.1% in Sweden, and 11 and 7% in Norway. In developing countries, the numbers are more favorable. As many as 49% of mothers breastfeed exclusively in Ethiopia, 13 and 46.4% in India, 14 and 27.7% in Iran. A study conducted in Peninsular Malaysia reported a rate of 14.5% [10].

The duration of exclusive breastfeeding continues monthly from 1 month to 6 months. Research in Sri Lanka found that the prevalence of exclusive breastfeeding for up to 6 months was 50.8% and up to 5 months or more was 81.3%. The average duration of exclusive breastfeeding is 6 months. The main reason for stopping early exclusive breastfeeding is that mothers think that breast milk alone is not enough for babies (52.9%). Items given to infants before 6 months were water (91.4%), fruit juice (83.9%), mashed rice (71.3%), and infant formula (16.1%). The majority of mothers (98.9%) know that the current recommendation for exclusive breastfeeding is 6 months. Only 27.7% of mothers could correctly define the term "exclusive breast-feeding." The majority of mothers (92.4%) know that babies should be breastfed while traveling, while 62.4% believe that formula feeding is an option. The percentage of mothers who know breast milk can be expressed and stored as 68.4%. 65.3% mother have information about breast milk can be stored at room temperature, while 48% and 12.1% know can be stored in refrigerator and freezer compartments. Meanwhile, 12.1%

of mothers said they were advised by health workers to start breastfeeding other than breast milk during the first 6 months. Of these mothers, 28 were advised by a doctor. Only 29 mothers (8.2%) started formula feeding in the first 6 months. The majority of babies (94.6%) were breastfed within 1 hour after delivery. Of them 77.7% of mothers believed that their baby was not allowed to finish the first breastfeeding, and 50.6% of mothers were advised by family members to stop exclusive breastfeeding early. Most commonly the family members referred to were their mother-in-law (55.9%) or their mother (44.7%), while 29.1% said their husband influenced them negatively. The majority of mothers (81.1%) have good family support. Some mothers feel that their family members have an encouraging attitude toward breastfeeding [11].

The prevalence of exclusive breastfeeding in Afar Ethiopia under 6 months is 55%. Infants whose mothers live in urban areas have knowledge about breastfeeding, are provided at health facilities, and are more likely to breastfeed exclusively than the referral group. In addition, mothers have a poor understanding of exclusive breastfeeding. Traditional beliefs, myths, and misconceptions about exclusive breastfeeding and lack of support from husbands and families were found to be barriers to proper exclusive breastfeeding practices [12].

The family plays a role in exclusive breastfeeding by supporting the mother in exclusive breastfeeding, supporting the mother to fulfill her nutrition by consuming nutritious foods, ensuring that the mother gets enough rest and creating a calm and peaceful home atmosphere.

2.4 Factors affecting exclusive breastfeeding

Breastfeeding is something natural but requires learning to be able to apply it. To be able to realize the success of breastfeeding requires strong support in achieving its sustainability. Among them, namely by improving the services provided to mothers by helping to increase the initiation of exclusive breastfeeding, consistent education and full support from the health system can help maintain the success of exclusive breastfeeding [13]. The International Confederation of Midwives provides support for exclusive breastfeeding in the form of collaborating with international organizations and government agencies engaged in the promotion and support of breastfeeding, ensuring scientific programs at international congresses to present breastfeeding including the development of HIV/AIDS, using communication media with midwives related to maintaining information on breastfeeding development and breastfeeding period, and ensuring documents related to care for mothers and their babies, which is part of the role of midwives in maintaining, supporting, and promoting breastfeeding [14].

There are ten (10) steps in successful breastfeeding, namely (1) having a policy from the hospital including the hospital providing support to mothers for breastfeeding by not promoting formula milk and using bottles and pacifiers, establishing standards of breastfeeding care practices, maintaining activities breastfeeding support, (2) having competent officers, including conducting training for officers in providing support to mothers for breastfeeding, evaluating the knowledge and skills of health workers, (3) providing pregnancy services that include discussing the importance of breastfeeding for mothers and babies, preparing mothers how to prepare food for the baby, (4) accuracy in providing maternal services after delivery includes encouraging the mother to immediately make skin contact between the mother and her baby after giving birth, helping the mother place the baby for continuous breastfeeding, (5) providing support to the mother for breastfeeding, including checking position, attachment and reflexes for sucking babies, providing breastfeeding support practices to mothers, helping mothers overcome problems that commonly occur in breastfeeding mothers, (6) giving supplements, including giving only milk, unless there is a medical/medication reason, and prioritizing giving milk assistance if needed, help the mother keep her safe if she wants formula food, (7) carry out in-patient care, including allowing the mother and baby to stay together for a day and a night, ensuring that the mother can stay with the baby even though she is sick, (8) caring about feeding, including helping mothers know when their babies are hungry, not limiting breastfeeding time, (9) bottles, pacifiers, and baby pacifiers, including explaining to mothers the use and risks of feeding using bottles, pacifiers, and baby pacifiers, and (10) exemption, including appointing mothers as a source of support for breastfeeding in the community, working with the community in improving breastfeeding support services [15].

Recommendations for increasing the practice of exclusive breastfeeding are increasing the habit of health professionals conducting breastfeeding counseling through training, involving husbands during counseling, and educating mothers and society as a whole to avoid traditional practices that hinder exclusive breastfeeding for up to 6 months [16]. From the results of other studies, it was found that the factors that influence the success of breastfeeding for up to 6 (six) months or exclusive breastfeeding at Cipto Mangkunkusumo Hospital are the mother's sense of confidence in milk production and the support of the family [17]. Educating mothers and society as a whole avoid traditional practices that hinder exclusive breastfeeding for up to 6 months [16]. From the results of other studies, it was found that the factors that influence the success of breastfeeding for up to 6 (six) months or exclusive breastfeeding at Cipto Mangkunkusumo Hospital are the mother's sense of confidence in milk production and the support of the family [17]. Several factors influence the practice of exclusive breastfeeding for 6 months, including the mother's knowledge about breastfeeding, family support, and health care providers who educate mothers about breastfeeding. A study reported that antenatal education can increase the practice of exclusive breastfeeding for 6 months with RR 2.16 (95% CI 1.05 to 4.43), while postnatal education can improve practice with RR 2.12 (95% CI 1, 03 to 4.37) [10].

2.5 Benefit of exclusive breastfeeding

Exclusive breastfeeding is beneficial for both mother and baby. Breastfeeding provides the baby with nutrients for growth, development, and boosting the immune system. There is some evidence to prove that exclusive breastfeeding for 6 months provides protection against gastrointestinal infections and iron deficiency anemia. Exclusive breastfeeding also makes women amenorrhea for 6 months postpartum and helps them avoid unplanned pregnancies that end in abortion. In addition, research evidence shows that breastfeeding improves sensory and cognitive development while protecting babies against chronic illnesses and respiratory infections (common cold, cough, or pneumonia) [3].

Benefits of breast milk for the infant are as follows:

- A lower rate of cot death, also known as sudden infant death syndrome
- A lower risk of ear infections, diabetes, and cancer in children.
- A quicker ability to fight disease and a better response to vaccinations

- A decrease in the number of orthodontic and dental issues (no bottle-related tooth decay).

- Improved psychomotor, emotional, and social growth.

- Benefits to mothers' health:

- Oxytocin, which is released during breastfeeding, helps to contract the uterus and reduce postpartum bleeding. Because of this, breastfeeding should begin immediately following birth and be continued frequently.

- Women who are nursing save energy; Even if they eat little, they can still make milk.

- The risk of ovarian and breast cancer is lower.

- Breastfeeding frequently helps prevent a second pregnancy and delays the return of menstruation. This helps children save space and iron stores.

- Breastfeeding as a means of delaying a new pregnancy. Breastfeeding can delay the return of ovulation and menstruation, making it an effective method for separating pregnancies. If the mother breastfeeds in the following manner, breastfeeding can provide effective protection against a subsequent pregnancy.

- She should breastfeed exclusively and frequently, night and day, whenever the baby desires it.

- She should breastfeed at least eight to ten times in a 24-hour period, with no break of more than 6 hours between feedings.

Breastfeeding is less effective for family planning when a baby is older than 6 months. Since a baby this age needs more than one food, breastfeeding can no longer be the only option. However, if the mother breastfeeds frequently, breastfeeding still provides some protection against a subsequent pregnancy. Every time she gives the baby complementary foods, she should breastfeed it. A mother who is unable to use any other method of family planning may benefit from this partial protection.

- A child's protection decreases after 1 year. Before breastfeeding, the child must now consume food to ensure adequate nutrition. However, if menstruation has not returned, frequent breastfeeding may still provide some protection.

- The woman becomes fertile once more when her periods return. Even if her baby is still under 6 months old, breastfeeding will not protect her. She requires a new method of family planning.

Menstruation returns prior to conception in the majority of women. Therefore, a woman's menstrual cycle is the primary indication that she is fertile once more. However, a small number of women ovulate and are able to conceive before returning to menstruation. When the baby is older than six months, this is more likely to occur.

- Breastfeed immediately after birth, within half an hour to one hour.
- Breastfeed whenever needed, eight to twelve times per day.
- One feeding lasts as long as you want.
- From the time a baby is 0 to about 6 months old, only breastfeed.
- Complementary foods can be started around the age of six months (the exact age varies).
- Beginning at 6 months of age, offer complementary foods to all children.
- Breastfeed until the child is two years old or older.

Calm your newborn by holding him or her against your skin right after birth. It will also keep baby warm and steady his or her breathing. Because baby will be awake and eager to eat within a few hours of birth, this is a great time to start breastfeeding first. Mother can get help with this from a midwife. Baby will be happier if mother feeds him whenever he is hungry and keeps him close to mother. During the first two days of life, a newborn may want to breastfeed frequently. She gets many small doses of colostrum from her frequent feedings, which helps her body remember to produce plenty of milk. Early breastfeeding is its name. Early breastfeeding involves placing the baby on their chest, smelling milk or breast milk, making eye contact with the mother, and the baby crawling up to feed [1].

2.6 What a health professional can do

Support the woman so that she does not need as many interventions during labor and delivery.

- Persuade the woman to try painkillers that would not stop her from breastfeeding. Medication that will eventually pass on to the baby transplacentally and have a sedative effect should be avoided whenever possible.
- From the moment the baby is born until the time the baby has finished eating, let the baby stay skin to skin with the mother.
- Allow mother and child to communicate at their own pace. Only provide assistance when you believe it is absolutely necessary or when the mother requests it. After the birth, postpone any routine procedures that can wait until the mother and baby are ready, which should be at least one to two hours. The baby's measurement and dressing are two examples.
- Only when absolutely necessary should mother and child be separated. Typically, the baby can be observed briefly while remaining close to its mother. The process can be disrupted by even a brief separation prior to the first feed.

- If the mother is unconscious or exhausted, assist the searching baby in receiving the first feed at the breast without the mother exerting any effort.

- During the first few days after delivery, encourage and assist the mother to have as much skin-to-skin contact as possible with her baby. It is possible to "re-enact" their interaction in the first few days or even weeks after birth at any time if it was disrupted for any reason.

- When the baby is learning to breastfeed, discourage the use of pacifiers and bottles during the initial stages of lactation. Some babies develop a preference for feeding with an artificial teat, which can make them less enthusiastic about breastfeeding.

- When the baby shows that it is ready, let it start eating [1].

3. Conclusion

The infants begin breastfeeding within the first hour of their birth and consume only breast milk for the first 6 months of their lives and no other foods or liquids, including water, are provided. Infants should be breastfed whenever they want to, throughout the day and night. Pacifiers, teats, and bottles should not be used. Exclusive breastfeeding is a form of mother's behavior in giving exclusive breastfeeding to her baby. The success of exclusive breastfeeding is influenced by many factors, both internal and external factors.

Author details

Imtihanatun Najahah
Poltekkes Kemenkes Mataram, Health Polytechnic of the Mataram Ministry of Health, Mataram, Indonesia

*Address all correspondence to: imtihanatun4a@gmail.com

References

[1] WHO. Breastfeeding [Internet]. 2022. Available from: https://www.who.int/health-topics/breastfeeding#tab=tab_1 [Accessed: October 10, 2022]

[2] Roesli U, Mengenal ASI. Eksklusif. Jakarta: Trubus Agriwidya; 2000

[3] Mufdlilah et al. Buku Pedoman pemberdayaan Ibu Menyusui Pada Programasi Eksklusif. Yogyakarta. 2017

[4] Semukasa et al. Six months of exclusive breastfeeding recommendation: How applicable is the universal exclusive breastfeeding recommendation policy? African Journal of Food, Agriculture Nutrition, and Development. Jul 2014;**14**(4)

[5] WHO. Essential Newborn Care and Breastfeeding. Regional Office for Europe. 2002. Available from: https://apps.who.int/iris/bitstream/handle/10665/107481/e79227.pdf

[6] Nasir M. Umur Sama, Kok Tinggi Bisa Beda? Kemenkes RI: Jakarta; 2012

[7] Pickering KL, Morrow AL, Palacios GMR, Schanler RJ. Protecting Infants through Human Milk Advancing the Scientific Evidence. Advance in Experimental Medicine and Biology. Vol. 554. New York 233 Spring Street: Kluwer Academic/Plenum Publishers; 2004

[8] Gibney JM, Margetts BM, Kearney JM, Arab L. Gizi Kesehatan Masyarakat. (Andry Hartono, Pentj). Jakarta: EGC; 2009

[9] Bloss E, Wainaina F, Bailey RC. Prevalence and predictors of underweight, stunting, and wasting among children aged 5 and under in Western Kenya. Journal of Tropical Pediatrics. 2004. School of Public Health and Tropical Medicine, Tulane University, New Orleans, LA, USA. Oxford University Press. 2004;**50**(5). all rights reserved

[10] Ananta Y et al. Exclusive breastfeeding rate and factors associated with infant feeding practices in Indonesia. Paediatrica Indonesiana. 2016;**56**(1)

[11] Yovita Ananta et al. Exclusive breastfeeding rate and factors associated with infant feeding practices in Indonesia, Paediatr Indones. Jan 2016;**56**(1)

[12] Tsegaye M et al. Level of exclusive breastfeeding practice in remote and pastoralist community, Aysaita woreda, Afar. Ethiopia. International Breastfeeding Journal. 2019;**14**:6

[13] Cross Barnet C, Augustyn MC, Gross S, Resnik A, Paige, D.). Long-term breastfeeding support: Failing mothers in need. Maternal Child Health Journal. 2012;**16**:1926-1932

[14] ICM. Breastfeeding [Internet]. 2018. Available from: 8atement-files/2018/04/breastfeeding--v2017-eng-breastfeeding.pdf [Accessed: January 10, 2019]

[15] WHO. The Ten Steps to Successful Breastfeeding (Review 2018). 2018. https://www.who.int/nutrition/bfhi/ten-steps/en/ [Accessed: February 2, 2019]

[16] Tiwabe T et al. Exclusive breastfeeding practice andassociated factors among mothers in Mottatown, East Gojjam zone, Amhara Regional State, Ethiopia, a cross-sectional study. 2015

[17] Dwinanda N, Syarif BH, Sjarif DR. Factors affecting exclusive breastfeeding in term infants. Paediatr Indones. Jan 2018;**58**(1)

Chapter 3

Breast Milk and Metabolic Programming: Short-Term and Long-Term Health Benefits

Carolina Roldão

Abstract

Nutrition plays a major role in the development of health and disease later in adulthood. Breastfeeding is considered a cornerstone of healthy infant nutrition. It provides energy and nutrients that will help preventing both undernutrition, overweight and obesity. The Developmental Origins of Health and Disease (DOHaD) theory suggests that breast milk may play a role in modulating epigenetic factors such as DNA methylation from early stages of the life cycle. Exclusively breastfeeding infants presented lower blood pressure and serum cholesterol in adult life and lower risk of obesity and metabolic disorders, such as diabetes, hypertension or cardiovascular disease. It is believed that these effects are associated with the nutritional differences between breast milk and infant formula, such as lower protein content and the presence of bioactive components in breast milk. Epigenetic mechanisms may be the cause for the so claimed protective effect of breast milk in relation to the development of many diseases.

Keywords: breast milk, breastfeeding, metabolic programming, epigenetic mechanism, DOHaD, bioactive compounds, macronutrients, infant formulas

1. Introduction

Breastfeeding is considered one of the keys elements in the promotion and protection of the health of infants worldwide. The European Society for Pediatric Gastroenterology, Hepatology and Nutrition (ESPGHAN) Committee on Nutrition described breastfeeding as the natural and advisable way of supporting the healthy growth and development of young children [1].

The World Health Organization (WHO) promotes the adoption of counseling guidelines to extend breastfeeding periods, suggesting that breastfeeding should begin within the first hour after birth, be exclusive for the first 6 months without any other liquids or solids, including water. After 6 months, breast milk alone is not sufficient and should be combined with appropriate complementary foods that are safe and adequate [2–6].

Breastfeeding is an essential aspect of healthy infant nutrition and growth, as it continues to supply energy and nutrients that help prevent undernutrition, overweight, and obesity [7–10].

The prevalence of breastfeeding has undergone changes over time, reaching its lowest point after World War II due to social and technological shifts affecting women's roles, income, education, and the widespread use and aggressive marketing of breast milk substitutes [8, 9]. However, starting in the 1970s, there was a resurgence of breastfeeding, particularly among employed women [8].

In response to the Innocenti Declaration, the World Health Organization (WHO) and UNICEF launched the Baby Friendly Hospital Initiative in 1992 [10, 11]. The program's objective is to protect, support, and promote breastfeeding in health facilities such as obstetrics, neonatology, and pediatrics services [11]. The aim is to provide new mothers and their infants with the information and confidence needed to initiate and continue breastfeeding. A baby-friendly facility complies with the International Code of Marketing of Breastmilk Substitutes by endorsing, supporting, and promoting breastfeeding while ensuring appropriate use of breast milk substitutes when necessary [11].

The European Region has the lowest breastfeeding rates, with only 14% of women breastfeeding their babies for up to 6 months according to data published in 2015. This highlights the importance of initiating breastfeeding within the first hour after birth to improve breastfeeding rates. Campaigns like the Baby Friendly Hospital Initiative should be encouraged [12]. Returning to the workplace can be a barrier to exclusive and continued breastfeeding. Maternity leave has been linked to better maternal and child health outcomes, with 40 of the world's 41 wealthiest countries offering paid maternity leave. However, the United States is the only country that does not provide paid maternity leave to employed mothers. The benefits of breastfeeding for both the infant and mother are well-documented and include a lower risk of respiratory infections, asthma, diarrhea, food allergies, diabetes, improved cognitive development, and a reduced risk of metabolic disease in adulthood [2, 13, 14].

The Developmental Origins of Health and Disease (DOHaD) theory suggests that breast milk may play a role in epigenetic regulation such as DNA methylation from early stages of life. Changes to the epigenome can lead to long-term development of metabolic disorders, linking external factors like nutrition and environment to the long-term health outcomes of early life phases [2, 15–17].

2. Metabolic programming

2.1 Epigenetic mechanism

The "first thousand days of life" from conception to age 2 has been the focus of attention for researchers worldwide. This period is considered critical for wellbeing and brain development, as the greatest amount of human growth occurs during this time when cells in the body are being formed and programmed. Studies have shown that insults during the crucial periods of pregnancy and lactation, such as malnutrition, stress, and air pollution exposure, increase the risk of chronic noncommunicable diseases (NCDs) such as obesity, cardiovascular disease, and diabetes throughout life. This leads to metabolic programming, developmental plasticity, and the concept of Developmental Origins of Health and Disease (DOHaD) [2].

The environment has a profound impact on organisms, as per the principle of modern biology. Darwin's Theory of Evolution suggests that through natural selection, the best DNA alleles are preserved across generations due to genetic variations caused by mutations in the DNA sequence. Currently, it is understood that the environment shapes the organism through epigenetic processes, which do not involve changes in the DNA sequence [18]. The idea of metabolic programming, which involves the impact of prenatal and postnatal metabolic events on adult health, has been established for about 40 years. This theory suggests that these events leave a "mark" in the body (or DNA) and result in cellular memory [9–11, 14, 19]. These physiological adaptations are possible due to the plasticity of cells, which is temporary in embryonic and fetal stages but persistent in cells like the immune system [20].

Epigenetics result in marks that play a significant role in shaping the risk of metabolic and non-communicable disorders. The DOHaD theory explains the connection between the nutritional and environmental conditions of pregnancy and early childhood, and the development of health and diseases [15–18]. NCDs usually appear in adulthood, due to the decreasing flexibility of cells and tissues over time. The likelihood of NCDs can be influenced by the body composition and diet of the mother before and during pregnancy, as well as the nutrition of the fetus and infant. Thus, early-life interventions have the potential to reduce later disease risk and affect future generations, while later interventions are expected to have only a minimal impact [16].

The concept of epigenetics refers to modifications that are passed down and affect gene expression, without altering the DNA sequence. These changes in the epigenome are achieved through three processes: DNA methylation, histone modifications, and noncoding RNA expression [2]. During DNA methylation, methyltransferases bind methyl groups to DNA at cytosine sites (CpG islands) during replication or de novo methylation. Methylation in promoter regions of DNA often results in inactive chromatin and silences gene transcription, impacting the expression of key genes for cell stability. Methylation of CpG dinucleotides at the 5′ promoter regions of genes results in stable silencing of transcription. Methylation patterns are established primarily during embryonic development or early postnatal life [2, 7, 20, 21].

The methylation of CpG dinucleotides results in the inactivation of gene transcription by RNA polymerase by making chromatin inaccessible for transcription. This affects the expression of genes crucial for maintaining cell homeostasis [2, 7]. The second mechanism is the modification of histones, which are proteins that help organize DNA by packaging it into nucleosomes. They negatively impact gene transcription by physically obstructing access and blocking the binding of transcription factors, making chromatin less accessible [2]. Histones regulate gene expression by controlling the access of transcription factors (TFs) to the DNA sequence, thereby altering the rate of transcription to messenger RNA (mRNA) [22].

The modification of histones in the amino-terminal region of the histone tails includes processes like acetylation, methylation, sumoylation, phosphorylation and ubiquitination. Acetylation is the most widely recognized modification, carried out by enzymes known as acetyltransferases (HATs) and deacetylases (HDACs). The acetylation of histones leads to the opening of chromatin, thereby enabling the transcription machinery to access the DNA [2].

In contrast, when chromatin is inactive, histone deacetylation reduces the attachment of transcription factors, hindering gene expression [22]. MicroRNAs (miRs), a type of small noncoding RNA, play a role in posttranscriptional regulation by either breaking down mRNA or blocking its translation into protein. These three epigenetic changes, DNA methylation, histone modification and microRNA regulation, shape the expression of multiple genes and drive metabolic programming [2].

3. The impact of breast milk components on metabolic programming

Breastfeeding is recognized to have significant short-term health benefits, and evidence is growing for its long-term consequences [17]. The first 6 months of life is a crucial period for the development of adiposity [23]. The composition of the nutritional environment during this time can contribute to the risk of certain diseases in adulthood, often through epigenetic changes. There is evidence to suggest that certain components of breast milk may directly impact epigenetic modifications [24, 25].

The composition of breast milk includes both macronutrients and micronutrients, and it changes regularly based on various factors such as the health of the mother and baby, maternal diet, environment, and genetics. These changes ensure that breast milk can adapt to the changing nutritional requirements of the growing infant [26, 27].

Moreover, breast milk has a distinct advantage in that it provides newborns with the necessary macronutrients and micronutrients through factors such as enzymes, immune components, and adipokines. Leptin, ghrelin, adiponectin, resistin, and obestatin are some of the most well-known adipokines. Adiponectin and leptin, in particular, are potent and widely studied appetite regulators that are linked to obesity. Research has demonstrated that the leptin present in breast milk helps control appetite and manage calorie intake. This finding has sparked further investigation into the impact of leptin on neonatal development, which was previously an under-researched area [28–31].

Over the years, numerous studies have explored the connections between breastfeeding and the regulation of infant appetite, as well as its correlation with a decreased risk of obesity and other chronic non-communicable diseases (NCDs). These relationships are due to the synergistic effects of various milk components, maternal characteristics, and breastfeeding patterns [32].

3.1 The role of leptin in the appetite regulation

Leptin, a bioactive compound found in breast milk, has a key impact on metabolic programming. It is generated by white adipose tissue based on the body's fat content, and it moves from adipose tissue into the bloodstream, where it binds to receptors in the hypothalamus and crosses the blood-brain barrier. Upon binding to the receptors, leptin influences the release of appetite-suppressing peptides, resulting in lower food intake and increased energy expenditure. With higher levels of leptin, energy expenditure is boosted through reduced food intake and increased heat production, while lower levels of leptin boost the growth of fat cells [30].

As a result, the amount of leptin in breast milk varies among infants, as it is dependent on the maternal adiposity and BMI (Body Mass Index). Mothers with low fat levels and low plasma concentrations of leptin produce milk with a low amount of leptin, resembling infant formulas (IFs), while obese mothers provide higher doses of leptin [25, 30].

Recently, it was discovered that leptin is produced not only by white adipose tissue, but also by the placenta and breast epithelium and secreted into breast milk [25, 30]. However, the contribution of each source to the total amount of leptin in breast milk is still unclear. A study on rats showed that gastric leptin is not fully functional during most of the lactation period due to immature stomachs. Additionally, leptin mRNA levels tend to be low during the first days of life and only start increasing after the fifteenth day of life [25].

Çağiran Yilmaz F et al., in cross-sectional study, assessed the relationship between the anthropometric measurements of the mothers (body weights and BMI) and leptin levels in breast milk and maternal serum, both were positively correlating in all months. The relationship between anthropometric measurements of infants, and the leptin levels in breast milk and maternal serum determined that the body weights of the infants and the breast milk leptin level in the assessed months were negatively correlated. In contrast, the length of the infants and leptin levels in breast milk and maternal serum were positive correlated [30].

Another similar study found that during the lactation period, breast milk leptin concentration correlated positively with maternal plasma leptin concentration and with maternal BMI. Breast milk leptin concentration at 1 month of lactation was negatively correlated with infant BMI at 18 and 24 months of age. When lactation occurred for a longer period (1 and at 3 months) was found a better negative correlation among milk leptin concentration and infant BMI at 12–24 months of age. It is concluded that infant body weight during the first 2 years may be influenced by milk leptin concentration during the first stages of lactation. These results seem to point out that milk leptin is an important factor that might explain, the major risk of obesity of formula-fed infants with respect to breast-fed infants [31].

Other appetite-regulating hormones, such as ghrelin and Peptide YY (PYY), are produced in the gastrointestinal tract. Ghrelin stimulates food intake, while PYY and leptin suppress appetite and increase metabolism. In addition, the ghrelin/PYY ratio is a more meaningful indicator of orexigenic drive, rather than ghrelin and PYY levels separately. Rapid weight gain in the early stages of life has been linked to a higher risk of adulthood obesity and cardiovascular disease [23].

The study by Fluiter, Kirsten S et al. aimed to investigate the impact of other appetite-regulating hormones (ARH) such as ghrelin, PYY, and leptin on the programming of adiposity. 297 term-born infants had their ghrelin, PYY, and leptin concentrations measured in their blood samples at 3 and 6 months of age, along with a measurement of their fat mass percentage. The results showed that ghrelin levels increased from age 3 to 6 months, while PYY levels decreased, leading to an increase in the ghrelin/PYY ratio over time. Meanwhile, leptin levels decreased from 3 to 6 months. Leptin levels at age 3 and 6 months were found to be related with the fat mass percentage at those same ages, as well as the gain in fat mass percentage from 1 to 6 months. Ghrelin at age 3 months correlated only with fat mass percentage at 6 months, while PYY and ghrelin/PYY ratio did not correlate. Among breastfeeding infants, both ghrelin and the ghrelin/PYY ratio at 3 months correlated with the increase in body fat percentage from 1 to 6 months. At 3 months, exclusively breastfeeding infants had lower levels of ghrelin and higher levels of PYY compared to those who were formula-fed. The increasing ghrelin/PYY ratio suggests a growing orexigenic drive, the ghrelin and leptin, but not PYY, correlated with more fat mass development during the first 6 months, suggesting that they might be involved in adiposity programming [23].

In another study, it was suggested that pre and neonatal overfeeding may affect the DNA methylation patterns in promoter regions of genes regulating food intake and body weight in the hypothalamus. When neonatal overfeeding was induced in rats, rapid weight gain was observed in the early stages, leading to a metabolic syndrome phenotype including obesity, hyperleptinemia, hyperglycemia, hyperinsulinemia, and an elevated insulin/glucose ratio. Low methylation levels of neuropeptide Y (NPY) were seen in both the overfed and control groups, while the gene proopiomelanocortin (POMC) showed increased methylation of CpG dinucleotides. The extent of DNA methylation was found to be inversely related to the ratios of POMC expression/leptin and POMC expression/insulin. These results indicate that a nutritionally-induced alteration of methylation patterns is crucial for regulating body weight and that overfeeding may be considered an epigenetic risk factor for obesity programming [25, 33]. These data suggest that the nutritional status affects methylation, and consequently, the regulatory mechanism of a gene promoter. Overfeeding has been identified as an epigenetic risk factor for programming obesity and consequent cardiovascular diseases [33].

Another study, rats were given physiological doses of leptin during lactation after being exposed to a high-fat diet, and it was found that their POMC promoter methylation was reduced. In contrast, the control group fed a high-fat diet and not supplemented with leptin showed increased POMC promoter methylation. There was also a negative correlation between DNA methylation and mRNA levels of POMC. This suggests that early supplementation with leptin can help regulate food intake, preventing excessive weight gain later in life. The findings indicate that gene promoter methylation may be a mechanism by which early life leptin supplementation can promote a healthy phenotype in adulthood [25].

The changes in the methylation status of the LEP gene are linked to perinatal conditions. The Dutch famine of 1944–1945 provides a prime example of this. Children of mothers who experienced undernutrition during the Dutch famine, either during the pre-conception period or late pregnancy, showed greater DNA methylation of the LEP gene. Additionally, LEP gene methylation was linked to the duration of breastfeeding, with a negative correlation between the DNA methylation of the LEP promoter and the length of breastfeeding. This lower methylation of the LEP gene may account for the higher levels of leptin in these infants and could be one of the ways in which breastfeeding helps protect against childhood obesity [25].

3.2 The role of adiponectin in the appetite regulation

Adipokines are secretory factors produced by adipocytes that play a role in regulating various metabolic processes, including lipid and glucose metabolism and energy homeostasis, as well as having anti-inflammatory effects [28, 29]. Adiponectin, in particular, is present in human milk at much higher concentrations than other appetite regulators, being forty times more abundant than leptin [29]. The levels of adiponectin in breast milk are positively correlated with those in the mother's bloodstream, and the mother's serum adiponectin levels are inversely linked to her body weight and BMI [29].

During pregnancy maternal serum adiponectin and breast milk adiponectin show an inverse relationship with infant adiposity, probably due the changes in maternal metabolism and adipose tissue deposition [28].

The impact of adiponectin on reducing childhood obesity is still a topic of debate. However, numerous studies have shown a negative correlation between maternal serum and breast milk adiponectin levels during pregnancy and infant adiposity development in the first year of life. Recently, adiponectin has gained attention as a potential clinical biomarker for obesity and related diseases in therapeutic approaches. Keeping in mind that adiponectin is not routinely measured, future studies are needed to verify which indicator - whether pre-pregnancy, early, mid- or late pregnancy weight status, or body fat - can be considered the best surrogate for adiponectin. Additionally, further human trials are needed in order to translate the observational research on the use of adiponectin as a clinical biomarker into therapeutic strategies in the future [28].

3.3 Macronutrients

The way an infant is fed (exclusive breastfeeding, milk formula or mixed feeding), the composition of their milk, and the amount they consume are crucial elements in ensuring optimal growth and development during the first 6 months of life, leading to long-term health benefits. Quick weight gain during the first 6 months can be a significant predictor of adverse metabolic outcomes in adulthood, such as a higher risk of obesity, central adiposity, and insulin resistance. However, it remains unclear if slow weight gain in breastfed infants is due to low caloric intake or the nutrient composition of breast milk (macronutrients) [34].

A cohort study tested the hypothesis that differential breast milk total calorie content or macronutrient contents may be associated with infancy growth. It was concluded breast milk of mothers exclusively breast feeding was more calorific with higher percentage fat, lower percentage carbohydrate and lower percentage protein. The higher breast milk total calorie content was associated with lower 12 months BMI/adiposity, and lower 3–12 months gains in weight/BMI. Breast milk percentage fat was inversely related to 3–12 months gains in weight, BMI and adiposity, whereas percentage carbohydrate was positively related to these measures. Breast milk percentage protein was positively related to 12-months BMI [34].

Infants who are fed breast milk tend to have lower levels of adiposity, suggesting that the composition of breast milk is optimal for their healthy growth. Breast milk has a higher proportion of lipids and a lower proportion of proteins and carbohydrates. Thus, infants fed breast milk with a lower percentage of fat felt less satiated and drank larger volumes of milk, hence gaining more weight [34].

3.3.1 Breast milk oligosaccharides

Lactose is the main sugar found in breast milk. Its high concentration, 6.7 g/100 ml, is higher than that of other species, reflecting the high nutritional needs of the human brain [35]. The unique nutritional value of breast milk is largely attributed to human milk oligosaccharides (HMOs), which are the third most abundant component after lactose and lipids. HMOs are complex sugars with diverse structures that are indigestible by infants [36].

HMOs are bioactive molecules that play a crucial role in infant health, with levels ranging from 1 to 10 g/l in mature milk and 15–23 g/l in colostrum [35, 37]. In mature milk, 35–50% of HMOs are fucosylated, 12–14% are sialylated, and 42–55% are non-fucosylated and neutral, respectively. The structures of oligosaccharides vary based on the presence of specific transferase enzymes expressed in the lactocytes. It has been hypothesized that the variation in HMO composition among mothers may enhance human survival, as pathogens exhibit different binding affinities according to specific structures of oligosaccharides [35]. HMOs also act as prebiotics, promoting the growth of beneficial bacteria such as Bifidobacteria and Bacteroides species [35, 36].

Throughout human life, the abundance of bifidobacteria decreases, going to 90% of the total colonic microbiota in breastfed infants to just 5% in adults, and declining even further in the elderly. A low abundance of bifidobacteria has been associated with gastrointestinal disorders such as irritable bowel syndrome. Supplementing with HMOs may be an effective strategy for modulating the gut microbiota and promoting the growth of beneficial bifidobacteria in adults [38].

HMOs have an anti-pathogenic effect against bacterium, virus, fungus and protozoan parasite. This is because HMOs can bind to pathogens and prevent pathogens from binding to receptors on the surface of epithelial cells and passing through the gastrointestinal tract, causing disease [36].

The impact of HMOs on gut barrier function has been largely underexplored. The intestinal epithelium the small intestine and colon are considered a key part of the innate immunity, serving as a physical barrier [36, 38].

The intestinal barrier is composed of a mucus layer that covers a single layer of intestinal epithelial cells, which separates bacteria from the underlying submucosa and is critical to maintaining gut homeostasis [38]. The intercellular junctional complexes regulate the passage of luminal nutrients, ions, and water and restrict bacterial entry, thereby controlling the barrier function of the epithelium. Microbes can indirectly affect epithelial permeability through their impact on host immune cells and the release of cytokines, either reducing or enhancing the barrier function. HMOs can influence the expression of intercellular junction proteins, reducing permeability and strengthening the barrier function of the epithelium [36, 38].

Currently, HMOs have been synthesized artificially as additives in infant milk formula for the infants who cannot be fed with breast milk. Thus, supporting the growth and providing protection against different diseases in early years life [36].

The HMOs that showed positive results were 2′-fucosylactose (2'-FL) and lacto-N-neo-tetraose (LNnT). A clinical study showed that IFs just with 2'-FL inhibited inflammatory cytokine production. IFs with 2′-FL and LNnT kept infants healthy whose parents had respiratory tract infections and bronchitis. Recently, it was found that the addition of 2′-FL and LNnT to IF could change the microbiota towards a similar microbiota of breastfed infants, by increasing the quantity of Bifidobacteria and decreasing the number of *Clostridium difficile* [36, 38].

Clinical studies have been conducted to investigate the impact of pre-pregnancy and postpartum maternal BMI on the composition of HMOs and its effect on infant growth [39, 40].

Results showed that maternal obesity was associated with lower levels of fucosylated and sialylated HMOs. Infants born to obese mothers had lower intake of these HMOs. Specific HMOs, including 3-fucosylactose, 3-sialylactose, 6-sialylactose, disyallylacto-N-tetraose, disyallylacto-N-hexaose, and total acidic HMOs, were positively related to infant growth during the first 6 months of life. This suggests that maternal obesity is linked to changes in HMO concentrations, which in turn may affect childhood adiposity [37, 41].

3.3.2 Breast milk lipids

Lipids, in the form of fat globules, are the main source of energy in breast milk, accounting for 44% of the total energy provided. They are produced in the endoplasmic reticulum of mammary epithelial cells and are surrounded by an outer membrane rich in bioactive compounds such as glycerophospholipids, sphingolipids, sphingomyelin, glycolipids, cholesterol, and glycosylated proteins. When these components are added to IFs, they have been linked to improved neurocognitive development and immune function [35].

The content of lipids, including long chain polyunsaturated fatty acids (LC-PUFAs), in breast milk is heavily influenced by the mother's diet. LC-PUFAs have several key biological effects, particularly on membrane functions, growth, immune response, and the functional development of the retina and cerebral cortex. This suggests that developing countries should consider supplementing IFs with alpha-linoleic and docosahexaenoic acid (DHA). Medium-chain monoglycerides have the ability to inactivate various pathogens in vitro, such as group B Streptococcus [34, 35].

The majority of breast milk arachidonic acid derives from maternal reserves, but the content of DHA depends on the maternal nutrition. For a daily DHA supply of 100 mg in exclusively breastfeeding infants, the mother should consume at least 200 mg/day of DHA [35].

A recent study reported an inverse association between fat intake at 2 years of age and body fat, assessed by bioelectrical impedance analysis at 20 years, also suggesting that early diet containing greater fat may benefit later body composition. It is believed that the content of omega 6 fatty acids and linoleic acid may explain this relationship [34].

Results of a recent systematic review showed a positive association between maternal BMI and the amount of fat in breast milk in term-born infants between 1 and 6 months postpartum. For each increase of 1 kg/m^2 in maternal BMI the concentration of fat in milk increased by 0.56 g/l [42].

The link between breastfeeding and obesity is well-established, but the mechanisms involved are unclear. Some studies have attempted to define some of the breast milk lipidome, identifying 300 lipid species and 700 lipid characteristics. However, more specific details on maternal genetics, health and diet are lacking from literature. Future research should to collat more maternal data, including dietary information as to understand the impact of the breast milk lipidome and it is consequences on infant health [43].

3.3.3 Breast milk proteins

Proteins are the third most important component in breast milk for the healthy growth and development of infants, providing not only nutrition but also performing several bioactive functions. Proteins act as carriers for other nutrients, such as lactoferrin, haptocorrin, alpha-lactalbumin, and beta-casein, and help promote intestinal development and nutrient absorption. The quantity and quality of protein in human milk are crucial in influencing infant growth and body composition. In fact, a high protein intake in infancy has been associated with increased weight gain and a higher risk of developing obesity later [35].

Breastfed infants' protein intake has served as a model for estimating protein needs in the first year of life. The protein content of breast milk depends on the stage of lactation and time since partum, with a high protein concentration during the first few weeks of lactation and a gradual decrease throughout the first year. Proteins are made up of amino acids that are linked together by peptide bonds. During digestion, proteins are broken down into simple amino acids and then absorbed. These absorbed amino acids are then used to build new proteins. The amount of protein intake may not accurately reflect the amount of amino acids used to synthesize new proteins because some breast milk proteins remain intact in the infant's feces. Despite a decrease in protein concentration during lactation, the nutritional value of breast milk remains constant to meet the growing infant's needs [44].

There is evidence to suggest a correlation between the presence of branched-chain amino acids (leucine, isoleucine, and valine) and aromatic amino acids (phenylalanine and tyrosine) in breast milk and an increased risk of childhood obesity. The maternal body mass index (BMI) is positively correlated with the amount of isoleucine, leucine, and aromatic amino acids consumed by infants. Infants who consume the highest amounts of these amino acids also show a positive association with their body composition [39].

4. Breastfeeding vs formula-fed infants

Breast milk has been shown to be the ideal source of nutrition for infants. However, most infants are fed human-milk substitutes. Cow's milk proteins are the unique source of proteins in most IFs but have a lower quality compared with breast milk, partly because of differences in their amino acid contents [41].

IFs have been designed to imitate the nutritional benefits of breast milk for infants unable to be breastfed. The aim is to provide similar outcomes for optimal growth, development, maturation of the immune system and programming of the metabolism system. Despite the ongoing improvement of IFs, the growth patterns and development of body composition still differ from those of breastfed infants and may result in a higher risk of obesity for formula-fed infants [41, 45].

The mechanism behind the protective effect of breastfeeding is not fully understood. Several mechanisms may account such as differences in appetite regulation, early growth patterns, circulating leptin, and the gut microbiome [44, 45].

The first few months of life are a crucial time for avoiding metabolic, cardiovascular, and obesity issues in the future. Infant growth and weight gain during the first half-year of life is a more accurate predictor of adolescent body composition compared to weight gain from 6 months to 2 years old. Early patterns of body fat also indicate future obesity, as obese adults tend to experience an earlier rise in body fat compared to non-obese adults [41].

Breastfed infants generally have a slower weight gain in the first year of life compared to formula-fed infants. Formula-fed newborns have a 22% higher risk of developing childhood obesity compared to breastfed infants. Breastfeeding has been shown to be associated with a 13% reduction in childhood overweight or obesity, which is strongly linked to adult obesity, despite declining rates of breastfeeding. Exclusive breastfeeding is more effective in preventing childhood obesity than the combination of breastfeeding and IFs (mixed feeding), and the mixed feeding is more effective than exclusive formula feeding [41].

Breast milk protein concentration decreases over the weeks of lactation, while the protein concentration in IFs remains constant. Research has demonstrated that formula-fed infants consume 66–70% more protein compared to breastfed infants in the first 6 months of life. The lower protein content in breast milk is believed to affect infants' growth, and reduced protein intake may prevent childhood obesity [44, 45].

Kouwenhoven et al. studied the short-term and long-term effects of a low-protein IFs (with 20% reduced protein content) on growth and body composition. Despite the lower protein levels, differences in growth, weight gain, and body composition still existed between formula-fed and breastfed infants. Formula-fed infants had significantly higher total fat mass, total fat-free mass, and fat-free mass index (FFMI) compared to breastfed infants up to 6 months of age. At 2 years old, significant differences in body composition were observed between the low-protein formula group and the breastfed reference group. Further research is necessary to examine the potential impact of higher protein intake on growth and body composition [45].

The exact mechanisms behind the impact of higher protein intake on growth and body composition are not yet understood. However, it is known that the anabolic hormones insulin and IGF-1 respond to changes in protein intake. No short-term correlations between insulin, glucose, the Homeostatic Model Assessment for Insulin Resistance (HOMA-IR), and body composition have been observed in the first year of life. However, these associations were evident at 2 years of age, indicating that decreased insulin sensitivity early in life may affect body composition later in life, rather than the other way around [32, 45].

The differences in growth and body composition between infants fed low-protein formula and those who are breastfed suggest the use of formula with even lower protein content than 1.7 g/100 kcal. A recent study showed that a formula containing only 1.43 g protein per 100 kcal resulted in a significantly lower weight gain rate compared to formulas with 1.9 g or 2.18 g protein/100 kcal during the first 4 months of life [45]. Although the investigators reported adequate growth, it was not possible to determine the safety of such a low-protein formula. Thus, further research is required to determine the safety and effectiveness of reducing protein intake to levels closer to that found in human milk [45].

The fat matrix of IFs changed in the early 20th century. Previously it was composed of cow's milk fat, later being constituted of a blend of vegetable oils.

This allows for a better mimicry of the mono- and polyunsaturated fatty acid (PUFA) profile found in breast milk. Formula is usually supplemented with higher levels of LC-PUFAs from the omega 3 and omega 6 families. The omega 3 LC-PUFAs have been linked to improved insulin sensitivity, reduced weight gain and adiposity, and improved lipid profiles. Postnatal supplementation with omega 3 PUFAs has been shown to reduce body fat deposition in adulthood and improve plasma lipid profile and glucose homeostasis. Similar benefits were observed with a low-omega-6 PUFA diet [41].

The main source of carbohydrates in standard IFs is lactose. Animal studies have shown that a high intake of carbohydrates in early life can have negative long-term effects, such as chronic hyperinsulinemia and adult-onset obesity [41].

Thus, although the mixture of HMOs found in breast milk cannot be replicated in IFs, adding prebiotics is a step towards mimicking their benefits. Currently, the prebiotics used in IFs mainly consist of a 9:1 mixture of short-chain galactooligosaccharides (scGOS) and long-chain fructooligosaccharides (lcFOS). However, the prebiotics commonly added to IFs have much simpler structures than HMOs and cannot reproduce all their benefits [41].

Recently, the availability of 2′FL and lacto-N-neotetraose (LNnT), has provided opportunities for the development of IFs that are similar to breast milk. Supplementation with these two HMOs did not result in any differences in weight, length, or BMI compared to non-supplemented IFs. However, it did result in a similar gut microbiota and metabolic programming to that of breastfed infants at 3 months of age [41].

Recently, it has been acknowledged that breast milk is a source of viable commensal and potentially probiotic bacteria such as Staphylococcus, Streptococcus, Bifidobacterium, and Lactobacillus. The composition of the breast milk microbiome is influenced by factors such as the maternal nutrition, gestational age and health status. The prevailing theory is that the bacteria reach the mammary gland through the lymphatic and circulatory systems, providing the infant with 107–108 bacterial cells per day through the consumption of approximately 800 ml of breast milk [41].

Probiotics are defined as 'live micro-organisms that, when administered in adequate amounts, confer a health benefit on the host'. The most commonly probiotics used in infant nutrition are strains of Bifidobacterium and Lactobacillus. The long-term impact of early consumption of probiotics on growth has been studied, with no effect observed from supplementation with *Lactobacillus rhamnosus* or *Lactobacillus fermentum* in the first months of life on growth at 2, 3, 5, and 13 years. Contrarily, the use of maternal probiotic supplementation with *L. rhamnosus* was seen to have an impact on the weight development of children. This was indicated by a slower rate of weight gain until the age of 2 to 4 years, particularly among children who became overweight later. This led to a lower body mass index until 7 years of age. The ESPGHAN Committee on Nutrition concluded in 2011 that supplementing healthy infants with currently evaluated probiotic formulas does not raise safety concerns regarding growth and adverse effects. However, due to high variability in responses, the relevance of supplementing IFs with probiotics remains unclear and the routine use of probiotic supplemented IFs is not currently mandatory [41].

Breastfeeding has been linked to a decreased risk of obesity, metabolic disorders such as diabetes, hypertension, and cardiovascular disease, as well as a lower likelihood of being overweight or obese in adulthood [25]. On the other hand, formula-fed infants have a higher risk of developing insulin resistance and type-2 diabetes later in life. They have been found to have higher levels of insulin secretion, indicated by higher concentrations of urinary C-peptide, as well as higher pre- and post-meal blood glucose levels. These elevated insulin levels may contribute to a greater buildup of subcutaneous fat. In comparison, breastfed infants have 3% lower insulin levels in adulthood than those who were formula-fed [41].

Early nutrition may also have an impact on cardiovascular risk factors and atherosclerosis in adulthood. Formula-fed infants may have higher blood pressure levels and an increased risk of atherosclerosis compared to breastfed infants. A prospective study of Mexican children found that exclusive and prolonged breastfeeding had a positive effect on later cardiovascular health, with lower levels of total cholesterol, LDL cholesterol, and triglycerides at age 4. However, at 4 and 8 weeks, formula-fed infants had lower levels of serum cholesterol, triglycerides, and transaminase (ALAT, ASAT, γGT) compared to breastfed infants. Despite these findings, the long-term impact of breastfeeding on the prevention of cardiovascular disease is still a matter of debate and more research is needed to fully understand the issue [41].

5. Conclusion

More and more evidence is showing that breast feeding confers protection to the infant against a range of diseases such as obesity, hypertension, dyslipidemia and cardiovascular disease.

This seems to be a result of early metabolic programming that we can find in the developmental origins of the health and disease hypothesis (DOHaD) theory. This DOHaD theory clarifies how the early life environment can impact the risk of chronic diseases from childhood to adulthood and witch the mechanisms epigenetics involved. Thus, there is a relationship between the Nutritional and environmental challenges prior to and during gestation, lactation, and early life and the health development of the infant. One where breast milk plays a key role. It is widely recognized that the mothers health and lifestyle has a big impact on offspring. The support and promotion of breastfeeding by healthcare professionals have the potential to increase breastfeeding prevalence before, during and after childbirth.

For the infants who need IF is possible adjust and further improve IF. However, is difficult to mimic breast milk or the art of breastfeeding because of its complexity and its effect on infant physiology.

Improving the functional effects of IF to reduce the gap between breastfed and formula-fed infants is crucial and has been the topic of great research over the past years. However, it is still under study which components should be added to IF and in which quantity.

Regarding metabolic health of infants, an improved IFs would consist in modulating all macronutrients. Decrease the quantity and improve their quality of the proteins, add lipids with size, structure and composition of the fat globule and balanced omega 3: omega 6 LC-PUFA ratio and to supplement with prebiotics, probiotics or synbiotics. The impact of breastfeeding on public's health is big as it will help with obesity and DNTs prevention and ensuring improvement of quality of life and sustainable living for current and future generations.

Acknowledgements

The author would like to acknowledge the editorial support, namely the constructive review of the manuscript and raised comments. The author also would like to acknowledge to Isabel Caçoilo e Joana Matos Silva for critical review of the manuscript.

Conflict of interest

The authors declare no conflict of interest.

Author details

Carolina Roldão
ICBAS School of Medicine and Biomedical Sciences, Porto, Portugal

*Address all correspondence to: carolinafroldao@outlook.pt

References

[1] Arslanoglu S, Corpeleijn W, Moro G, Braegger C, Campoy C, Colomb V, et al. Donor human milk for preterm infants: Current evidence and research directions. Journal of Pediatric Gastroenterology and Nutrition. 2013;**57**(4):535-542

[2] Lisboa PC, Miranda RA, Souza LL, Moura EG. Can breastfeeding affect the rest of our life? Neuropharmacology [Internet]. 2021;**200**(August):108821. DOI: 10.1016/j.neuropharm.2021.108821

[3] Qian J, Wu T, Lv M, Fang Z, Chen M, Zeng Z, et al. The value of mobile health in improving breastfeeding outcomes among perinatal or postpartum women: Systematic review and meta-analysis of randomized controlled trials. JMIR mHealth and uHealth. 2021;**9**(7):1-12

[4] Cordero MJA, Sánchez Lòpez AM, Baños NM, Villar NM, Ruiz ME, Rodrìguez EH. Lactancia materna como prevención del sobrepeso y la obesidad en el niño y el adolescente; revisión sistemática. Nutrición Hospitalaria. 2015;**31**(2):606-620

[5] Lewkowitz AK, López JD, Stein RI, Rhoades JS, Schulz RC, Woolfolk CL, et al. Effect of a home-based lifestyle intervention on breastfeeding initiation among socioeconomically disadvantaged African American women with overweight or obesity. Breastfeeding Medicine. 2018;**13**(6):418-425

[6] De Nutrição C, Amil J, Porto D. Alimentação e nutrição do lactente. Acta Pediátrica Portuguesa. 2012;**43**(5):S17-S40

[7] Cordero MJA, Baños NM, García LB, Villar NM, Barrilao RG, López AMS. Lactancia materna como método para prevenir alteraciones cardiovasculares en la madre y el niño. Nutrición Hospitalaria. 2015;**31**(5):1936-1946

[8] Sarafana S, Abecasis F, Tavares A, Soares I, Gomes A. Aleitamento materno: evolução na última década. Acta Pediátrica Portuguesa [Internet]. 2006;**1**(37):9-14. Available from: http://www.spp.pt/Userfiles/File/App/Artigos/7/20080424104556_APP_Vol_37_N1.pdf#page=21

[9] Aguiar H et al. Aleitamento Materno: A importância de intervir. Acta Médica Portuguesa. 2011;**24**:889-896

[10] Kislaya I, Braz P, Dias CM, Loureiro I. Evolução do aleitamento materno em Portugal: dados dos Inquéritos Nacionais de Saúde entre 1995-2014. Repositório Científico do Instituto Nacional de Saúde [Internet]. 2018;**2014**:1-3. Available from: http://repositorio.insa.pt/handle/10400.18/6110

[11] Unicef Portugal. A Iniciativa Amiga dos Bebés tem como missão proteger, promover e apoiar o aleitamento materno. Lisbon, Portugal: UNICEF Portugal; 2022. Available from: https://www.unicef.pt/o-que-fazemos/o-nosso-trabalho-em-portugal/iniciativa-amiga-dos-bebes/a-iniciativa-amiga-dos-bebes/

[12] Tudela J, Martínez M, Valdivia R, Romo J, Portillo M, Rangel R. Enhanced reader.pdf. Nature. 2010;**388**:539-547

[13] Shamir R. The benefits of breast feeding. Nestle Nutrition Institute Workshop Series [Internet]. 2016;**86**:67-76. Available from: https://www.karger.com/Article/FullText/442724

[14] Agostoni C, Braegger C, Decsi T, Kolacek S, Koletzko B, Michaelsen KF, et al. Breast-feeding: A commentary by

the ESPGHAN committee on nutrition. Journal of Pediatric Gastroenterology and Nutrition. 2009 Jul;**49**(1):112-125

[15] Bianco-Miotto T, Craig JM, Gasser YP, Van Dijk SJ, Ozanne SE. Epigenetics and DOHaD: From basics to birth and beyond. Journal of Developmental Origins of Health and Disease. 2017;**8**(5):513-519

[16] Godfrey KM, Costello P, Lillycrop K. Development, epigenetics and metabolic programming Europe PMC funders group. Nestle Nutrition Institute Workshop Series [Internet]. 2016;**85**:71-80. Available from: https://www.ncbi.nlm.nih.gov/pmc/articles/PMC4880042/pdf/emss-68148.pdf

[17] Hartwig FP, De Mola CL, Davies NM, Victora CG, Relton CL. Breastfeeding effects on DNA methylation in the offspring: A systematic literature review. PLoS One. 2017;**12**(3):1-18

[18] Ganu RS, Harris RA, Collins K, Aagaard KM. Early origins of adult disease: Approaches for investigating the programmable epigenome in humans, nonhuman primates, and rodents. ILAR Journal. 2012;**53**(3-4):306-321

[19] Koletzko B, Brands B, Demmelmair H. The early nutrition programming project (EARNEST): 5 Y of successful multidisciplinary collaborative research. The American Journal of Clinical Nutrition. 2011;**94**(6):1749-1753

[20] Langley-Evans SC. Nutrition in early life and the programming of adult disease: A review. Journal of Human Nutrition and Dietetics. 2015;**28**(s1):1-14

[21] Burdge GC, Hanson MA, Slater-Jefferies JL, Lillycrop KA. Epigenetic regulation of transcription: A mechanism for inducing variations in phenotype (fetal programming) by differences in nutrition during early life? British Journal of Nutrition [Internet]. 2007;**97**(6):1036-1046. DOI: 10.1017/S0007114507682920

[22] Wadhwa P, Buss C, Entringer S, Swanson J. Developmental origins of health and disease: Brief history of the approach and current focus on epigenetic mechanisms. Seminars in Reproductive Medicine [Internet]. 2009;**27**(05):358-368. Available from: http://www.thieme-connect.de/DOI/DOI?10.1055/s-0029-1237424

[23] de Fluiter KS, Kerkhof GF, van Beijsterveldt IALP, Breij LM, van Vark-van der Zee LC, Mulder MT, et al. Appetite-regulating hormone trajectories and relationships with fat mass development in term-born infants during the first 6 months of life. European Journal of Nutrition [Internet]. 2021;**60**(7):3717-3725. DOI: 10.1007/s00394-021-02533-z

[24] Verduci E, Banderali G, Barberi S, Radaelli G, Lops A, Betti F, et al. Epigenetic effects of human breast milk. Nutrients [Internet]. 2014;**6**(4):1711-1724. Available from: http://www.mdpi.com/2072-6643/6/4/1711

[25] Palou M, Picó C, Palou A. Leptin as a breast milk component for the prevention of obesity. Nutrition Reviews [Internet]. 2018;**76**(12):875-892. Available from: https://academic.oup.com/nutritionreviews/advance-article/doi/10.1093/nutrit/nuy046/5114480

[26] Sinkiewicz-Darol E, Adamczyk I, Łubiech K, Pilarska G, Twarużek M. Leptin in human milk—One of the key regulators of nutritional programming. Molecules [Internet]. 2022;**27**(11):3581. Available from: https://www.mdpi.com/1420-3049/27/11/3581

[27] Vieira Borba V, Sharif K, Shoenfeld Y. Breastfeeding and autoimmunity: Programing health from the beginning. American Journal of Reproductive Immunology. 2018;**79**(1):1-11

[28] Mohamad M, Loy S, Lim P, Wang Y, Soo K, Mohamed H. Maternal serum and breast milk adiponectin: The association with infant adiposity development. International Journal of Environmental Research and Public Health [Internet]. 2018;**15**(6):1250. Available from: http://www.mdpi.com/1660-4601/15/6/1250

[29] Gridneva Z, Kugananthan S, Rea A, Lai CT, Ward LC, Murray K, et al. Human milk adiponectin and leptin and infant body composition over the first 12 months of lactation. Nutrients. 2018;**10**(8):1125

[30] Çağiran Yilmaz F, Özçelik AÖ. The relationships between leptin levels in maternal serum and breast milk of mothers and term infants. Annals of Medicine [Internet]. 2021;**53**(1):1310-1316. DOI: 10.1080/07853890.2021.1964037

[31] Miralles O, Sánchez J, Palou A, Picó C. A physiological role of breast milk leptin in body weight control in developing infants*. Obesity [Internet]. 2006;**14**(8):1371-1377. Available from: http://doi.wiley.com/10.1038/oby.2006.155

[32] Gridneva Z, Tie WJ, Rea A, Lai CT, Ward LC, Murray K, et al. Human milk casein and whey protein and infant body composition over the first 12 months of lactation. Nutrients. 2018;**10**(9):1332

[33] Plagemann A, Harder T, Brunn M, Harder A, Roepke K, Wittrock-Staar M, et al. Hypothalamic proopiomelanocortin promoter methylation becomes altered by early overfeeding: An epigenetic model of obesity and the metabolic syndrome. Journal of Physiology [Internet]. 2009;**587**(20):4963-4976. Available from: http://doi.wiley.com/10.1113/jphysiol.2009.176156

[34] Prentice P, Ong KK, Schoemaker MH, Van Tol EAF, Vervoort J, Hughes IA, et al. Breast milk nutrient content and infancy growth. Acta Paediatrica, International Journal of Paediatrics. 2016;**105**(6):641-647

[35] Mosca F, Giannì ML. Human milk: Composition and health benefits. La Pediatria Medica e Chirurgica. 2017;**39**(2):155

[36] Zhang S, Li T, Xie J, Zhang D, Pi C, Zhou L, et al. Gold standard for nutrition: A review of human milk oligosaccharide and its effects on infant gut microbiota. Microbial Cell Factories [Internet]. 2021;**20**(1):108. Available from: https://microbialcellfactories.biomedcentral.com/articles/10.1186/s12934-021-01599-y

[37] Saben JL, Sims CR, Abraham A, Bode L, Andres A. Human milk oligosaccharide concentrations and infant intakes are associated with maternal overweight and obesity and predict infant growth. Nutrients [Internet]. 2021;**13**(2):446. Available from: https://www.mdpi.com/2072-6643/13/2/446

[38] Šuligoj T, Vigsnæs LK, Van den Abbeele P, Apostolou A, Karalis K, Savva GM, et al. Effects of human milk oligosaccharides on the adult gut microbiota and barrier function. Nutrients [Internet]. 2020;**12**(9):2808. Available from: https://www.mdpi.com/2072-6643/12/9/2808

[39] Saben JL, Sims CR, Pack L, Lan R, Børsheim E, Andres A. Infant intakes of human milk branched chain amino acids

are negatively associated with infant growth and influenced by maternal body mass index. Pediatric Obesity [Internet]. 2022;**17**(5):e12876. Available from: https://onlinelibrary.wiley.com/doi/10.1111/ijpo.12876

[40] Lagström H, Rautava S, Ollila H, Kaljonen A, Turta O, Mäkelä J, et al. Associations between human milk oligosaccharides and growth in infancy and early childhood. The American Journal of Clinical Nutrition [Internet]. 2020;**111**(4):769-778. Available from: https://academic.oup.com/ajcn/article/111/4/769/5735195

[41] Lemaire M, Le Huërou-Luron I, Blat S. Effects of infant formula composition on long-term metabolic health. Journal of Developmental Origins of Health and Disease. 2018;**9**(6):573-589

[42] Daniel AI, Shama S, Ismail S, Bourdon C, Kiss A, Mwangome M, et al. Maternal BMI is positively associated with human milk fat: A systematic review and meta-regression analysis. The American Journal of Clinical Nutrition [Internet]. 2021;**113**(4):1009-1022. Available from: https://academic.oup.com/ajcn/article/113/4/1009/6155850

[43] George AD, Burugupalli S, Paul S, Mansell T, Burgner D, Meikle PJ. The role of human milk lipids and lipid metabolites in protecting the infant against non-communicable disease. International Journal of Molecular Sciences MDPI. 2022;**23**(14):7490

[44] Haschke F, Haiden N, Thakkar SK. Nutritive and bioactive proteins in breastmilk. Annals of Nutrition & Metabolism. 2017;**69**(2):17-26

[45] Kouwenhoven SMP, Muts J, Finken MJJ, van Goudoever JB. Low-protein infant formula and obesity risk. Nutrients [Internet]. 2022;**14**(13):2728. Available from: https://www.mdpi.com/2072-6643/14/13/2728

Chapter 4

Polyamines in Human Milk and Their Benefits for Infant Health

Nelly C. Muñoz-Esparza, Oriol Comas-Basté, Edgar M. Vásquez-Garibay, M. Teresa Veciana-Nogués, M. Luz Latorre-Moratalla and M. Carmen Vidal-Carou

Abstract

Breastfeeding is the gold standard for infant nutrition in the first six months of life when feeding choices determine growth and development. However, human milk is a complex and highly variable fluid that, in addition to nutrients, contains several bioactive components, including polyamines (putrescine, spermidine, and spermine), and constitutes the first exogenous source of these compounds for infants. Active in various cellular processes, polyamines are involved in the growth and maturation of the gastrointestinal tract and the development of the immune system and therefore play an important role in the first year of life. This chapter reviews the impact of polyamines on infant growth and health, the polyamine content in human milk and how it is influenced by factors related to both the mother-child dyad and breastfeeding itself. In addition, a comparative analysis of human milk and infant formulas in terms of polyamine content and profile is presented.

Keywords: polyamines, human milk, breastfeeding, infant, infant formulas

1. Introduction

The first 1000 days of life, from conception to 23 months postpartum, constitute the most important period of growth and development for the human body and brain. Therefore, early food choices play a crucial role in health in infancy and later in life [1, 2]. Widely accepted as the gold standard for human nutrition in the first six months of life, breast milk satisfies all the infant's nutritional requirements for optimal growth and development [3–5]. According to the World Health Organization (WHO) and United Nations Children's Fund (UNICEF), breastfeeding should begin within the first hour after birth, continue as the exclusive source of nutrition during the first semester of life, and ideally be extended until the infant is at least two years of age [3].

Human milk is a complex and highly variable fluid that, in addition to nutrients, contains other substances such as nucleotides, hormones, growth factors, immunoglobulins, oligosaccharides, cytokines, and antibodies, which participate in the development of the immune system and provide protection against infectious

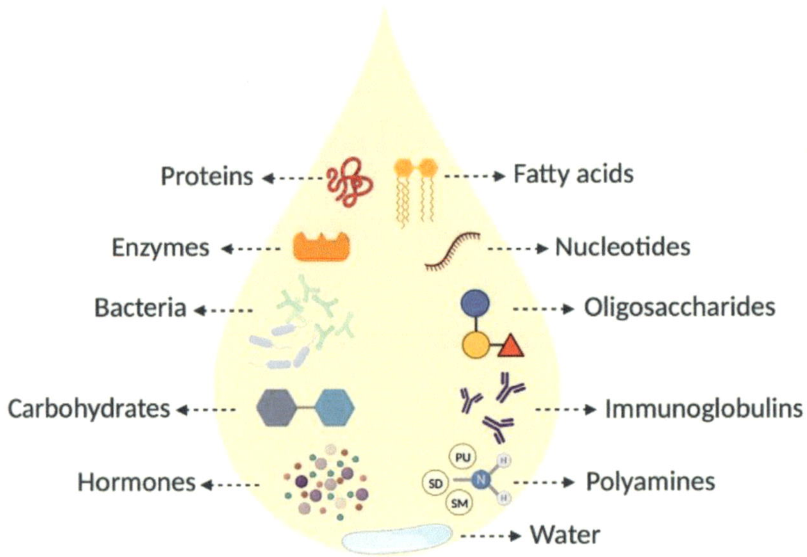

Figure 1.
Qualitative composition of human milk.

diseases (**Figure 1**) [5–9]. Although human milk has been described as sterile, it is now known to harbor a complex community of bacteria that help establish the infant's gut microbiota, with an impact on future health (e.g., by helping to prevent allergies, asthma, and obesity) [10–12]. Among the bioactive compounds found in human milk are the polyamines putrescine, spermidine, and spermine [9, 13, 14], which are synthesized in the mammary gland during pregnancy and lactation and are associated with hormonal regulation of lactogenic processes [15].

Several studies have shown that growth patterns and body composition differ between infants fed with human milk and infant formulas [16–18]. For example, infants that are exclusively breastfed accumulate more fat (both in grams and percentage) during the first four months of life, whereas those that are formula-fed acquire more lean mass and gain weight more rapidly, a tendency associated with a higher risk of developing overweight and obesity later in life [16, 18–21]. Likewise, differences in growth have also been described between exclusive and partially breastfed infants [18, 22, 23]. It has been suggested that the unique composition of human milk in terms of nutrients, protein concentration, and qualitative characteristics may explain these differences in growth and the beneficial effects of breastfeeding [21].

2. Polyamines: biochemical properties and functions

Polyamines are low molecular weight nitrogenous compounds found in all living organisms [24–26]. Putrescine (1,4-butane diamine), spermidine (N-(3-aminopropyl)-1,4-butane diamine), and spermine (N,N-bis(3-aminopropyl)-1,4-butane diamine) are characterized by the presence of two or more amino groups (**Figure 2**). Due to their structure, they are relatively stable compounds, capable of withstanding both acidic and alkaline conditions and establishing hydrogen bonds

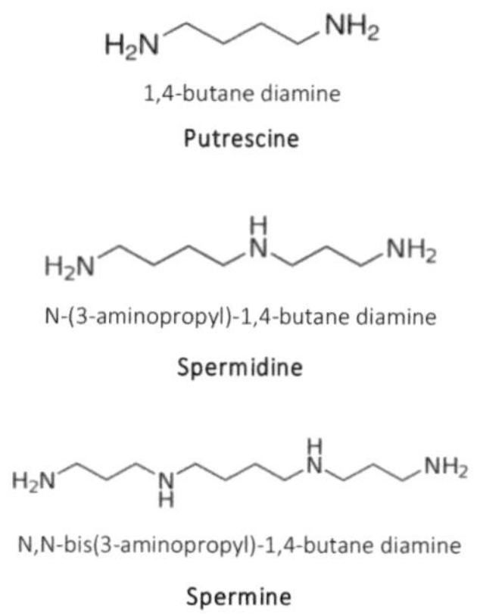

Figure 2.
Chemical structure of polyamines.

with hydroxyl solvents such as water and alcohol. At physiological pH, polyamines are fully protonated in the organism and can bind strongly to biomolecules such as DNA, RNA, ATP, proteins, and phospholipids, stabilizing their negative charges and, in many cases, modulating their function [27, 28]. In the cell, polyamines are stored mainly in the cytosol and nucleus, which participate in DNA transcription and RNA translation [24, 29].

In humans, polyamines play an essential role in regulating several cellular processes, such as cell growth and differentiation, and protein and nucleic acid synthesis [25, 30]. In addition, polyamines participate in the modulation of the immune response, ionic channels (e.g., acting as blockers of potassium channels), and cell apoptosis [24, 25, 31, 32]. Another important feature of polyamines is their antioxidant capacity, described as comparable to that of recognized antioxidants such as α-tocopherol, ascorbyl palmitate, and octyl gallate [33]. Polyamines exert antioxidant effects mainly through the mechanism of metal chelation, which prevents the formation of hydroperoxides and secondary oxidation compounds [33]. Spermine is the polyamine with the highest antioxidant capacity, as its chemical structure has the largest number of positive charges, followed by spermidine [33]. Additionally, polyamines are reported to protect DNA against oxidative damage by eliminating free radicals, especially in lipophilic media [33, 34].

The three polyamines can be found in a wide variety of animal and plant foods, but with qualitative and quantitative variation [25, 35]. For newborns, human breast-milk is the first exogenous source of these compounds [9, 24, 26].

2.1 Cellular homeostasis of polyamines

Cellular homeostasis of polyamines in the body is strongly regulated and depends on the balance between their endogenous synthesis, dietary intake, and catabolism [25, 29, 36]. **Figure 3** schematically depicts the metabolic routes of polyamine synthesis, interconversion, and catabolism.

The de novo synthesis of polyamines begins with the formation of putrescine from the amino acid ornithine by the action of the enzyme ornithine decarboxylase (ODC). Next, spermidine is obtained from putrescine by the action of spermidine synthase, which catalyzes the addition of a propylamine group from the

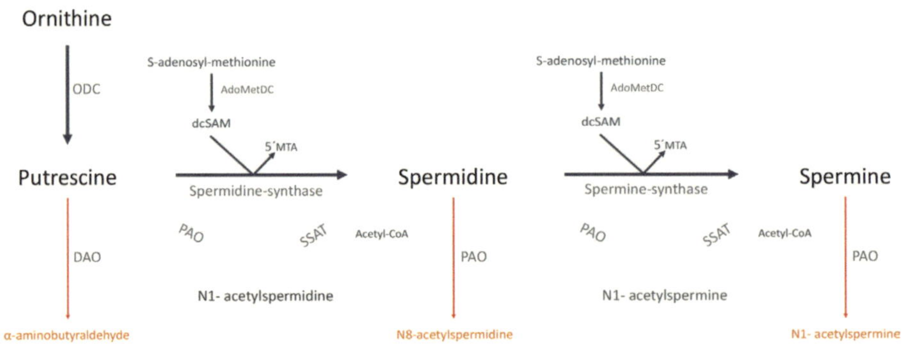

Figure 3.
De novo synthesis, interconversion, and catabolism of polyamines in the body. ODC: ornithine decarboxylase, AdoMetDC: S-adenosyl-L-methionine-decarboxylase; dcSAM: decarboxylated S-adenosyl-methionine, 5′MTA: 5′-methylthioadenosine, SSAT: spermidine/spermine N1-acetyl-transferase, PAO: polyamine oxidase Acetyl-CoA: Acetyl coenzyme-A. Adapted from Munoz-Esparza et al. [26].

decarboxylation of S-adenosyl-methionine. Finally, spermine synthase transforms spermidine into spermine by adding a second propylamine group [29, 37]. In addition to de novo formation, polyamines may arise from interconversion reactions, a cyclical process that controls polyamine turnover and maintains intracellular homeostasis (**Figure 3**). The interconversion begins with the acetylation of spermine or spermidine by the action of spermidine/spermine N1-acetyltransferase (SSAT) and with the participation of acetyl coenzyme-A. Subsequently, polyamine oxidase (PAO) removes a propylamine group to generate putrescine from the acetylated metabolite of spermidine, or spermidine from the acetylated metabolite of spermine [24–26, 38].

The principal source of exogenous polyamines is food [24, 26]. Dietary polyamines are absorbed in the small intestine, mainly in the duodenum and the first segment of the jejunum, either through transcellular absorption mechanisms involving transporters or passively through the paracellular route, the latter being more common [24, 28, 30, 39]. Although not much information exists about polyamine transporters in mammalian cells, two transmembrane transporters from the family of solute carriers (SLC) have been identified [30, 40]. Exogenous polyamines are incorporated into the cell via the carnitine transporter SLC22A16, whereas SLC3A2 is responsible for the excretion of acetylated polyamines, especially putrescine and spermidine [30, 39].

3. The role of polyamines in infant health

Polyamines participate in different biological processes in the first years of life, promoting the growth and maturation of the gastrointestinal tract and the development of the immune system [7, 41–45]. Thus, it has been postulated that polyamine requirements may be higher during the neonatal and infant stages when the rate of cell growth is more rapid [46, 47].

Several studies have shown that oral administration of polyamines in animal models induces morphological and biochemical modifications in the intestine. For example, the administration of spermine and spermidine in mice increased protein expression and modified the activity of disaccharidases, markers of small intestinal maturation [42, 43, 48]. Biol-N'garagba et al. [49] proposed that postnatal changes in glycoprotein fucosylation in the intestinal maturation process largely depend on polyamine intake. They demonstrated in mice that oral administration of 10 μmol/day of spermine and spermidine increased the activity of α-1,2-fucosyltransferase, causing a higher concentration of α-1,2-fucoproteins in the brush border membrane [49]. Other authors have reported biochemical changes associated with the maturation of the small intestine, such as the increased activity of alkaline phosphatase and glutamyl-transferase gamma [44, 48].

At the morphological level, Sabater-Molina et al. [44] demonstrated that a physiological dose of polyamines significantly increased crypt depth in the small intestine of newborn piglets compared to the control group. In addition, Pérez-Cano et al. [7] reported that spermine and spermidine administered to newborn rats were associated with increased gut weight and length, indicating a more mature gut structure.

Regarding the immune response, animal model studies indicate that oral administration of spermine and spermidine in the postnatal period induces the maturation of intestinal immune cells and increases concentrations of immunoglobulin A [7, 42, 43, 50]. Ter Steege et al. [50] demonstrated that the intake of spermine increased the percentage of intraepithelial lymphocytes (CD4, CD5, and CD54) and the expression levels of these antibodies. Likewise, Pérez-Cano et al. [7] observed that daily supplementation with spermidine and spermine significantly increased the maturation of CD8 intraepithelial lymphocytes and the number of natural killer cells are related to greater innate immunity.

During the first months of life, the intestine is more permeable to macromolecules, a state associated with a higher propensity to develop allergies [43]. Dandrifosse et al. [51] reported that spermine administration in rats increased pancreatic protease activity, which improved protein digestion and reduced the likelihood of allergenicity. It is well established that breastfed infants have a lower risk of developing food allergies than those fed infant formula [52]. This tendency is mainly attributed to the presence of polyamines in human milk and other bioactive compounds, such as immunoglobulins, growth factors, nucleotides, and cytokines [7, 52]. In support of this effect, Peulen et al. [53] reported that a higher spermine content in human milk during the first month postpartum was associated with a lower incidence of allergy at five years of age. Furthermore, intestinal maturation, promoted by polyamines, involves a reduction in intestinal permeability, limiting the passage of antigens from the lumen into the bloodstream, thus lowering the risk of allergy in the infant [7, 41, 45]. Consequently, supplementing infant formulas with polyamines has been described as important for allergy prevention [7, 43, 48, 53].

Finally, in addition to their role in intestinal maturation and immunity, polyamines have also been associated with changes in the microbiota [15, 54]. For example, studies in newborn mice found that administering an infant formula supplemented with polyamines significantly impacted the composition and activity of the intestinal microbiota, resulting in a significant increase in the number of *Bifidobacteria* species compared to the control group. These bacteria have a biological role in the relationship between the host mucosa and the microbiota, immune regulation, and the control of inflammation. Also observed was an increase in the concentration of the bacterium *Akkermansia muciniphila*, a common species of intestinal microbiota that promotes the development of innate and adaptive immune responses [15, 54].

4. Polyamine content and profile in human milk

As mentioned, human milk has a substantial content of polyamines, serving as the first dietary source of these compounds for infants. However, in the last three decades, several studies have investigated polyamines in human milk, reporting a wide variability of contents, with total polyamine concentrations ranging between 25.7 nmol/dL and 948.5 nmol/dL (**Table 1**). Explanations for this broad divergence include cohort heterogeneity, the uniqueness of each mother-child dyad, and the

	Lactation phase	Total polyamines	Putrescine	Spermidine	Spermine	References
Full-term human breast milk	1st week	396.1	20.5	185.4	190.2	[55]
		713.3	82.4	457.5	173.4	[14]
	1st month	861.5	61.5	351.2	448.8	[55]
		881.0	21.0	352.0	508.0	[15]
		25.7	2.9	12.4	10.4	[47]
		790.5	18.0	389.5	382.9	[57]
	2 months	819	90.0	385.0	344.0	[41]
		145.8	Nd	73.6	72.2	[55]
		659.1^{+}	85.3^{+}	414.0^{+}	159.8^{+}	[56]
		567.7*	73.0*	348.6*	146.1*	[56]
		506.9°	34.1°	243.7°	206.2°	[9]
		876.6♦	50.0♦	407.7♦	418.9♦	[9]
		756.1	30.0	381.0	345.1	[57]
	3 months	562.3	30.4	285.7	246.2	[57]
	4 months	745	79.0	316.0	350.0	[41]
		429.0°	30.3°	206.2°	192.5°	[9]
		788♦	51.0♦	357.8♦	379.2♦	[9]
		508.3	29.6	239.9	238.8	[57]
	5 months	448.2	19.0	229.7	199.5	[57]
	6 months	618	87.0	298.0	233.0	[41]
		405.6°	35.0°	192.5°	178.1°	[9]
		708.6♦	49.8♦	379.2♦	279.6♦	[9]
	Mean	557	24.0	220.0	313.0	[13]
Preterm human breast milk	1st week	948.5	165.6	615.2	167.7	[14]
	1st month	82.2	5.8	46.2	30.2	[47]

*Nd: not detected. Milk from mothers with +normal weight and *obesity. Average: does not specify month of lactation. The milk sample corresponds to °foremilk and ♦hindmilk.*

Table 1.
Mean contents of polyamines in human breast milk (nmol/dL) reported in the literature.

different phases of lactation at which samples were taken (from the first week to six months of life) [9, 13, 15, 41, 47, 55–57].

Studies disagree about the main polyamine in human milk, some indicating spermidine [14, 41, 47, 56], and others spermine [13, 15, 55]. In two recent studies, Muñoz-Esparza et al. [9, 57] found that spermidine and spermine predominated, being detected in similar proportions. In contrast, putrescine is unanimously described as a minor polyamine in human milk (**Table 1**).

5. Influence of the mother-child dyad and lactation on the polyamine content in human milk

It has been suggested that the polyamine content in human milk may be influenced by multiple factors associated with the lactation process and the individuality of each mother–child dyad (**Figure 4**). Thus, concentrations may be affected by genetics, ethnicity, nutritional status, and maternal dietary intake [13, 15, 47, 56, 58]. Gomez-Gallego et al. [15] reported that the polyamine content in human milk varies according to the geographical region, being higher in Spanish and Finnish versus Chinese and South African mothers. Likewise, Muñoz-Esparza et al. [9, 57] found higher concentrations of polyamines in breast milk samples from Spanish compared to Mexican mothers (**Table 1**). These differences could potentially be explained by the link between geographical regions and factors such as ethnic origin, genetics, and maternal dietary patterns. The influence of the diet on polyamine levels in human milk has been investigated in only two studies. Atiya-Ali et al. [14] reported a positive association between the maternal intake of polyamines and concentrations in breast milk. Thus, higher consumption of vegetables in lactating mothers was significantly associated with higher spermidine contents in breast milk, whereas fruits, mainly oranges, were correlated with higher levels of putrescine. It was also observed that the polyamine content in breast milk increased in obese mothers participating in a nutritional intervention, correlating with higher consumption of vegetables and fruits [56]. It should be noted that spermidine is the major polyamine in most vegetables and fruits, although putrescine predominates in citrus fruits [25, 35]. Further research is needed to shed light on the association between maternal polyamine intake and the content in breast milk, for which information is still scarce. Finally, regarding

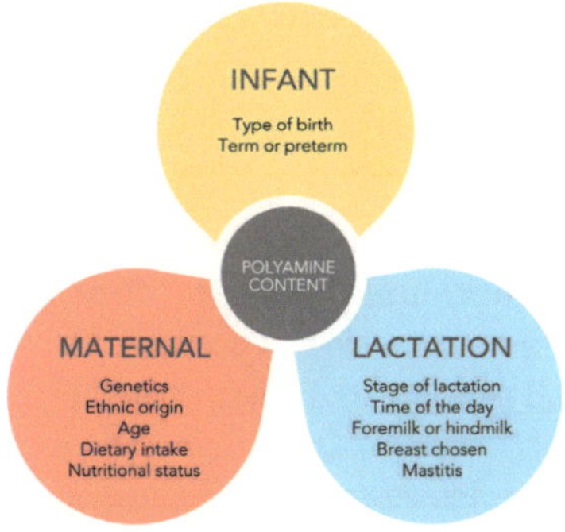

Figure 4.
Factors influencing the content of polyamines in human milk. Adapted from Muñoz-Esparza et al. [9].

the nutritional status of the mother, Atiya-Ali et al. [56] reported lower polyamine concentrations in the milk of mothers with obesity compared to those of normal weight without exploring the underlying reasons.

The type of birth may also affect the constituents of breast milk. Two studies found a higher polyamine content in the milk of mothers of premature versus term newborns [14, 47]. Another potentially influential factor is the type of delivery. Gómez-Gallego et al. [15] reported that mothers who delivered their babies by cesarean section, as opposed to natural birth, produced milk with a significantly lower polyamine content, the same trend being observed by Muñoz-Esparza et al. [9]. Again, more research is needed, not only to confirm these results but also to analyze why the type of birth can affect polyamine concentrations.

Regarding breastfeeding, two studies carried out in 1992 by Romain et al. [41] and Pollack et al. [55] with breast milk samples from North American and Belgian mothers, respectively, found a progressive decrease in polyamines during the lactation period, with contents being up to 28% lower after six months. More recently, a reduction in polyamine content during the first semester of lactation was also described in milk samples from Mexican and Spanish mothers [9, 57]. In both studies, a significant decrease in spermidine (around 30%) and spermine (25%) was found, whereas putrescine remained practically unchanged during this period [9, 57]. According to Plaza-Zamora et al. [47], the higher polyamine content in human milk produced at the beginning of lactation could be related to the high cell growth rate and differentiation during the first months of life. In addition, the increasing catalytic activity of the PAO enzyme in breast milk along the lactation period could be responsible for the progressive reduction of polyamine concentrations [59]. On the other hand, the polyamine content in human milk may not only depend on the lactation phase but can also vary within a feed. Muñoz-Esparza et al. [9] found significantly higher concentrations (up to twofold), particularly of spermidine and spermine, in the hindmilk produced at the end of the feed compared to the foremilk, regardless of the month of lactation. The fact that hindmilk remains in the mammary gland for longer in the presence of active endo- and exopeptidases (enzymes responsible for breaking down milk peptides) could lead to a higher content of free amino acids [60, 61]. Sadelhoff et al. [61] reported that hindmilk has a higher content of arginine, an amino acid precursor of ornithine and, therefore, a key substrate for the endogenous synthesis of polyamines [37, 40]. The finding that the polyamine content is higher in hindmilk is further evidence of the importance of full feeds for infants so that they may benefit from all the nutrients available in human milk.

Finally, it has also been proposed that certain infections, such as mastitis, can potentially modify the polyamine content of breast milk and lead to the appearance of other biogenic amines [62]. Perez et al. [62] reported higher concentrations of putrescine and the presence of tyramine and histamine in the milk of mothers with mastitis compared to healthy mothers. Likewise, Muñoz-Esparza et al. [57] detected abnormally high putrescine concentrations (up to 183 nmol/dL) in a breast milk sample, as well as the unusual presence of histamine (170 nmol/dL) and cadaverine (2680 nmol/dL), which may have been due to mastitis in the mother, although the infection was not corroborated. Perez et al. [62] suggested that the increase in putrescine concentrations, and the appearance of other amines, could be largely attributed to the aminogenic activity of the infectious bacteria (e.g., staphylococcal, streptococcal, and/or corynebacterial species) responsible for the inflammatory process of the mammary gland that gives rise to mastitis.

6. Polyamine content and profile in infant formulas

The WHO recommends that infants be fed exclusively with human milk in the first six months of life and that breastfeeding should continue until two years of age with suitable complementary feeding [3]. However, feeding with infant formulas during the first year of life remains a common practice, either in combination with breastfeeding or as the sole food [63].

Infant formulas	Total polyamines	Putrescine	Spermidine	Spermine	References
First formula	136.0	94.0	27.0	15.0	[41]
	213.0	192.0	10.0	11.0	[41]
	20.5	1.8	18.7	Nd	[55]
	313.3	80.4	188.2	44.7	[55]
	78.4	23.9	39.4	15.1	[13]
	333.6	17.6	213.0	103.0	[14]
	441.3	359.6	51.6	30.1	[68]
	2599	964.0	923.0	712.0	[69]
	15.7	Nd	15.7	Nd	[57]
	59.5	36.9	22.6	Nd	[57]
	80.5	36.8	43.7	Nd	[57]
Follow-on formula	83.3	13.7	56.5	13.1	[13]
	354.1	11.0	280.0	63.1	[14]
	1970	749.0	482.0	739.0	[69]
	77.4	41.4	36.0	Nd	[57]
	67.6	35.2	32.4	Nd	[57]
	110.4	58.4	52.0	Nd	[57]
Preterm formula	144.4	105.7	21.5	17.2	[55]
	649.9	154.5	433.1	62.3	[14]
	128.9	40.8	27.0	61.1	[57]
	290.9	Nd	228.2	62.7	[57]
	72.5	39.1	33.4	Nd	[57]
Soy-based formula	361.0	84.0	233.0	44.0	[41]
	385.0	64.0	278.0	43.0	[41]
	381.9	74.0	307.9	Nd	[57]
	254.3	51.9	202.4	Nd	[57]
	378.5	74.9	303.6	Nd	[57]
Rice-based formula	206.5	190.3	16.2	Nd	[57]
	242.2	194.0	48.2	Nd	[57]
	360	306.3	53.7	Nd	[57]

Nd: not detected.

Table 2.
Mean contents of polyamines in infant formulas (nmol/dL) reported in the literature.

Infant formulas or human milk substitutes are designed to replace breast milk, either partially or totally [64]. In 1977, the nutritional composition of formulas was established by the Nutrition Committee of the European Society of Pediatric Gastroenterology, Hepatology and Nutrition (ESPGHAN) to achieve products that match human milk as closely as possible and cover all infant nutritional requirements [64]. To benefit infant health and nutrition, the formulation of these preparations has been modified over the years based on new knowledge about the composition of human milk and according to the updated standards of ESPGHAN and the American Academy of Pediatrics [65–67].

Table 2 shows the contents of putrescine, spermidine, and spermine in different types of infant formulas reported in the literature [13, 14, 41, 55, 57, 68, 69]. In general, both polyamine content and profile are highly variable among studies.

The polyamine contents of infant formulas for special medical use, made from vegetable proteins such as soy and rice, have only been analyzed in two studies [41, 57], detecting only putrescine and spermidine. Soy-based formulas stood out for their high concentrations of spermidine (202.4–307.9 nmol/dL), while putrescine was the major polyamine in the rice-based formulas (190.3–306.3 nmol/dL). As in formulas made from cow's milk, the amount and type of polyamines in those based on vegetable protein are related to the content in the raw material. Accordingly, various authors have described spermidine as the major polyamine in soybeans and putrescine in rice [35, 70–73]. In addition, various factors, such as the conditions of cultivation, the environment, and harvesting, can potentially modify the final polyamine content in vegetables and, consequently, in derived products such as infant formulas [35, 74–76].

Regardless of the great variability of polyamines in infant formulas and human milk, the polyamine content is much lower in the former (up to 60 times lower). Furthermore, the polyamine profile also differs between spermidine and spermine, predominating in human milk and putrescine in infant formulas. These data indicate that infant formulas should be improved in terms of qualitative and quantitative polyamine content to achieve a closer match with the composition of human milk.

7. Conclusion

Polyamines are relatively underrecognized as bioactive components of human milk, even though their physiological effects on the growth and maturation of the gastrointestinal tract and the development of the infant's immune system have been extensively studied. Breast milk is the first exogenous source of polyamines in humans, and the content can be influenced by various factors related to the mother–child dyad and the lactation process itself. The geographical region, closely linked to maternal dietary patterns, seems to strongly influence the polyamine concentrations in human milk, mainly spermidine and spermine. If these findings are confirmed in further studies, promoting polyamine-rich foods in the maternal diet would be a useful strategy to increase concentrations in breast milk. On the other hand, polyamine levels clearly decrease along the lactation period, thought to be an adaptation to the decreasing requirements of the infant as the growth rate slows. It should also be highlighted that the levels of polyamines, mainly spermidine and spermine, change within a single feed, up to twofold higher in the hindmilk provided at the end of the feed compared to the foremilk. This information supports the importance of the infant fully emptying the breast to take advantage of all the nutrients available in human milk, including polyamines. Analysis of infant formulas reveals a clear difference in polyamine content and profile compared to human milk, with much lower levels, especially of spermidine and spermine. Therefore, these products need to be reformulated to achieve a profile that more closely resembles human breast milk.

Conflict of interest

The authors declare no conflict of interest.

Author details

Nelly C. Muñoz-Esparza[1,2,3]*, Oriol Comas-Basté[1,2]*, Edgar M. Vásquez-Garibay[3], M. Teresa Veciana-Nogués[1,2], M. Luz Latorre-Moratalla[1,2] and M. Carmen Vidal-Carou[1,2]

1 Department of Nutrition, Food Sciences and Gastronomy, Faculty of Pharmacy and Food Sciences, Food and Nutrition Torribera Campus, University of Barcelona (UB), Santa Coloma de Gramenet, Spain

2 Research Institute of Nutrition and Food Safety of the University of Barcelona (INSA·UB), Santa Coloma de Gramenet, Spain

3 Human Nutrition Institute, University of Guadalajara, Guadalajara, Mexico

*Address all correspondence to: nelly.munoz@academicos.udg.mx and oriolcomas@ub.edu

References

[1] Consales A, Morniroli D, Vizzari G, Mosca F, Giannì ML. Nutrition for infant feeding. Nutrients. 2022;**27**:1823. DOI: 10.3390/nu14091823

[2] Pietrobelli A, Agosti M. Nutrition in the first 1000 days: Ten practices to minimize obesity emerging from published science. International Journal of Environmental Research and Public Health. 2017;**14**:1491. DOI: 10.3390/ijerph14121491

[3] WHO. Infant and Young Feeding. Model Chapter for Textbooks for Medical Students and Allied Health Professionals. Geneva: Organization WH; 2009

[4] Mosca F, Giannì ML. Human milk: Composition and health benefits. La Pediatria Medica e Chirurgica. 2017;**39**:155. DOI: 10.4081/pmc.2017.155

[5] Garwolińska D, Namieśnik J, Kot-Wasik A, Hewelt-Belka W. Chemistry of human breast milk—A comprehensive review of the composition and role of milk metabolites in child development. Journal of Agricultural and Food Chemistry. 2018;**66**:11881-11896. DOI: 10.1021/acs.jafc.8b04031

[6] Carr LE, Virmani MD, Rosa F, Munblit D, Matazel KS, Elolimy AA, et al. Role of human milk bioactives on infants' gut and immune health. Frontiers in Immunology. 2021;**12**:1-17. DOI: 10.3389/fimmu.2021.604080

[7] Pérez-Cano FJ, González-Castro A, Castellote C, Franch À, Castell M. Influence of breast milk polyamines on suckling rat immune system maturation. Developmental and Comparative Immunology. 2010;**34**:210-218. DOI: 10.1016/j.dci.2009.10.001

[8] Andreas NJ, Kampmann B, Mehring L-DK. Human breast milk: A review on its composition and bioactivity. Early Human Development. 2015;**91**:629-635. DOI: 10.1016/j.earlhumdev.2015.08.013

[9] Muñoz-Esparza NC, Vásquez-Garibay EM, Guzmán-Mercado E, Larrosa-Haro A, Comas-Basté O, Latorre-Moratalla ML, et al. Influence of breastfeeding factors on polyamine content in human milk. Nutrients. 2021;**29**:3016. DOI: 10.3390/nu13093016

[10] Gomez-Gallego C, Garcia-Mantrana I, Salminen S, Collado MC. The human milk microbiome and factors influencing its composition and activity. Seminars in Fetal & Neonatal Medicine. 2016;**21**:400-405. DOI: 10.1016/j.siny.2016.05.003

[11] Fitzstevens JL, Smith KC, Hagadorn JI, Caimano MJ, Matson AP, Brownell EA. Systematic review of the human milk microbiota. Nutrition in Clinical Practice. 2017;**32**:354-364. DOI: 10.1177/0884533616670150

[12] Moossavi S, Sepehri S, Robertson B, Bode L, Goruk S, Field CJ, et al. Composition and variation of the human milk microbiota are influenced by maternal and early-life factors. Cell Host & Microbe. 2019;**25**:324-335.e4. DOI: 10.1016/j.chom.2019.01.011

[13] Buts JP, De Keyser N, De Raedemaeker L, Collette E, Sokal EM. Polyamine profiles in human milk, infant artificial formulas, and semi-elemental diets. Journal of Pediatric Gastroenterology and Nutrition. 1995;**21**:44-49

[14] Atiya Ali M, Strandvik B, Sabel K-G, Palme Kilander C, Strömberg R,

Yngve A. Polyamine levels in breast milk are associated with mothers' dietary intake and are higher in preterm than full-term human milk and formulas. Journal of Human Nutrition and Dietetics. 2014;**27**:459-467. DOI: 10.1111/jhn.12156

[15] Gómez-Gallego C, Kumar H, García-Mantrana I, du Toit E, Suomela J-P, Linderborg KM, et al. Breast milk polyamines and microbiota interactions: Impact of mode of delivery and geographical location. Annals of Nutrition & Metabolism. 2017;**70**:184-190. DOI: 10.1159/000457134

[16] Giannì ML, Roggero P, Orsi A, Piemontese P, Garbarino F, Bracco B, et al. Body composition changes in the first 6 months of life according to method of feeding. Journal of Human Lactation. 2014;**30**:148-155. DOI: 10.1177/0890334413516196

[17] Giugliani ERJ. Growth in exclusively breastfed infants. The Journal of Pediatrics. 2019;**95**:79-84. DOI: 10.1016/j.jped.2018.11.007

[18] Rodríguez-Cano AM, Mier-Cabrera J, Muñoz-Manrique C, Cardona-Pérez A, Villalobos-Alcázar G, Perichart-Perera O. Anthropometric and clinical correlates of fat mass in healthy term infants at 6 months of age. BMC Pediatrics. 2019;**19**:60. DOI: 10.1186/s12887-019-1430-x

[19] Butte NF, Wong WW, Hopkinson JM, Smith EO, Ellis KJ. Infant feeding mode affects early growth and body composition. Pediatrics. 2000;**106**:1355-1366. DOI: 10.1542/peds.106.6.1355

[20] Gale C, Logan KM, Santhakumaran S, Parkinson JRC, Hyde MJ, Modi N. Effect of breastfeeding compared with formula feeding on infant body composition: A systematic review and meta-analysis. The American Journal of Clinical Nutrition. 2012;**95**:656-669. DOI: 10.3945/ajcn.111.027284

[21] Patro-Gołąb B, Zalewski BM, Polaczek A, Szajewska H. Duration of breastfeeding and early growth: A systematic review of current evidence. Breastfeeding Medicine. 2019;**14**:218-229. DOI: 10.1089/bfm.2018.0187

[22] Muñoz-Esparza NC, Vásquez-Garibay EM, Guzmán-Mercado E, Larrosa-Haro A, Comas-Basté O, Latorre-Moratalla ML, et al. Influence of the type of breastfeeding and human milk polyamines on infant anthropometric parameters. Frontiers in Nutrition. 2022;**8**:1-7. DOI: 10.3389/fnut.2021.815477

[23] Jia N, Gu G, Zhao L, He S, Xiong F, Chai Y, et al. Longitudinal study of breastfeeding and growth in 0-6 month infants. Asia Pacific Journal of Clinical Nutrition. 2018;**27**:1294-1301. Available from: https://search.informit.org/doi/10.3316/ielapa.035725110718556

[24] Larqué E, Sabater-Molina M, Zamora S. Biological significance of dietary polyamines. Nutrition. 2007;**23**:87-95. DOI: 10.1016/j.nut.2006.09.006

[25] Kalač P. Health effects and occurrence of dietary polyamines: A review for the period 2005-mid 2013. Food Chemistry. 2014;**161**:27-39. DOI: 10.1016/j.foodchem.2014.03.102

[26] Muñoz-Esparza NC, Latorre-Moratalla ML, Comas-Basté O, Toro-Funes N, Veciana-Nogués MT, Vidal-Carou MC. Polyamines in food. Frontiers in Nutrition. 2019;**2019**:6. DOI: 10.3389/fnut.2019.00108

[27] Handa AK, Fatima T, Mattoo AK. Polyamines: Bio-molecules with diverse

functions in plant and human health and disease. Frontiers in Chemistry. 2018;**6**:1-18. DOI: 10.3389/fchem.2018.00010

[28] Hirano R, Shirasawa H, Kurihara S. Health-promoting effects of dietary polyamines. Medical Science. 2021;**9**:8. DOI: 10.3390/medsci9010008

[29] Moinard C, Cynober L, de Bandt JP. Polyamines: Metabolism and implications in human diseases. Clinical Nutrition. 2005;**24**:184-197. DOI: 10.1016/j.clnu.2004.11.001

[30] Bae DH, Lane DJR, Jansson PJ, Richardson DR. The old and new biochemistry of polyamines. Biochim Biophys Acta—General Subjects. 2018;**1862**:2053-2068. DOI: 10.1016/j.bbagen.2018.06.004

[31] Ruiz-Cano D. Implicaciones de las poliaminas en la salud infantil. Archivos Argentinos de Pediatría. 2012;**110**:244-250. Available from: http://www.sap.org.ar/docs/publicaciones/archivosarg/2012/v110n3a10.pdf

[32] Hofer SJ, Simon AK, Bergmann M, Eisenberg T, Kroemer G, Madeo F. Mechanisms of spermidine-induced autophagy and geroprotection. Nature Aging. 2022;**2**:1112-1129. DOI: 10.1038/s43587-022-00322-9

[33] Toro-Funes N, Bosch-Fusté J, Veciana-Nogués MT, Izquierdo-Pulido M, Vidal-Carou MC. In vitro antioxidant activity of dietary polyamines. Food Research International. 2013;**51**:141-147. DOI: 10.1016/j.foodres.2012.11.036

[34] Farriol M, Segovia-Silvestre T, Venereo Y, Orta X. Antioxidant effect of polyamines on erythrocyte cell membrane lipoperoxidation after free-radical damage. Phyther Research. 2003;**17**:44-47. DOI: 10.1002/ptr.1073

[35] Muñoz-Esparza NC, Costa-Catala J, Comas-Basté O, Toro-Funes N, Latorre-Moratalla ML, Veciana-Nogués MT, et al. Occurrence of polyamines in foods and the influence of cooking processes. Food. 2021;**10**:1752. DOI: 10.3390/foods10081752

[36] Sagar NA, Tarafdar S, Agarwal S, Tarafdar A, Sharma S. Polyamines: Functions, metabolism, and role in human disease management. Medical Science. 2021;**9**:44. DOI: 10.3390/medsci9020044

[37] Miller-Fleming L, Olin-Sandoval V, Campbell K, Ralser M. Remaining mysteries of molecular biology: The role of polyamines in the cell. Journal of Molecular Biology. 2015;**427**:3389-3406. DOI: 10.1016/j.jmb.2015.06.020

[38] Minois N, Carmona-Gutierrez D, Madeo F. Polyamines in aging and disease. Aging. 2011;**3**:716-732. DOI: 10.18632%2Faging.100361

[39] Ramos-Molina B, Queipo-Ortuño MI, Lambertos A, Tinahones FJ, Peñafiel R. Dietary and gut microbiota polyamines in obesity- and age-related diseases. Frontiers in Nutrition. 2019;**6**:1-15. DOI: 10.3389/fnut.2019.00024

[40] Lenis YY, Elmetwally MA, Maldonado-Estrada JG, Bazer FW. Physiological importance of polyamines. Zygote. 2017;**25**:244-255. DOI: 10.1017/S0967199417000120

[41] Romain N, Dandrifosse G, Jeusette F, Forget P. Polyamine concentration in rat milk and food, human milk, and infant formulas. Pediatric Research. 1992;**32**:58-63. DOI: 10.1203/00006450-199207000-00011

[42] Buts J-P, De Keyser N, Kolanowski J, Sokal E, Van Hoof F. Maturation of

villus and crypt cell functions in rat small intestine. Digestive Diseases and Sciences. 1993;**38**:1091-1098. DOI: 10.1007/BF01295726

[43] Dandrifosse G, Peulen O, Khefif NE, Deloyer P, Dandrifosse AC, Grandfils C. Are milk polyamines preventive agents against food allergy? The Proceedings of the Nutrition Society. 2000;**59**:81-86. DOI: 10.1017/S0029665100000100

[44] Sabater-Molina M, Larqué E, Torrella F, Plaza J, Lozano T, Muñoz A, et al. Effects of dietary polyamines at physiologic doses in early-weaned piglets. Nutrition. 2009;**25**:940-946. DOI: 10.1016/j.nut.2009.01.017

[45] Gómez-Gallego C, Frias R, Pérez-Martínez G, Bernal MJ, Periago MJ, Salminen S, et al. Polyamine supplementation in infant formula: Influence on lymphocyte populations and immune system-related gene expression in a Balb/cOlaHsd mouse model. Food Research International. 2014;**59**:8-15. DOI: 10.1016/j.foodres.2014.01.066

[46] Gallego G, Carlos RB, Gaspar BC, José M, Conesa P, Darío PC, et al. Papel de las poliaminas en la alimentación. Importancia de las poliaminas en la alimentación infantil. Archivos Latinoamericanos de Nutrición. 2008;**58**:117-125. Available from: http://ve.scielo.org/scielo.php?script=sci_arttext&pid=S0004-06222008000200001&lng=es&tlng=pt

[47] Plaza-Zamora J, Sabater-Molina M, Rodríguez-Palmero M, Rivero M, Bosch V, Nadal JM, et al. Polyamines in human breast milk for preterm and term infants. The British Journal of Nutrition. 2013;**110**:524-528. DOI: 10.1017/S0007114512005284

[48] Peulen O, Gharbi M, Powroznik B, Dandrifosse G. Differential effect of dietary spermine on alkaline phosphatase activity in jejunum and ileum of unweaned rats. Biochimie. 2004;**86**:487-493. DOI: 10.1016/j.biochi.2004.06.002

[49] Ngaragba M-C, Greco S, George P, Hugueny I, Louisot P. Polyamine participation in the maturation of glycoprotein fucosylation, but not sialylation, in rat small intestine. Pediatric Research. 2002;**51**:625-634. DOI: 10.1203/00006450-200205000-00014

[50] Ter Steege JCA, Buurman WA, Forget P-P. Spermine induces maturation of the immature intestinal immune system in neonatal mice. Journal of Pediatric Gastroenterology & Nutrition. 1997;**25**:332-340. Available from: http://journals.lww.com/00005176-199709000-00017

[51] Dandrifisse G, Forget G, Romain N, Deloyer P, Wery I. Maturation précoce de línte stine du rat par la spermine: résultats et perspectives. In: Quemener JM, editor. Les polyamines: chimie, biologie, médecine. 1991. pp. 237-247

[52] Matsumoto N, Yorifuji T, Nakamura K, Ikeda M, Tsukahara H, Doi H. Breastfeeding and risk of food allergy: A nationwide birth cohort in Japan. Allergology International. 2020;**69**:91-97. DOI: 10.1016/j.alit.2019.08.007

[53] Peulen O, Dewé W, Dandrifosse G, Henrotay I. The relationship between spermine content of human milk during the first postnatal month and allergy in children. Public Health Nutrition. 1998;**1**:181-184. DOI: 10.1079/PHN19980028

[54] Gómez-Gallego C, Collado MC, Ilo T, Jaakkola U-M, Bernal MJ, Periago MJ,

et al. Infant formula supplemented with polyamines alters the intestinal microbiota in neonatal BALB/cOlaHsd mice. The Journal of Nutritional Biochemistry. 2012;**23**:1508-1513. DOI: 10.1016/j.jnutbio.2011.10.003

[55] Pollack PF, Koldovský O, Nishioka K. Polyamines in human and rat milk and in infant formulas. The American Journal of Clinical Nutrition. 1992;**56**:371-375. DOI: 10.1093/ajcn/56.2.371

[56] Ali MA, Strandvik B, Palme-Kilander C, Yngve A. Lower polyamine levels in breast milk of obese mothers compared to mothers with normal body weight. Journal of Human Nutrition and Dietetics. 2013;**26**:164-170. DOI: 10.1111/jhn.12097

[57] Muñoz-Esparza NC, Comas-Basté O, Latorre-Moratalla ML, Veciana-Nogués MT, Vidal-Carou MC. Differences in polyamine content between human milk and infant formulas. Food. 2021;**10**:2866. DOI: 10.3390/foods10112866

[58] Löser C. Polyamines in human and animal milk. The British Journal of Nutrition. 2000;**84**:55-58. DOI: 10.1017/S0007114500002257

[59] Bjelakovic L, Kocic G, Bjelakovic B, Najman S, Stojanović D, Jonovic M, et al. Polyamine oxidase and diamine oxidase activities in human milk during the first month of lactation. Iranian Journal of Pediatrics. 2012;**22**:218-222

[60] Nielsen SD, Beverly RL, Dallas DC. Peptides released from foremilk and hindmilk proteins by breast milk proteases are highly similar. Frontiers in Nutrition. 2017;**2017**:4. DOI: 10.3389/fnut.2017.00054

[61] Van Sadelhoff J, Mastorakou D, Weenen H, Stahl B, Garssen J, Hartog A. Short communication: Differences in levels of free amino acids and total protein in human foremilk and Hindmilk. Nutrients. 2018;**10**:1828. DOI: 10.3390/nu10121828

[62] Perez M, Ladero V, Redruello B, del Rio B, Fernandez L, Rodriguez JM, et al. Mastitis modifies the biogenic amines profile in human milk, with significant changes in the presence of histamine, putrescine and spermine. PLoS One. 2016;**11**:e0162426. DOI: 10.1371/journal.pone.0162426

[63] Libuda L, Bolzenius K, Alexy U. Breastfeeding trends in healthy infants since 1990—Results of the DONALD study. European Journal of Clinical Nutrition. 2017;**71**:1016-1018. DOI: 10.1038/ejcn.2017.106

[64] Koletzko B, Baker S, Cleghorn G, Neto UF, Gopalan S, Hernell O, et al. Global standard for the composition of infant formula: Recommendations of an ESPGHAN coordinated international expert group. Journal of Pediatric Gastroenterology and Nutrition. 2005;**41**:584-599. DOI: 10.1097/01.mpg.0000187817.38836.42

[65] Moreno-Villares JM. Actualización en fórmulas infantiles. An Pediatría Contin. 2011;**9**:31-40. Available from: https://linkinghub.elsevier.com/retrieve/pii/S169628181170004X

[66] Lönnerdal B. Infant formula and infant nutrition: Bioactive proteins of human milk and implications for composition of infant formulas. The American Journal of Clinical Nutrition. 2014;**99**:712S-717S. DOI: 10.3945/ajcn.113.071993

[67] De Almagro García MC. Nuevos ingredientes en fórmulas infantiles. Beneficios sanitarios y funcionales. Nutrición Hospitalaria. 2017;**2017**:34. DOI: 10.20960/nh.1564

[68] Gómez-Gallego C, Recio I, Gómez-Gómez V, Ortuño I, Bernal MJ, Ros G, et al. Effect of processing on polyamine content and bioactive peptides released after in vitro gastrointestinal digestion of infant formulas. Journal of Dairy Science. 2016;**99**:924-932. DOI: 10.3168/jds.2015-10030

[69] Spizzirri UG, Puoci F, Iemma F, Restuccia D. Biogenic amines profile and concentration in commercial milks for infants and young children. Food Additives and Contamination Part A. 2019;**36**:337-349. DOI: 10.1080/19440049.2018.1563306

[70] Nishimura K, Shiina R, Kashiwagi K, Igarashi K. Decrease in polyamines with aging and their ingestion from food and drink. Journal of Biochemistry. 2006;**139**:81-90. DOI: 10.1093/jb/mvj003

[71] Cipolla BG, Havouis R, Moulinoux JP. Polyamine contents in current foods: A basis for polyamine reduced diet and a study of its long term observance and tolerance in prostate carcinoma patients. Amino Acids. 2007;**33**:203-212. DOI: 10.1007/s00726-007-0524-1

[72] Toro-Funes N, Bosch-Fuste J, Latorre-Moratalla ML, Veciana-Nogués MT, Vidal-Carou MC. Biologically active amines in fermented and non-fermented commercial soybean products from the Spanish market. Food Chemistry. 2015;**173**:1119-1124. DOI: 10.1016/j.foodchem.2014.10.118

[73] Byun BY, Bai X, Mah JH. Occurrence of biogenic amines in Doubanjiang and tofu. Food Science and Biotechnology. 2013;**22**:55-62. DOI: 10.1007/s10068-013-0008-x

[74] Glória MBA, Tavares-Neto J, Labanca RA, Carvalho MS. Influence of cultivar and germination on bioactive amines in soybeans (*Glycine max* L. Merril). Journal of Agricultural and Food Chemistry. 2005;**53**:7480-7485. DOI: 10.1021/jf0509310

[75] Ponce De León C, Torija E, Matallana MC. Utilidad en la alimentación de algunas semillas germinadas: brotes de soja y trigo. Boletín de la Real Sociedad Española de Historia Natural. Sección Biología. 2013;**107**:47-55

[76] Menéndez AB, Calzadilla PI, Sansberro PA, Espasandin FD, Gazquez A, Bordenave CD, et al. Polyamines and legumes: Joint stories of stress, nitrogen fixation and environment. Frontiers in Plant Science. 2019;**10**:1-15. DOI: 10.3389/fpls.2019.01415

Chapter 5

Technological Advances in Infant Formula Ingredients

Roberta Claro da Silva and Md. Jannatul Ferdaus

Abstract

The best source of nutrients for babies is breast milk. However, the baby formula offers a crucial alternative to nursing when it is not practical or viable to meet the growing child's nutritional needs. Bovine milk has traditionally been used as a primary component in baby formula production. It is then prepared with additional nutrients and bioactive substances to resemble the makeup of human breastmilk closely. Bovine-based baby formula is the most accessible type of formula, but it is not appropriate for all newborns; thus, alternatives, including those based on caprine milk, soy, and rice protein, are becoming more readily available. The composition of baby formula made from soy, rice, caprine milk, and cow's milk is thoroughly examined in this chapter. In addition, we cover the literature that is currently available on nutrient bio-accessibility and features of protein functioning that are pertinent to baby formula.

Keywords: infant formula, ingredients, advance technology, fatty acids, macronutrients, prebiotics and probiotics

1. Introduction

Human milk (HM) plays a crucial role in newborns' healthy growth and development of gastrointestinal (GI) tracts and immune systems. Therefore, breast milk is the best and only naturally designed food for babies [1]. In addition to the nutritional components, HM also contains essential physiologically active elements that help to reduce malnutrition risk. Sometimes, preterm babies do not get an adequate amount of their mother's milk [2]. In that case, milk from the donor or HM bank is needed, which is not always available in many countries. However, infant formula is required to maintain a newborn's normal physical, mental, and immunological development when breast milk is not available [3]. Therefore, it is formulated as a complete substitute for mother's milk to support an infant's necessary nutritional needs under 6 or 12 months [3]. Generally, infant formulas are prepared as a powder for bottle feeding, which is mixed with purified and sterile water [4]. The rehydrated mixture needs to be homogenized for adequate absorption in the infant's stomach. Formulas are made with different ratios of 6 basic food components, which are carbohydrates, proteins, fats, vitamins, minerals, and prebiotics and probiotics [3]. Manufacturers claim that formulas are identical to the HM. Bovine milk (BM) is the primary source of proteins (whey and casein) in most infant formulas [5]. In addition, some manufacturers also use soy protein [6]. However, almost half of the calories in formulas made with cow's milk come from a specific blend of fats designed to be easily absorbed by the body. Palm olein, soy, coconut, high-oleic sunflower, and safflower oils are frequent sources of fat [7]. Many infant formulas include omega fatty acids, which are long-chain polyunsaturated fatty acids (LCPUFAs) [8]. Studies reported that 20% of energy in a formula comes from carbohydrates or sugar. In milk-based products, lactose is the primary source of carbohydrates. The main benefit of lactose is that it is tolerable for almost all babies regardless of having protein allergy [9].

In the past half-century, there have been tremendous breakthroughs in infant formulas. During the middle of the 20th century, formula-fed infants typically received cow milk-based or homemade formulations with evaporated milk, sugar, and water [10]. However, technological advancements have changed formula preparation and nutritional compositions [11]. As a result, different formulas for different target groups are available in the market to support the infant's dietary needs with special conditions. For example, there are currently soy, lactose-free, rice starch formulations and formulas for preterm babies and infants with specific disorders, such as metabolic problems [12]. As more constituents of HM are identified and their physiological functions described, new formulas continue to be developed, and established formulas are continually modified. Nevertheless, hormones, immunological components, and enzymes analyzed in breast milk cannot be added to infant formulas.

This chapter reviews the application of technologies in infant formulations. There are many challenges that manufacturers need to encounter during the preparation of formulas. Most of these challenges are nutrition related, to be specific, the improvement of the nutritional benefits of infant formulations. For example, there were many limitations in the past to increasing the level or fortifying the formulas with macronutrients (carbohydrates, proteins, and fats), bioactive compounds, and prebiotics or probiotics.

2. Protein

The first year of an infant's life is a crucial time of rapid growth and development. Between birth and weaning, development and growth are required for long-term health [13]. Protein is a macronutrient that is necessary for the development of organ systems and bodily structures, as well as the regulation of several physiological processes. Protein synthesis must occur quickly to sustain the infant's rapid development. As a result of their fast growth, babies and early children have more significant protein needs per kilogram of body weight than any other age group [14]. In babies, the protein synthesis and turnover rate are disproportionately high to their body weight. During the first month of life, infants require around 3.5 times more protein per kilogram of body weight than adults [15]. HM includes more than 400 proteins that may be roughly categorized into three groups: caseins, whey proteins, and mucins, which are found in the milk fat globule membrane (MFGM). Although it varies across mothers and throughout lactation, the macronutrient content of HM is consistent among populations, despite nationality and race variability [16]. Throughout the first year of breastfeeding, the total protein content and concentrations of different proteins in HM fluctuate to meet the demands of the newborn. Regardless of the moment of birth, protein levels in human milk drop throughout the first 4–6 weeks [17, 18]. HM is dominated by whey; however, the ratio of whey to casein fluctuates throughout lactation, from 90/10 in colostrum to 60/40 in mature HM.

Protein content in mature, full-term milk is expected to be between 0.9 and 1.2 g/dl on average [18, 19]. Significant levels of α-lactalbumin, lactoferrin, IgA (Immunoglobulin A), osteopontin (OPN), and lysozyme are found in the whey fraction. After intake, these proteins are swiftly degraded into amino acids that may be absorbed and used [20]. Many of these proteins have both bioactive and non-nutritive activities. For example, α-lactalbumin is needed for lactose production and Ca and Zn ion binding [21]. Casein aids calcium and phosphorus in bulk formation. Lactoferrin and lysozyme inhibit the spread of potentially dangerous germs, protecting newborns from disease. The IgA antibody eliminates microorganisms and protects the intestinal mucosa [20].

2.1 Cow's milk formula and allergy

Cow's milk is an excellent source of protein for the baby. It includes crucial amino acids for the healthy growth of the body and mental health [15]. For example, while cow's milk has a protein level of 5 g/100 kcal, human milk has a protein content of just 1.5 g/100 kcal [18]. However, GI resistance to infant formulas manufactured with cow's milk occurs frequently during the first several months of life. Lactose intolerance may also be impacted by sensitivity to milk protein, lactose, or both [9]. A cow's milk allergy is a consistently unpleasant response to one or more milk proteins mediated by IgE and/or non-IgE pathways (CMA) [6]. Within one to two hours after consumption, gastrointestinal, respiratory, and cutaneous symptoms may manifest as IgE-mediated reactions. A skin rash or dermatitis as well as gastrointestinal (GI) symptoms like diarrhea, mucous stools, vomiting, and stomach discomfort may also be present [22]. Immune system-related, non-IgE mediated reactions can take up to 48 hours to develop but are immune system-delayed. Infants with ongoing issues may wheeze, become irritable, or underperform [22]. The majority of CMA cases occur in the first year of life, and hypoallergenic formula is the dietary treatment if the kid is not breastfed. For treating CMA, particularly in infants and young children, extensively hydrolyzed cow's milk formula (eHF) with confirmed hypo-allergenicity can be advised [23]. Amino acid-based formulas (AAF) can also be recommended, particularly for patients with more severe symptoms or in patients who are not responding to the eHF. They offer 90% of infants with CMA effective therapy [24]. Infants with CMA, who cannot tolerate or prefer eHF should use soy- and hydrolyzed rice-based formulas (HRFs).

CMA is widespread, but it is frequently improperly diagnosed because of its ambiguous indications [23]. The baby and the parents will suffer; thus, it will be advantageous to prevent CMA. A partly hydrolyzed formula (pHF) is one method to stop CMA in newborns. Using a combination of thermal processing and enzymatic hydrolysis reduces the protein's molecular weight and peptide lengths, which is created to lessen protein sensitivity [15]. pHFs typically have a molecular weight of around 5000 Da (range: 3–10,000 Da), whereas raw cow's milk-based formula (CMF) has peptides ranging from 14,000 Da to 67,000 Da [15]. Sensitivity has been reported in around fifty percent of newborns with CMA; hence, pHF should not be used for treatment. The hypoallergenic formulation has been thoroughly hydrolyzed and includes no peptides with a molecular weight of more than 5000 Da [25]. The majority of recommendations call for pHFs to protect at-risk non-breastfed babies against allergy illnesses, namely, atopic dermatitis (AD) and CMA. However, according to epidemiological research, almost 50% of newborns who later acquired allergies did not belong to the at-risk category. This is because the non-at-risk population is substantially more significant than the at-risk group. There is a 15% chance that non-at-risk infants may acquire allergies [26]. According to evaluation, formulas that have been partly hydrolyzed are secure, well-tolerated, and promote healthy newborn growth. In addition, in comparison to intact proteins, partly hydrolyzed formulas are easier to digest and hasten the transit time in premature newborns [27].

2.2 Soy-based infant formula

Infant formulas containing soy have already been used for over a century. Despite few indicators, soy-based formula accounts for around 20% of the U.S. formula market [28]. Available formulas using extracted soy protein are currently devoid of cow milk protein and lactose and offer 67 kcal/dL [29]. The protein consists of a soy isolate supplemented with L-methionine, L-carnitine, and taurine to produce a protein level of 1.65 to 1.90 g/dL [6]. Among the several heat-stable components in soy formula, phytoestrogens are particularly important to health. Phytoestrogens include numerous categories of non-steroidal estrogens, such as isoflavones, often found in legumes, with soybeans having the most significant concentration [6]. Concerns about isoflavones' possible adverse effects on reproductive development, neurobehavior, immunological performance, and hormone levels have been expressed [30]. However, the latest soy research indicates that phytoestrogens can lead to a reduced risk of coronary artery disease, cancer, and menopausal symptoms, all of which might be extra benefits of eating a soy-based diet at an early age [31]. Researchers are particularly concerned about the nutritional features of soy, especially as soy is the primary source of nutrition for many newborns for a minimum of six months during their growth. However, gas chromatography and mass spectrometry (GS/MS) were the traditional techniques for evaluating the isoflavone content of soy [28]. Recently, it was discovered that high-performance liquid chromatography (HPLC) was quicker, required less preparation time, and cheaper equipment.

Consequently, HPLC has been utilized in most research investigating the phytoestrogens content of soy formula [28]. Multiple experiments have extracted isoflavones from soy formula and compared these quantities to those found in the human milk collected following soy eating by the mother [6, 28, 32]. The decreased isoflavone content may give the advantages without causing as many of the dangers associated with high soy formula intake.

2.3 Hydrolyzed rice in infant formula

Formulas containing hydrolyzed rice have been used for decades in Europe, but they are still not widely accessible worldwide. A recent meta-analysis of 11 clinical trials using hydrolyzed rice formula in babies with CMA presented no cross-reactivity [33]. Another meta-analysis study of seven trials indicated that typically developing children and those with CMA could compensate for lost ground in height and weight. A skin prick test revealed rice-specific IgE levels in 4% of newborns in a multicenter trial of 100 infants with confirmed CMA; however, these infants showed no symptoms [25]. For children allergic to rice, hydrolysis of rice protein in the formula changes its allergenic characteristics and avoids an immunological response, as evidenced by negative Western blotting results [34]. Hydrolyzed rice formula's unpleasant flavor and limited availability are two drawbacks that might impair the formula's effectiveness in improving adherence. However, the taste scores of partially hydrolyzed rice formulas are comparable to those of soy formulas and are just as effective in treating CMA [27].

In choosing a formula substitute, factors like symptom intensity, preferences, cost, and effectiveness should be taken into account because all replacements to CMFs are nutritionally appropriate. Both substantially hydrolyzed formula and rice formula must be taken into consideration when nursing kids, who are allergic to CMF and soy-based formula. The effectiveness of HRFs as a choice for babies with CMA and soy allergy was investigated in a trial of 18 children, who were given SF but later experienced allergic responses after two to eighteen months of supplementation [34]. Skin prick test findings revealed that 8 and 2 children reacted to rice and rice hydrolysate, respectively. At the same time, 7 infants had antibodies in response to rice according to their serology tests [35].

3. Carbohydrates

Early childhood is a time of high-speed development. Babies who do not get enough nutrients and calories cannot maintain their predicted growth and maturation throughout this time; therefore, better nutrition is crucial. During such a critical phase, dietary carbohydrates, mainly lactose, are an essential primary source of food-derived energy [36]. Moreover, sugar and polysaccharides are some other significant sources of energy. Lactose is the primary carbohydrate source in baby formula made from caprine and bovine milk (BM). These formulas contain around 7–7.5 g of lactose per 100 mL. BM and caprine milk (CM) primarily include lactose, which has a mass of 44–56 g/L and 32–50 g/L, respectively [36]. Since many decades back, lactose intolerance has been acknowledged as a widespread issue affecting most adults and children. Although lactose intolerance symptoms are seldom fatal, they can cause severe pain and negatively impact the quality of life [37]. Therefore, the goal of treatment is to reduce or eliminate lactose, the provoking ingredient, either by removing it from the diet or by "predigesting" it with an additional lactase-enzyme replacement whose diarrhea may be exacerbated by formulas containing lactose while benefiting from formulas devoid of lactose [37]. However, the particular need for lactose has not been established, and formulations with decreased or no lactose have become more popular recently.

The growing worry about newborn lactose intolerance has been the key factor behind the rise in the usage of formulas that incorporate different carbohydrate groups [9]. Glycemic and non-glycemic are the two main kinds of carbohydrates. In newborn and follow-up formulas, some permitted glycemic carbohydrates, such as pre-cooked starch, gelatinized starch, corn syrup solids (CSS), and maltodextrin, are frequently used as substitute sugar [38]. Glycemic carbohydrates are digested and absorbed in the small intestine, followed by a rise in blood glucose [39]. A reduced-sweet saccharide polymer made of D-glucose molecules primarily connected linearly with α-1,4 bonds, where maltodextrin also contains a complex structure with α −1,6 linkages [40]. Maltodextrin is used as the primary source of sugars in non-allergenic infant formula. It has a nearly equivalent energy content to lactose of 4 kcal/g with a dextrose equivalent (DE) of $\leq$20 [41]. In baby formula made with soy and rice protein, maltodextrins are often used as the primary carbohydrate source [42]. That is why newborns with genetic lactose intolerance may consume these infant formulas. In the lactose-free formula, glucose syrup or dried glucose syrup may also be used when DE $\leq$ 32 [36]. In addition, other lactose-free formulas based on animal milk protein have been prepared by membrane screening or enzymatic hydrolysis. As a result, up to 30% of the total carbohydrates in baby formulas may contain pre-cooked or gelatinized starches [43]. This makes baby formula intended for babies with gastroesophageal reflux viscous. Additionally, they are frequently added to infant formulas that contain hydrolyzed proteins because this process raises the osmolarity of the formula.

Human milk oligosaccharides (HMOs) are hypothesized to have prebiotic effects by acting as nutrients for good bacteria like bifidobacteria. Compared to human milk, which includes 5–15 g/L of oligosaccharides, BM only contains 0.03–0.12 g/L of these sugars [44, 45]. In comparison to BM, CM has an oligosaccharide content that is over ten times higher and includes molecules that are functionally more comparable to HMOs. 2′-Fucosyllactose (20FL) and Lacto-N-neotetrose (LNnT), two structurally isoforms of HMOs, have been created by microbial fermentation for inclusion in the newborn formula [46]. Moreover, as an alternative to mimic many of the positive benefits of HMOs, producers are now adding non-digestible carbohydrates such as fructooligosaccharides (FOS) and galactooligosaccharides (GOS) to newborn formula [47].

4. Lipids

Lipid content in breast milk is significantly more different compared to the other macronutrients. In matured milk, lipid concentrations range from 3.5 to 4.5/100 g, although they vary depending on the mother's duration of nursing and throughout each meal [3]. High levels of medium-chain fatty acids (MCFA) and triacylglycerols are present in breast milk fat, which is dissolved by a phospholipid membrane. Lipids provide 40–50% of a newborn's energy needs and are the main energy source in baby formula [48]. The key ingredients of infant formula are long-chain fatty acids (LCFA), which are emulsified with dairy proteins, and soy lecithin (SL), which lacks sphingomyelin [16]. The amount of lipid hydrolysis products in the intestine are altered by changes in the sphingomyelin content and saturation level of phospholipids, which ostensibly influences the advantage of the certain gut microbiome [49].

The lipid content of baby formula must fall between the range of 4.4–6.0 g/100 kcal [36]. Due to significant changes in their fatty acid profiles from HM, which has a higher proportion of unsaturated fatty acids (C18:1, C18:2, and C18:3) and LCPUFAs (C20:4 and C22:6), BM and CM are not suitable as the only source of lipids in infant formula [36]. In newborn formula manufactured from BM and CM, vegetable oils are combined in a way comparable to human milk because of these discrepancies. The LCPUFAs, for example, arachidonic acid (ARA) (C20:4ω6) and docosahexaenoic acid (DHA) (C22:6ω3), are not present in the blends of vegetable oils [50]. Infant formulas are presently required by EU law to include 20–50 mg/100 kcal DHA [51]. Fish oils, microbe oil, and egg-yolk-produced lipids are all acceptable sources of LCPUFAs to add to baby formula. However, using unfractionated fish oil is not recommended since it contains eicosapentaenoic acid (EPA), which is hostile to the actions of ARA [52]. Triglyceride structure in baby formula is crucial because it influences lipid hydrolysis and, in turn, the bioavailability of fatty acids. The precise esterification of fatty acids to glycerol at the outer sn-1 and sn-3 and inner sn-2 locations of a triglyceride is known as triglyceride synthesis. Over 70% of the palmitic acid (C16:0) in HM is found at the sn-2 position on the triglyceride backbone. Because of this, structured triglycerides containing 17–25% palmitic acid and more than 40% of it esterified at the sn-2 position have been created by enzymatic procedures [53]. When added to the newborn formula, these structured triglycerides have been linked to altered intestinal microbiota, decreased colic incidence, enhanced bone growth, and lower intestinal inflammation.

During the manufacturing process, infant formula often goes through a homogenization stage. Consequently, globules are created in plant-based oil (approximately 0.4–0.5 μm), which are then solidified by protein [3]. Casein and whey proteins served as stabilizers in baby formula made from BM and CM, whereas soy and hydrolyzed rice proteins serve as the main emulsifiers of fat globules in formulas made from soy and rice, respectively [3, 54]. It has been reported that the characteristics of the lipid/water (L/W) interface and the globules' diameter influence how easily newborn formula digest. Consequently, efforts have been made to alter the structure of the L/W interface. One method involves adding BM's phospholipids to baby formula to change its concentration [20]. On the other hand, palmitic acid is abundant in human and animal milk, making up around 70% and 45%, respectively. However, less than 20% of vegetable oils are esterified with palmitic acid at the sn-2 position [50]. Compared to newborn formulas containing milk fat or β-palmitate, formulas using just plant-based oils had a lower percentage of palmitic acid in the sn-2 place of triglycerides. According to Prosser et al., who studied the fatty acid profile of a CM-based formula product in which goat milk accounted for 55% of the total fat and a vegetable oil mix for the rest, this blend provided the necessary fatty acids profile for the babies [55].

5. Prebiotics and probiotics

Probiotics in formula help infants maintain a healthy proportion of microbes in their gut and inhibit the development of "unfriendly" microorganisms that may otherwise cause illness and irritation [56]. Probiotics and prebiotics are included in baby formula to establish good gastrointestinal bacteria similar to those of breastfed babies in order to support optimal growth and minimize illnesses. Breastfeeding newborns have a higher proportion of bifidobacteria in their gut microbial population and a lower number of pathogens than those who are formula-fed [57]. Prebiotics are indigestible components of some foods that promote the development of probiotics in the digestive system. Prebiotics may be found naturally in foods, including human milk, fruits, and vegetables. Probiotics are live microorganisms that mimic the microflora typically present in the body and are included in certain meals. Probiotics are useful for better digestion since they assist in moving food through the gastrointestinal tract, maintaining a healthy digestive system [58]. Numerous substances included in human milk influence the infant's gut flora. Although it is impossible to trace breastfeeding's effects on the gut microbiota to a single substance, mounting research suggests that human milk oligosaccharides play a key role. Human milk oligosaccharides (HMOs), which have distinct nutritional and functional qualities, are a common and significant group of components [46]. Prebiotic oligosaccharides (OS), which are essentially missing in cow's milk, are the third most common substance in a mother's milk, which is made with complex combination of glycan [57].

The presence of growth factors (HMOs) in HM and their absence in baby formula have been cited as the main reasons why breastfed babies have a large proportion of bifidobacteria in GI microflora as opposed to formula fed babies [59]. Because of this, prebiotics are usually added to baby formula today to improve its functional qualities. Infant formula has been supplemented with oligosaccharides more often in recent years, primarily a combination of fructo and galacto-oligosaccharides (FOS) (GOS) and polydextrose [57]. Prebiotic functions have been reported to enhance immunity and resemble the bifidogenic action of HMOs [60]. Breastfed babies have a predominance of Bifidobacterium and Lactobacillus in their feces. However, by producing organic acids, hence reducing the level of pH, Bifidobacterium and Lactobacillus may prevent the development of harmful microbes in the intestine. In addition, these gut microflorae emulate harmful microorganisms for resources and epithelial attachment sites [61]. Recent research on prebiotics in a formula examined if adding probiotics or prebiotic FOS to the milk-based formula would alter the fecal bacteria of babies compared to breastfed infants. On the other hand, the fortification of the GOS/FOS combination to newborn formula was shown to have an influencing impact on the proliferation of Bifidobacterium and the digestion characteristics of the whole GI microflora [57].

Moreover, 1,3-olein-2-palmitin (OPO), a triacylglycerol that may be produced from plant-based oil (palm oil) and added to baby formula, is the most prevalent in HM. OPO may smooth and boost the frequency of stools in newborns without causing diarrhea and raising the percentage of Bifidobacterium in feces. However, it is uncertain how prebiotics and OPO may affect feeding results comparable to breast milk [62].

6. Bioactive compounds

An increasing number of research indicates that the numerous components in human milk, referred to as functional or bioactive components, cause the short- and long-term advantages of breastfeeding [18, 46, 63]. These bioactive compounds include various components such as macronutrients, nucleotides, minerals, and Igs [64]. Due to the essential nutrients and bioactive components in HM that are lacking or not present in sufficient quantity in the newborn formula, ingesting human milk has more health advantages than feeding infant formula. Human milk is utilized as a model for potentially adding new bioactive compounds to baby formula. There is little proof that one baby formula is superior to another, and most commercially available infant formulas are nutritionally equivalent [3]. However, potential sources of such bioactive components must be investigated. They may be added to baby formulas in order to make them equal to the HM. Due to rigorous regulations on baby formula content in many nations, this is not a simple task [20]. Clinical studies in newborns are necessary to assess changes in nutritional content, but they are expensive and time-consuming. Including bioactive components necessitates that they are both safe and provide the recipient babies with clear advantages. The ingredients' cost, quality, and origins will also impact whether it is practical to use them.

6.1 α-lactalbumin

In cow's milk, just 3.5% of the total protein is α-lactalbumin (α-La), while it makes up 22% in HM. The homology of the amino acid patterns of BM and HM α-La is quite close (73.9%), and they both have a similar length [65]. Since it contains relatively large amounts of tryptophan (Trp) and cysteine (Cys), α-La has primarily been used to supplement baby formula. Bioactive peptides from α-La are a significant source and may impact GI health. The presence of Trp and Cys, which are thought to be the source of these advantages, is supported by evidence [20]. In addition to serving as a nutrient, α-La contains a unique calcium receptor and another for iron and zinc, making it easier for the body to absorb [63]. By preventing pathogens from adhering to the intestine because lactosamine, which is required for its adherence, is absent when α-La is lactosylated, it may reduce the risk of contamination. It has been anticipated that several peptides produced from α-La when it is digested will have biological effects [65]. Data comparing the development of breastfed and formula-fed (α-La enriched) newborns showed that children's growth trends were identical. According to these clinical investigations, α-La, a source abundant in essential amino acids, may serve as an appropriate dietary component [20].

6.2 Lactoferrin

In different research studies, lactoferrin (LF) was initially discovered in cow's milk and later from HM. Bovine lactoferrin (BLF), with a weight of 80 kDa and peptides that are quite comparable to those of human lactoferrin (HLF), has around 70% sequence similarity [20]. LF has versatile components, which have a role in the immune system and as an anti-inflammatory. It is widely recognized that lactoferrin has iron-binding properties and is the first line of defense against microbial contamination. It is extraordinarily resistant to proteolytic enzymes, allowing it to perform all these activities [63]. Additionally, LF may have biological effects that are not caused by the interaction of its receptor. Similar bioactive characteristics exist in commercially added LF and HLF. It was discovered that the prevalence of respiratory infections dropped while hematocrit rose when LF was added to the newborn formula [66]. However, since BLF does not attach to HLF receptors, enhanced lactoferrin did not increase iron absorption. However, equivalent bioactivity has been shown in both in vitro and animal models, including improved growth, similar effects against a variety of pathogenic organisms, and antioxidant activity [21]. In research, formulas enhanced with BLF at levels comparable to those found in mature HM were given to healthy newborns to assess their development and tolerance [63]. The study found that breastfed newborns grew at the same rate as formula-fed infants. Nowadays, BLF is widely accessible and comparatively proteolysis resistant. In a previous research, commercial BLF was added to baby formula and investigated its outcomes comparing with HLF in an intestinal enterocyte model [20]. In addition, Similar to the HLF, market-available BLF has been demonstrated to enhance cell proliferation. However, the findings revealed no appreciable impact on the microbiota of feces, pathogens, or iron status [63]. Synthesized LF sometimes contains lipopolysaccharides, which likewise have a strong attraction for LF receptors and inhibit their roles as a bioactive compound. Studies conducted in vitro on the bioactivity of BLF without the presence of lipopolysaccharides produced encouraging findings [20].

6.3 Milk fat globule membrane

The milk fat globule membrane (MFGM) is made of lipids and proteins, which surround the fat globule released by the alveolar epithelial cells of humans and other animals [67]. MFGM and its components are a significant source of bioactive substances. Because of their nutritional, physiological, and health advantages, they have recently attracted the attention of nutritionists in baby feeding. In addition, clinical research studies on humans and animals have shown benefits for immunological and GI health and cognitive function [20]. A whey protein concentrate high in MFGM may thus aid in guarding against diarrhea of both bacterial and viral origin [68]. In addition, several proteins in MFGM have been demonstrated to have inhibitory effects against different infections. Since the MFGM fraction is now marketed, it could be possible to include it in a newborn formula [69]. Clinical studies on MFGM are required to investigate impacts on essential outcomes in newborns because in vitro experiments have shown bioactivities and because the components of the bovine MFGM are comparable to those in human milk. In randomized controlled research in Peru, babies aged 6 to 8 months were given supplemental food containing bovine MFGM twice daily for six months. The incidence of diarrhea, especially bloody diarrhea, was shown to be lower [70]. Young babies were given MFGM-based or conventional formula from 6 weeks up to 6 months of age in a recent experiment in Sweden. Babies who had been breastfed were also used as a comparison group. However, results showed no difference in cognitive scores between the formula-fed and breastfed groups [71]. This implies that adding MFGM to baby formula may provide formula-fed babies with nutrients that assist brain development.

6.4 Polyunsaturated fatty acids

PUFAs have been introduced to baby formula to serve as bioactive components that promote eye and brain development. PUFAs like docosahexaenoic acid (DHA) and arachidonic acid (ARA), present in human milk, are crucial for forming the proteins that make up plasma membranes [20]. Globally, human milk produced by mothers is estimated to include an average amount of DHA and ARA of 0.32% and 0.47% of total fatty acids, respectively [72]. Due to the sluggish and ineffective elongation and desaturation processes, which result in a relatively low conversion rate, DHA and ARA are substituted for the formula's corresponding n-6 and n-3 precursors. The membranes of the cells in the central nervous system and retina are structural components made up entirely of DHA and ARA. While DHA builds up throughout the first few years of life, the infant's brain must develop normally [73]. Together, DHA and ARA make up around 25% of the total fatty acids profile in the brain, and they are both essential for a baby's neurological development [20]. Newborns who are breastfed or given formulas without PUFA supplements have lower amounts of DHA and ARA in plasma or red blood cells than infants fed formulas with PUFA supplements. Upper respiratory infections are less common in infants given formula supplemented with DHA and ARA. Compared to a baby formula containing ARA, the lack of ARA impacts circulating T lymphocytes, macrophages, and B cells activation markers. Clinical studies have been conducted to evaluate the effectiveness of adding DHA and ARA to infant formula [74]. Infants who consumed formulas lacking LCPUFAs had significantly lower concentrations of DHA and ARA in their plasma and red blood cells compared to breastfed infants [48]. These results were compared to those of babies who received formula with DHA and ARA, and it was found that they have a satisfactory amount of these LCPUFAs. Moreover, it has been demonstrated that breastfed infants have far higher quantities of DHA in their brains than newborns who are given formula.

7. Technology of infant formula production

Infant formula was first made using customized cow's milk around the start of the 20th century, but more modern formulas have come to closely resemble HM as a result of advances in our understanding of infant nutrition and production technology.

The amounts of essential nutrients are the primary distinctions between HM and BM. LCPUFAs and choline are crucial elements that must be included in formulas [3]. The sterilized combination of required ingredients is then homogenized and evaporated before spray-drying. Thermal processes, such as component rearrangement, may take place throughout any step of this process [75].

Using a ribbon blender, the raw and dried materials collected from the vendor are combined in bulk until the ingredients are evenly redistributed everywhere in the mixture. Next, the ingredients are sorted via a fine mesh to remove large and unwanted particles. The powder is subsequently moved from the screened material to the packing line, which is then shifted to a filler hopper [3]. After that mixture is fed further into the can-filling chamber from the filler hopper, noble gas is used to rinse the cans. The dry blending method has several benefits, one of which is that it consumes less energy and needs less financial investment for the infrastructure, the machinery, and the operation [76]. Because the powder-forming technique does not include the use of any water, the potential for microbial contamination is drastically reduced.

Currently, the wet mixing-spray drying procedure is the most commonly used technique for making powdered baby formula. One benefit of this drying method is that all quality parameters may be more successfully controlled than they can be with the dry mix method [77]. Water-soluble components are mixed with milk in a high-shear mixer before being added to the mixture. Once fully hydrated, the mixture is then kept in a tank. Minerals that may dissolve in water are incorporated into the blend after being individually hydrated in warm water. To add oil-soluble vitamins to the mixture, they must first be dissolved in oil [76]. Evaporation, which uses less energy than spray drying, is, therefore, a required stage in the water removal process. In vacuum evaporators, evaporation is always performed. As a result, the components are shielded from heat damage since the pressure is lowered, allowing boiling to occur at a lower temperature. A continuous multiple-effect evaporator, often of the tubular form, concentrates milk before it is dried [77]. The drying method is to blame for the variation in maximum concentrations that might occur during evaporation. Milk is often dried using a hot air stream or a roller dryer. Both systems need to have the application modified for industrial usage. Because roller-dried goods are less soluble in water, spray drying is often used for baby formula. A solution is sprayed into a compartment with heated air flowing within it in the form of tiny droplets according to the drying concept. Expanding the surface area enables quick mass transfer. Before being exposed to the hot air in the chamber, evaporated milk must first be divided into tiny droplets. Different types of drying chambers exist. They typically consist of a cylindrical cone that is tilted between 40 and 60°, allowing the powder to escape the chamber by gravity. Additionally, the bottoms of these compartments are flat so that suction or scraper devices may be added to remove the powder. There are certain spray drying chambers with fixed nozzles. For the comparatively big milk droplets to be released in counterflow to the drying air, they are utilized in low spray towers and are situated in a lower location inside the chamber. The milk is released from the stationary nozzle in the identical airflow direction. In the chamber, generally, the air temperature range is between 170 and 250° C, whereas the formula mixture has a temperature below 100° C. Due to the fast heat transfer caused by the temperature differential, quick and homogenized drying is accomplished. However, the drying procedure might be carried out in phases, with each step having a distinct time-temperature profile to limit the destruction of delicate items, such as baby formula [77].

8. Conclusion

In conclusion, baby formula is still undergoing modifications, and these changes often lead to products with properties and compositions that are more similar to those of human milk. New formula is also being created to satisfy the demands of newborns who have specific nutritional requirements. Data show that formulas with PUFAs added in quantities comparable to those in human milk may help the visual system's development. According to many studies, bioactive compounds in formula promote the development of the immunological and gastrointestinal systems. According to multiple studies, catch-up growth was higher in newborns given this novel formula than in those fed regular term-infant formulas. Formulas for preterm infants are created to satisfy the demands of a population at risk of developing growth and nutritional deficits. The complex components of human milk and the unique dietary requirements of various groups of newborns will continue to be characterized by researchers via continuing investigations. It is necessary to conduct lengthy research with large newborn cohorts to ascertain if the biochemical effects of formula changes are related to functional results.

Conflict of interest

The authors declare no conflict of interest.

Author details

Roberta Claro da Silva* and Md. Jannatul Ferdaus
Department of Family and Consumer Sciences, College of Agriculture and Environmental Sciences, North Carolina A&T State University, Greensboro, NC, USA

*Address all correspondence to: rcsilva@ncat.edu

References

[1] Chong HY, Tan LT, Law JW, Hong KW, Ratnasingam V, Ab Mutalib NS, et al. Exploring the potential of human Milk and formula Milk on infants' gut and health. Nutrients. 2022;**14**(17):3554. DOI: 10.3390/nu14173554

[2] Underwood MA. Human milk for the premature infant. Pediatric Clinics. 2013;**60**(1):189-207. DOI: 10.1016/j.pcl.2012.09.008

[3] Martin CR, Ling PR, Blackburn GL. Review of infant feeding: Key features of breast milk and infant formula. Nutrients. 2016;**8**(5):279. DOI: 10.3390/nu8050279

[4] Losio MN, Pavoni E, Finazzi G, Agostoni C, Daminelli P, Dalzini E, et al. Preparation of powdered infant formula: Could product's safety be improved? Journal of Pediatric Gastroenterology and Nutrition. 2018;**67**(4):543. DOI: 10.1097%2FMPG.0000000000002100

[5] Davoodi SH, Shahbazi R, Esmaeili S, Sohrabvandi S, Mortazavian A, Jazayeri S, et al. Health-related aspects of milk proteins. Iranian Journal of Pharmaceutical Research: IJPR. 2016;**15**(3):573. DOI: 10.22037/ijpr.2016.1897

[6] Bhatia J, Greer F, Committee on Nutrition. Use of soy protein-based formulas in infant feeding. Pediatrics. 2008;**121**(5):1062-1068. DOI: 10.1542/peds.2008-0564

[7] Schwingshackl L, Bogensberger B, Benčič A, Knüppel S, Boeing H, Hoffmann G. Effects of oils and solid fats on blood lipids: A systematic review and network meta-analysis. Journal of Lipid Research. 2018;**59**(9):1771-1782. DOI: 10.1194/jlr.P085522

[8] Qawasmi A, Landeros-Weisenberger A, Leckman JF, Bloch MH. Meta-analysis of long-chain polyunsaturated fatty acid supplementation of formula and infant cognition. Pediatrics. 2012;**129**(6):1141-1149. DOI: 10.1542/peds.2011-2127

[9] Heine RG, AlRefaee F, Bachina P, De Leon JC, Geng L, Gong S, et al. Lactose intolerance and gastrointestinal cow's milk allergy in infants and children–common misconceptions revisited. World Allergy Organization Journal. 2017;**10**(1):1-8. DOI: 10.1186/s40413-017-0173-0

[10] Fomon SJ. Infant feeding in the 20th century: Formula and beikost. The Journal of Nutrition. 2001;**131**(2):409S-420S. DOI: 10.1093/jn/131.2.409S

[11] Spalinger J, Nydegger A, Belli D, Furlano RI, Yan J, Tanguy J, et al. Growth of infants fed formula with evolving nutrition composition: A single-arm non-inferiority study. Nutrients. 2017;**9**(3):219. DOI: 10.3390/nu9030219

[12] Chen M, Sun Q. Current knowledge in the stabilization/destabilization of infant formula emulsions during processing as affected by formulations. Trends in Food Science & Technology. 2021;**109**:435-447. DOI: 10.1016/j.tifs.2021.01.036

[13] Vail B, Prentice P, Dunger DB, Hughes IA, Acerini CL, Ong KK. Age at weaning and infant growth: Primary analysis and systematic review. The Journal of Pediatrics. 2015;**167**(2):317-324. DOI: 10.1016/j.jpeds.2015.05.003

[14] Tang M. Protein intake during the first two years of life and its association with growth and risk of overweight. International Journal of Environmental Research and Public Health. 2018;**15**(8):1742. DOI: 10.3390/ijerph15081742

[15] Nutten S. Proteins, peptides and amino acids: Role in infant Nutrition. Nestle Nutrition Institute Workshop Series. 2016;**86**:1-10. DOI: 10.1159/000442697

[16] Lee H, Padhi E, Hasegawa Y, Larke J, Parenti M, Wang A, et al. Compositional dynamics of the milk fat globule and its role in infant development. Frontiers in Pediatrics. 2018;**6**:313. DOI: 10.3389/fped.2018.00313

[17] Gridneva Z, Tie WJ, Rea A, Lai CT, Ward LC, Murray K, et al. Human milk casein and whey protein and infant body composition over the first 12 months of lactation. Nutrients. 2018;**10**(9):1332. DOI: 10.3390/nu10091332

[18] Ballard O, Morrow AL. Human milk composition: Nutrients and bioactive factors. Pediatric Clinics. 2013;**60**(1): 49-74. DOI: 10.1016/j.pcl.2012.10.002

[19] Kunz C, Lönnerdal B. Re-evaluation of the whey protein/casein ratio of human milk. Acta Paediatrica. 1992;**81**(2):107-112. DOI: 10.1111/j.1651-2227.1992.tb12184.x

[20] Almeida CC, Mendonça Pereira BF, Leandro KC, Costa MP, Spisso BF, Conte-Junior CA. Bioactive compounds in infant formula and their effects on infant nutrition and health: A systematic literature review. International Journal of Food Science. 2021;**2021**:31. DOI: 10.1155/2021/8850080

[21] Skolnick J, Chou C, Miklavcic J. Insights into novel infant Milk formula bioactives. Nutrition and Dietary Supplements. 2020;**12**:11-19. DOI: 10.2147/nds.s192099

[22] Walsh J, Meyer R, Shah N, Quekett J, Fox AT. Differentiating milk allergy (IgE and non-IgE mediated) from lactose intolerance: Understanding the underlying mechanisms and presentations. British Journal of General Practice. 2016;**66**(649):e609-e611. DOI: 10.3399/bjgp16X686521

[23] Vandenplas Y, Brough HA, Fiocchi A, Miqdady M, Munasir Z, Salvatore S, et al. Current guidelines and future strategies for the management of cow's milk allergy. Journal of Asthma and Allergy. 2021;**14**:1243-1256. DOI: 10.2147/JAA.S276992

[24] Saeed F, Ullah Khan A, Mushtaq Z, Afzaal M, Niaz B, Hussain M, et al. Amino acid profile and safety assessment of infant formula available in local market, Pakistan. International Journal of Food Properties. 2021;**24**(1):533-543. DOI: 10.1080/10942912.2021.1900241

[25] D'Auria E, Salvatore S, Acunzo M, Peroni D, Pendezza E, Di Profio E, et al. Hydrolysed formulas in the Management of Cow's Milk allergy: New insights, pitfalls and tips. Nutrients. 2021;**13**(8):2762. DOI: 10.3390/nu13082762

[26] Verduci E, Di Profio E, Cerrato L, Nuzzi G, Riva L, Vizzari G, et al. Use of soy-based formulas and cow's milk allergy: Lights and shadows. Frontiers in Pediatrics. 2020;**8**:591988. DOI: 10.3389/fped.2020.591988

[27] Kipfer S, Goldman RD. Formula choices in infants with cow's milk allergy. Canadian Family Physician. 2021;**67**(3):180-182. DOI: 10.46747/cfp.6703180

[28] Badger TM, Gilchrist JM, Pivik RT, Andres A, Shankar K, Chen JR, et al. The health implications of soy infant formula. The American Journal of Clinical Nutrition. 2009;**89**(5):1668S-1672S. DOI: 10.3945/ajcn.2009.26736U

[29] Singh P, Kumar R, Sabapathy SN, Bawa AS. Functional and edible uses of soy protein products. Comprehensive Reviews in Food Science and Food Safety. 2008;**7**(1):14-28. DOI: 10.1111/j.1541-4337.2007.00025.x

[30] Dinsdale EC, Ward WE. Early exposure to soy isoflavones and effects on reproductive health: A review of human and animal studies. Nutrients. 2010;**2**(11):1156-1187. DOI: 10.3390/nu2111156

[31] Wroblewski Lissin L, Cooke JP. Phytoestrogens and cardiovascular health. Journal of the American College of Cardiology. 2000;**35**(6):1403-1410

[32] Testa I, Salvatori C, Di Cara G, Latini A, Frati F, Troiani S, et al. Soy-based infant formula: Are phyto-oestrogens still in doubt? Frontiers in Nutrition. 2018;**5**:110. DOI: 10.3389/fnut.2018.00110

[33] Picaud JC, Pajek B, Arciszewska M, Tarczón I, Escribano J, Porcel R, et al. An infant formula with partially hydrolyzed whey protein supports adequate growth and is safe and well-tolerated in healthy, term infants: A randomized, double-blind, equivalence trial. Nutrients. 2020;**12**(7):2072. DOI: 10.3390/nu12072072

[34] Fiocchi A, Restani P, Bernardini R, Lucarelli S, Lombardi G, Magazzù G, et al. A hydrolysed rice-based formula is tolerated by children with cow's milk allergy: A multi-Centre study. Clinical & Experimental Allergy. 2006;**36**(3):311-316. DOI: 10.1111/j.1365-2222.2006.02428.x

[35] Reche M, Pascual C, Fiandor A, Polanco I, Rivero-Urgell M, Chifre R, et al. The effect of a partially hydrolysed formula based on rice protein in the treatment of infants with cow's milk protein allergy. Pediatric Allergy and Immunology. 2010;**21**(4p1):577-585. DOI: 10.1111/j.1399-3038.2010.00991.x

[36] Stephen A, Alles M, de Graaf C, Fleith M, Hadjilucas E, Isaacs E, et al. The role and requirements of digestible dietary carbohydrates in infants and toddlers. European Journal of Clinical Nutrition. 2012;**66**:765-779. DOI: 10.1038/ejcn.2012.27

[37] Heyman MB, Committee on Nutrition. Lactose intolerance in infants, children, and adolescents. Pediatrics. 2006;**118**(3):1279-1286. DOI: 10.1542/peds.2006-1721

[38] Ackerman DL, Craft KM, Townsend SD. Infant food applications of complex carbohydrates: Structure, synthesis, and function. Carbohydrate Research. 2017;**437**:16-27. DOI: 10.1016/j.carres.2016.11.007

[39] Gromova LV, Fetissov SO, Gruzdkov AA. Mechanisms of glucose absorption in the small intestine in health and metabolic diseases and their role in appetite regulation. Nutrients. 2021;**13**(7):2474. DOI: 10.3390/nu13072474

[40] Hofman DL, Van Buul VJ, Brouns FJ. Nutrition, health, and regulatory aspects of digestible maltodextrins. Critical Reviews in Food Science and Nutrition. 2016;**56**(12):2091-2100. DOI: 10.1080/10408398.2014.940415

[41] Call L, Stoll B, Oosterloo B, Ajami N, Sheikh F, Wittke A, et al. Metabolomic signatures distinguish the impact of formula carbohydrates on disease outcome in a preterm piglet model

of NEC. Microbiome. 2018;**6**(1):1-5. DOI: 10.3390/nu12113465

[42] Young B. Variation in infant formula macronutrient ingredients is associated with infant anthropometrics. Nutrients. 2020;**12**(11):3465. DOI: 10.3390/nu12113465

[43] Clouard C, le Bourgot C, Respondek F, Bolhuis JE, Gerrits WJJ. A milk formula containing maltodextrin, vs. lactose, as main carbohydrate source, improves cognitive performance of piglets in a spatial task. Scientific Reports. 2018;**8**(1):9413. DOI: 10.1038/s41598-018-27796-1

[44] Plaza-Díaz J, Fontana L, Gil A. Human milk oligosaccharides and immune system development. Nutrients. 2018;**10**(8):1038. DOI: 10.3390/nu10081038

[45] Mank M, Hauner H, Heck AJ, Stahl B. Targeted LC-ESI-MS2 characterization of human milk oligosaccharide diversity at 6 to 16 weeks post-partum reveals clear staging effects and distinctive milk groups. Analytical and Bioanalytical Chemistry. 2020;**412**(25):6887-6907. DOI: 10.1007/s00216-020-02819-x

[46] Hegar B, Wibowo Y, Basrowi RW, Ranuh RG, Sudarmo SM, Munasir Z, et al. The role of two human milk oligosaccharides, 2′-fucosyllactose and lacto-N-neotetraose, in infant nutrition. Pediatric Gastroenterology, Hepatology & Nutrition. 2019;**22**(4):330-340. DOI: 10.5223/pghn.2019.22.4.330

[47] Verkhnyatskaya S, Ferrari M, de Vos P, Walvoort MT. Shaping the infant microbiome with non-digestible carbohydrates. Frontiers in Microbiology. 2019;**10**:343. DOI: 10.3389/fmicb.2019.00343

[48] Gianni ML, Roggero P, Baudry C, Fressange-Mazda C, Galli C, Agostoni C, et al. An infant formula containing dairy lipids increased red blood cell membrane omega 3 fatty acids in 4 month-old healthy newborns: A randomized controlled trial. BMC Pediatrics. 2018;**18**(1):1-8. DOI: 10.1186/s12887-018-1047-5

[49] Nejrup RG, Licht TR, Hellgren LI. Fatty acid composition and phospholipid types used in infant formulas modifies the establishment of human gut bacteria in germ-free mice. Scientific Reports. 2017;**7**(1):1-1. DOI: 10.1038/s41598-017-04298-0

[50] Delplanque B, Gibson R, Koletzko B, Lapillonne A, Strandvik B. Lipid quality in infant nutrition: Current knowledge and future opportunities. Journal of Pediatric Gastroenterology and Nutrition. 2015;**61**(1):8-17. DOI: 10.1097/MPG.0000000000000818

[51] Bocquet A, Briend A, Chouraqui JP, Darmaun D, Feillet F, Frelut ML, et al. The new European regulatory framework for infant and follow-on formulas: Comments from the Committee of Nutrition of the French Society of Pediatrics (CN-SFP). Archives de Pédiatrie. 2020;**27**(7):351-353

[52] Pal A, Metherel AH, Fiabane L, Buddenbaum N, Bazinet RP, Shaikh SR. Do eicosapentaenoic acid and docosahexaenoic acid have the potential to compete against each other? Nutrients. 2020;**12**(12):3718. DOI: 10.3390/nu12123718

[53] Innis SM, Dyer R, Nelson CM. Evidence that palmitic acid is absorbed assn-2 monoacylglycerol from human milk by breast-fed infants. Lipids. 1994;**29**(8):541-545. DOI: 10.1007/BF02536625

[54] Chen W, Liang G, Li X, He Z, Zeng M, Gao D, et al. Effects of soy proteins and hydrolysates on fat globule coalescence and meltdown properties of ice cream. Food Hydrocolloids. 2019;**94**:279-286. DOI: 10.1016/j.foodhyd.2019.02.045

[55] Prosser CG, Svetashev VI, Vyssotski MV, Lowry DJ. Composition and distribution of fatty acids in triglycerides from goat infant formulas with milk fat. Journal of Dairy Science. 2010;**93**(7):2857-2862. DOI: 10.3168/jds.2009-2946

[56] Fabiano V, Indrio F, Verduci E, Calcaterra V, Pop TL, Mari A, et al. Term infant formulas influencing gut microbiota: An overview. Nutrients. 2021;**13**(12):4200. DOI: 10.3390/nu13124200

[57] Vandenplas Y, Greef ED, Veereman G. Prebiotics in infant formula. Gut Microbes. 2014;**5**(6):681-687. DOI: 10.4161/19490976.2014.972237

[58] Mugambi MN, Musekiwa A, Lombard M, Young T, Blaauw R. Synbiotics, probiotics or prebiotics in infant formula for full term infants: A systematic review. Nutrition Journal. 2012;**11**(1):1-32. DOI: 10.1186/1475-2891-11-81

[59] Boudry G, Charton E, Le Huerou-Luron I, Ferret-Bernard S, Le Gall S, Even S, et al. The relationship between breast milk components and the infant gut microbiota. Frontiers in Nutrition. 2021;**8**:629740. DOI: 10.3389/fnut.2021.629740

[60] Borewicz K, Suarez-Diez M, Hechler C, Beijers R, de Weerth C, Arts I, et al. The effect of prebiotic fortified infant formulas on microbiota composition and dynamics in early life. Scientific Reports. 2019;**9**(1):1-3. DOI: 10.1038/s41598-018-38268-x

[61] Giovannini M, Verduci E, Gregori D, Ballali S, Soldi S, Ghisleni D, et al. Prebiotic effect of an infant formula supplemented with galacto-oligosaccharides: Randomized multicenter trial. Journal of the American College of Nutrition. 2014;**33**(5):385-393. DOI: 10.1080/07315724.2013.878232

[62] Zhu B, Zheng S, Lin K, Xu X, Lv L, Zhao Z, et al. Effects of infant formula supplemented with prebiotics and OPO on infancy fecal microbiota: A pilot randomized clinical trial. Frontiers in Cellular and Infection Microbiology. 2021;**11**:650407. DOI: 10.3389/fcimb.2021.650407

[63] Lönnerdal B. Infant formula and infant nutrition: Bioactive proteins of human milk and implications for composition of infant formulas. The American Journal of Clinical Nutrition. 2014;**99**(3):712S-717S. DOI: 10.3945/ajcn.113.071993

[64] Poonia A. Bioactive compounds, nutritional profile and health benefits of colostrum: A review. Food Production, Processing and Nutrition. 2022;**4**(1):1-21. DOI: 10.1186/s43014-022-00104-1

[65] Layman DK, Lönnerdal B, Fernstrom JD. Applications for α-lactalbumin in human nutrition. Nutrition Reviews. 2018;**76**(6):444-460. DOI: 10.1093/nutrit/nuy004

[66] García-Montoya IA, Cendón TS, Arévalo-Gallegos S, Rascón-Cruz Q. Lactoferrin a multiple bioactive protein: An overview. Biochimica et Biophysica Acta (BBA)-General Subjects. 2012;**1820**(3):226-236. DOI: 10.1016/j.bbagen.2011.06.018

[67] Nieto-Ruiz A, Diéguez E, Sepúlveda-Valbuena N, Herrmann F, Cerdó T, López-Torrecillas F, et al. The effects of an infant formula enriched with milk fat globule membrane, long-chain polyunsaturated fatty acids and synbiotics on child behavior up to 2.5 years old: The COGNIS study. Nutrients. 2020;**12**(12):3825. DOI: 10.3390/nu12123825

[68] Brink LR, Chichlowski M, Pastor N, Thimmasandra Narayanappa A, Shah N. In the age of viral pandemic, can ingredients inspired by human milk and infant nutrition be repurposed to support the immune system? Nutrients. 2021;**13**(3):870. DOI: 10.3390/nu13030870

[69] da Silva RC, Colleran HL, Ibrahim SA. Milk fat globule membrane in infant nutrition: A dairy industry perspective. Journal of Dairy Research. 2021;**88**(1):105-116. DOI: 10.1017/S0022029921000224

[70] Zavaleta N, Kvistgaard AS, Graverholt G, Respicio G, Guija H, Valencia N, et al. Efficacy of an MFGM-enriched complementary food in diarrhea, anemia, and micronutrient status in infants. Journal of Pediatric Gastroenterology and Nutrition. 2011;**53**(5):561-568. DOI: 10.1097/MPG.0b013e318225cdaf

[71] Li X, Peng Y, Li Z, Christensen B, Heckmann AB, Stenlund H, et al. Feeding infants formula with probiotics or milk fat globule membrane: A double-blind, randomized controlled trial. Frontiers in Pediatrics. 2019;7:347. DOI: 10.3389/fped.2019.00347

[72] Salem N Jr, Van Dael P. Arachidonic acid in human milk. Nutrients. 2020;**12**(3):626. DOI: 10.3390/nu12030626

[73] Innis SM. Perinatal biochemistry and physiology of long-chain polyunsaturated fatty acids. The Journal of Pediatrics. 2003;**143**(4):1-8. DOI: 10.1067/s0022-3476(03)00396-2

[74] Miller MR, Seifert J, Szabo NJ, Clare-Salzler M, Rewers M, Norris JM. Erythrocyte membrane fatty acid content in infants consuming formulas supplemented with docosahexaenoic acid (DHA) and arachidonic acid (ARA): An observational study. Maternal & Child Nutrition. 2010;**6**(4):338-346. DOI: 10.1111/j.1740-8709.2009.00230.x

[75] Lee HM, Yang SY, Han J, Kim YK, Kim YJ, Rhee MS, et al. Optimization of spray drying parameters and food additives to reduce glycation using response surface methodology in powdered infant formulas. Food Science and Biotechnology. 2019;**28**(3):769-777. DOI: 10.1007/s10068-018-0524-9

[76] Montagne D-H, Van Dael P, Skanderby M, Hugelshofer W. Infant formulae–powders and liquids. In: AY T, editor. Dairy Powders and Concentrated Products. Chichester: Wiley-Blackwell; 2009. pp. 313-350. DOI: 10.1002/9781444322729.ch9

[77] Jiang YJ, Guo M. Processing Technology for Infant Formula. Sawston, Cambridge: Human Milk Biochemistry and Infant Formula Manufacturing Technology, Elsevier Ltd; 2014. pp. 211-229. DOI: 10.1533/9780857099150.2.211

Section 2

Infant Feeding Overview and Perspectives

Chapter 6

Infant Nutrition and Feeding in the First 2 Years of Life

Prince Kwabena Osei and Alex Kojo Anderson

Abstract

Infant feeding is the practice of feeding children who are below two years of age. The World Health Organization recommends that infants be exclusively breastfed for the first 6 months of life, followed by continued breastfeeding and gradual introduction of complementary foods. Breastfeeding is beneficial for both the mother and the infant. Breast milk is safe, sterile, and contains antibodies that protect infants against many childhood illnesses. In the US, infants who are not breastfed have a 21% higher risk of post-neonatal infant mortality. It is recommended that mothers who cannot breastfeed exclusively feed their infants with breast milk for at least four months before introducing complementary foods. Infant formula cannot be an absolute substitute for human breast milk, and the use of infant formula must be the last option to feed infants if mothers cannot breastfeed. Although breast milk continues to be an important source of nutrition for growing infants, at six months and beyond breast milk becomes insufficient to provide all the nutrient needs of infants. Therefore, infants must be introduced to complementary foods in addition to breast milk. Complementary foods should provide sufficient energy, protein, essential fats, oils, and particularly, micronutrients to meet the nutritional needs of infants.

Keywords: breast milk, infant-formula, complementary-foods, exclusive, breastfeeding

1. Introduction

Infant feeding (IF) is the practice of feeding infants who are below two years of age [1]. The food choices parents/caregivers make for feeding infants could have both short and long-term health consequences on them [1, 2]. What we feed infants, when, and how they are fed during the first two years of their lives are essential for the following reasons [3, 4]:

- Infants who are below two years of age are vulnerable to irreversible damage to brain formation that serves as a foundation for the development of cognitive, motor, and socio-emotional skills

- Infants are at risk of irreversible growth retardation

 IntechOpen

- The risk of developing chronic diseases like cardiovascular diseases, diabetes, and other chronic diseases later in the life span is linked to infant nutrition in the early stages of the life cycle
- Infants are at risk of mortality from common childhood illnesses

This chapter reviews and presents knowledge from several scientific research studies and evidence on policies, programs, recommendations, and the challenges of infant nutrition at different stages of the first two years of life. The chapter provides the reader with an overview of the current situation of infant food choices from birth through two years of age. The chapter is divided into four different sections. The first section discusses prelacteal feeds and the health benefits of human breast milk and exclusive breastfeeding [5–7]. In the second section, the benefits of breastfeeding and infant formula feeding are discussed and compared [8–11]. Under certain circumstances, women may not be able to breastfeed their newborns. Many myths are associated with the appropriate timelines to feed infants with breast milk and when to introduce complementary foods. The timelines and alternative food choices available to mothers for feeding their infants during complementary feeding are discussed in the third section [12–15]. Methods for the expression of breast milk are discussed in the fourth section [16].

1.1 Prelacteal feeds

Prelacteal feeds are substances (mixtures and concoctions) such as honey, sugar water, dates, herbal tea and concoction, and fruit juice, among others that are given to newborns before the onset of breastfeeding within 1 to 3 days after birth [5]. The practice of giving prelacteal feeds to newborns is more common in developing countries than in developed countries [5–7, 17, 18]. The most usual reasons for giving prelacteal feeds are that newborns need them for their health and to fulfill traditional/cultural norms and practices [19]. In addition, some mothers give prelacteal feeds because of delayed lactation. However, this practice is inappropriate and unhealthy because it could be a potential source of infection in newborns, thereby affecting their health [5]. When babies are born, their intestines are sterile, and the introduction of prelacteal feeds may be a source of harmful microorganisms that may hurt their health [20]. Furthermore, the initiation of exclusive breastfeeding could be affected negatively by the introduction of prelacteal feeds to newborns after delivery, and therefore they may not benefit from the full immunological benefits of colostrum [5, 21]. More so, the early introduction of prelacteal feeds could lead to poor feeding of infants and increased risk of mortality [7]. For example, prelacteal feeding accounted for 45% of neonatal mortality, 30% of diarrheal mortality, and 18% of acute respiratory deaths globally [4]. Currently, the practice of prelacteal feeding is a predominant problem in low- and middle-income countries in Africa and Asia [19].

1.2 The human breast milk

1.2.1 Lactation

During pregnancy, between weeks 16 and 22, the production of breast milk begins in the mammary gland in the breasts [22, 23]. The process of producing and releasing

Hormone	Stimulation	Function
Prolactin	Suckling, stress, & sleep	Promotes milk production
Oxytocin	Suckling or nipple stimulation	Promotes the ejection of milk from the milk gland

Table 1.
Hormonal control of lactation.

milk from the breast is called lactation [24]. Lactation is controlled by two main hormones; prolactin and oxytocin [23]. The functions and sources of stimulation for the release of these hormones are listed in **Table 1** [23]:

1.2.2 Colostrum

The first milk that is produced in the breast after birth is called colostrum and it typically lasts up to 5 days [23, 24]. Colostrum must be a newborn's first food after delivery [23]. It is thick and yellowish milk high in calories, essential nutrients, and antibodies [25]. Lactoferrin is a primary protein in colostrum and has antimicrobial activity [21]. In many societies, it is perceived that colostrum is dirty and contains germs or diseases because of its yellowish color [26]. This is untrue. Rather colostrum is rich in energy and several nutrients that are important for the health of newborn babies in their early days [26]. The health benefits of colostrum for newborn babies are listed below [22–24, 27]:

- The yellowish color of colostrum is due to the high carotene content. Carotene functions as an antioxidant to protect the newborn against inflammation
- Colostrum is rich in immunoglobulins that are involved in building the immune system of the newborn against infections
- It contains special protein compounds like κ-casein, α-lactalbumin, lactoferrin, haptocorrin, and lysozyme that fight against infections
- Colostrum contains enzymes like Bile Salt Stimulated Lipase (BSSL), which allows for effective lipid digestibility, and better utilization of triglycerides, cholesterol, and fat-soluble vitamins
- It contains growth factors that promote growth and development
- Colostrum functions as a laxative to facilitate the defecation of a newborn's first stool, known as meconium, which aids the preparation of the newborn's gastro-intestinal tract for mature breast milk
- Colostrum is high in energy and contains all the essential nutrients required for the growth of infants in the early days after birth

Following colostrum comes transitional milk which is much thinner and whiter than colostrum [1, 23]. It provides the baby with more calories and typically lasts for a few days after colostrum [21]. Mature breast milk is usually produced from the

10th day and is the type of milk that would be produced to feed infants until they are weaned from their mother's milk [24].

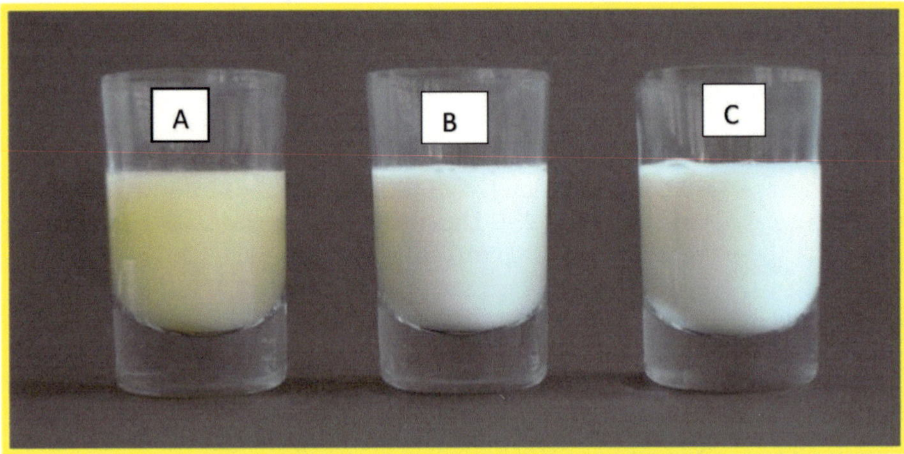

A = colostrum, B = transitional milk, C = mature milk
Adapted from: https://myaloo.com/blogs/news/colostrum-the-true-super-food

1.2.3 Mature human breast milk

The production of mature breast milk continues as long as the mother is comfortable with breastfeeding, nurses the infant or expresses her milk, and it is important to mention that infants do not need any other source of nutrition apart from breastmilk, from when they are born until they are six months old [28]. Breast milk is the ideal food for the growth and development of infants [1]. It is made up of approximately 87% water, 1% protein, 4% lipid, and 7% carbohydrate, in addition to many minerals like calcium, phosphorus, magnesium, potassium, sodium, and vitamins [24]. The nutritional composition of breast milk is dynamic and changes within a feed, time of the day, and as an infant grows [29]. Breast milk contains two types of proteins: whey and casein [22, 30]. Over time, the ratio of casein and whey proteins changes [29]. Whey is high in immunoglobulins and easier to digest, whereas casein helps babies feel full longer [30]. Human milk is more than food and cannot be substituted with any other infant foods because it contains immune factors that cannot be found in other foods like infant formula [10, 31]. The following are the main benefits of breast milk for infants:

- Breast milk is safe, and sterile and provides all the energy and nutrients required by infants for the first six months of their lives for optimal growth [1]. In addition, breast milk provides up to half or more of a child's nutritional needs during the second half of the first year, and up to one-third during the second year of life [29]

- Breast milk contains antibodies that protect infants against many childhood illnesses and breastfed infants are more likely to have fewer cases of colds and other infections than infants who are not breastfed [25]

- Research has shown that breastfed infants are less likely to become obese later in life because formula-fed infants usually have a higher calorie intake than infants who are fed breast milk [10, 32]

- Breast milk is easier for infants to digest and this helps to prevent diarrheal diseases as well as allergenic and autoimmune responses [21].
- Breastmilk helps reduce the incidence of infant mortality. Infants who are not breastfed have a 21% risk of post-neonatal infant mortality [4].
- Children who are not breastfed and fed with infant formula without docosahexaenoic acid/arachidonic acid supplementation are likely to develop autism [11].

1.3 Exclusive breastfeeding

When babies are born, mothers must be supported by lactation support groups and professionals, Baby-Friendly Hospital, and breastfeeding education and resources to help initiate breastfeeding [3, 31]. Mothers must also be supported to have safe sleep practices [33]. Exclusive breastfeeding is the practice of giving only breast milk to infants as the sole source of nourishment until they are six months old, except for medications or vitamin and mineral supplements when there is a need [3, 34]. The World Health Organization (WHO) recommends that infants be exclusively breastfed until approximately six months of age, followed by continued breastfeeding and gradual introduction of complementary foods [4]. Breastfeeding is recommended to continue until a baby is at least 2 years old, and beyond, as long as it's mutually desired by the mother and infant [3]. Breastfeeding offers myriad of benefits for mothers including:

- Reducing the risk of cancers like breast cancer, ovarian cancer, and endometrial cancer [9].
- Improves cardiovascular health and prevents diseases like high blood pressure and high cholesterol [9].
- Mothers who breastfeed recover faster from childbirth [29].
- Breastfeeding produces the hormone oxytocin that aids the contraction of the uterus to return to its normal size [29].
- It increases both physical and emotional bonding between mother and baby [9].
- It helps to promote weight loss [35].

1.3.1 Factors affecting exclusive breastfeeding

Many factors are associated with the discontinuation of exclusive breastfeeding by mothers before six months [9]. Studies have shown that mothers with early breastfeeding difficulties are more likely to discontinue exclusive breastfeeding, and the commonest reason for the inability of many mothers to exclusively breastfeed their infants is insufficient milk production [36, 37]. Some mothers also believe that breast milk is never sufficient to meet the nutritional needs of their infants [37]. Others discontinue breastfeeding due to busy work schedules, the illness of the infant, or the mother [37]. Hence, despite the enormous benefits of exclusive breastfeeding to both infants and their mothers, studies have shown that many mothers are unable to feed their infants exclusively [9]. Globally, only 40% of infants aged 0–6 months are exclusively breastfed [9]. In the US, the breastfeeding initiation rate is approximately 84% [38]. However, the rate drops drastically by 6 months of age to 57% and by one year, only 35% of infants receive breast milk [38]. Despite these challenges, mothers could be supported to exclusively breastfeed their infants. Mothers must be educated about the importance of breast milk and exclusive breastfeeding. They must be supported by families, peers, and any other support groups that can empower them to feed their infants exclusively [4, 37, 38].

1.4 Overcoming breastfeeding problems

It is not uncommon for some mothers to experience some physiological challenges in their pursuit to feed their infants with breast milk [39]. For instance, after the delivery of a newborn, it is normal for a mother's breast to become heavy and tender [40]. However, this could lead to engorgement if the milk is not adequately removed, which is associated with severe pain and discomfort [40, 41]. Some infants may bite the nipples of their mother when they start teething and this could lead to sores on the nipples and in some cases, mastitis, which is the inflammation of breast tissues may occur [42]. Details of some of these physiological breastfeeding problems are discussed below:

1.4.1 Nipple soreness

For many mothers, there is no clear cause of nipple soreness. However, factors such as improper feeding techniques and lack of proper care of nipples [40]. Also, some infants often bite on the nipples of their mothers when they start teething [43]. For such infants, giving something cold and wet to chew on a few minutes before breastfeeding can help avoid this problem [43].

1.4.2 Breast engorgement

The gradual buildup of blood and milk in the breast a few days after birth without the milk being removed could lead to breast engorgement [41]. When a breast is engorged, it becomes swollen, hardened, and very painful [41]. The nipple may not stick out well to allow the infant to latch on it correctly [40]. To prevent engorgement, mothers must relax in a comfortable position when breastfeeding [43]. Mothers must also try to feed their infants more often or express their breast milk manually or with a breast pump [43]. Discomfort that comes with breast engorgement could be alleviated by taking warm showers and applying warm compresses on the breast [43].

1.4.3 Clogged milk duct

The milk duct can become plugged when breast milk is not completely drained from the breasts in successive breastfeeding sessions [40]. This could happen if the infant does not feed regularly or the mother skips feeding [40]. To remove the plug, the milk duct area can be massaged by putting gentle pressure [40].

1.4.4 Mastitis

This condition usually occurs within the first 12 weeks after birth [42]. It occurs when there is either the obstruction of the breast milk ducts, nipple cracks or there is infection by microorganisms like *Escherichia coli*, streptococci, and staphylococci [42]. Breasts become reddish, and tender, and mothers could develop fever [43]. To prevent mastitis, the breasts must be emptied with the appropriate breastfeeding technique [43]. Also, if pain becomes unbearable, the mother will need to be evaluated by an International Board-Certified Lactation Consultant (IBCLC or a physician).

1.5 When should a baby or a mother not breastfeed

Although breastfeeding is recommended as the optimal nutrition for the infant, it is a personal choice and if a mother is not comfortable with it or has medical contraindications, may choose not to breastfeed [9]. However, under the circumstances listed below, mothers and newborns may be advised not to breastfeed [3, 9, 42, 44]:

- Mother has HIV infection and AIDS
- Mother has active tuberculosis
- Mother has T-cell leukemia or any other cancer and is receiving chemotherapy
- Mother is a drug addict or heavy user of alcohol
- Mother is exposed to environmental pollutants
- Infant has galactosemia and cannot metabolize lactose

2. Infant formula feeding

Although infant formula has an important role in infant feeding, it cannot be said to be an absolute substitute for breast milk, and the use of infant formula must be the last option to feed infants in early life if mothers cannot breastfeed [1, 10]. Extensive evidence has shown that human breast milk contains many bioactive compounds and substances that support the building of the immune system and brain development of infants which cannot be found in infant formula and other human milk substitutes [45]. Infant formula processing companies only try to mimic the composition of human breast milk hence, the health benefits of breast milk cannot be equated to infant formula [10, 25, 45]. It is recommended that mothers who cannot do exclusive breastfeeding feed their infants breast milk for at least four months before introducing infant formula [4, 9]. However, if mothers cannot breastfeed their infants, they are advised to use infant formula and other appropriate human milk substitutes, which are mainly intended to be an effective substitute for breast milk [45].

2.1 Types of infant formula

There are three main categories of infant formulas. These are cow milk-based formula, soy-based formula, and specialized formula [45]. The distinctions between these types of formulas are in terms of nutrition, energy content, taste, the bioavailability of nutrients, and cost [45]. The cow milk-based formula is the commonest type of formula for feeding most infants in many countries [46]. Raw cow's milk naturally contains high amounts of fats, minerals, and protein compared to human breast milk [47]. Hence, in the processing of cow milk-based formulas, the nutrients in raw cow's milk are diluted to levels similar to that of human breast milk [46]. Soy-based formulas are produced from soy milk and are usually intended to be given to infants with galactosemia or congenital lactase deficiency [45]. Due to soy allergies, it is recommended that mothers pay attention to signs of soy allergies like skin rashes and diarrhea during the introduction of soy-based formulas, especially to infants who are less than six months old [45]. Specialized formulas are mainly synthesized from protein hydrolysate and amino acids and are intended for infants who cannot tolerate cow's milk or soy-based formulas [46]. Finally, there is no brand of infant formula that is best for all infants. Only infant formula specifically made for infants within a certain age category must be selected for feeding infants, and the infant formula selected must meet the FDA standards regarding the nutritional composition of the type of formula [27]. The health benefits of human breast milk over infant formulas are summarized in **Table 2** [4, 9, 22, 27, 29].

2.2 Complementary feeding and infant food choices

At six months of age, breastmilk continues to be an important source of nutrition but is insufficient to provide all the nutrient needs of infants [4]. Therefore, infants must be introduced to other foods in addition to breastmilk, to keep up with their growing needs for energy and nutrients. This process of introducing other foods is called complementary feeding [13]. Complementary feeding must begin after six months when breast milk alone is no longer enough to meet all the nutritional needs of infants, and therefore other sources of food are needed [3]. The American Academy of Pediatrics and the World Health Organization recommend introducing complementary foods at approximately 6 months of age [4, 48]. The introduction of complementary foods before 4 months of age may be too early for many health reasons [49]. Firstly, infants at this time are not developmentally ready for solid complementary foods [1, 48, 49]. The gut of an infant is more permeable at this stage and gastrointestinal

Nutrient factor	Breast milk	Infant formula
Carbohydrates	Rich in lactose and oligosaccharides	Some formulas do not have lactose and oligosaccharides
Fats & oils	Rich in omega 3 and cholesterolAll fats and oils are highly digestible and absorbed.Milk composition is adjusted to the infant's needs.	No DHADigestion and absorption are usually not incompleteMilk composition cannot be adjusted to the infant's needs.
Proteins	Soft easily digestible whey protein.Contains growth factorsLactoferrin for intestinal health, lysozyme	Casein proteins are hard to digest.No growth factorsNo Lactoferrin and lysozyme
Minerals	Iron, zinc, and calcium are better absorbed	Iron, zinc, and calcium are not well absorbed
Immune boosters	Contains White Blood Cells	No live White Blood Cells
Enzymes and hormones	Rich in digestive enzymes and hormones	No digestive enzymes and hormones

Table 2.
Comparison of breast milk and infant formula.

colonization of microflora is not fully established [50]. Also, infants may be infected and suffer from respiratory and diarrheal illnesses because their immune system is still developing [49]. More so, the early introduction of complementary foods could put undue stress on many of the developing internal organs of infants such as the immature renal and digestive systems [49]. Infants could also develop food allergies [13]. Lastly, infants who are introduced to complementary foods early are unlikely to be fed sufficient amounts of breastmilk which is the ideal food for infants until six months old [13]. Furthermore, many infants are at high risk of undernutrition after six months of age [3]. This is because feeding infants at this age with the right foods in the right amounts could be a challenge for many mothers [37]. Studies have shown that infants after six months are highly at risk of stunting, being underweight, and wasting, as well as food-borne illnesses [1, 3, 4, 51]. Hence, the World Health Organization recommends complementary feeding must be timely, adequate, safe, and properly fed [3, 4]. That is, complementary foods must provide sufficient energy, protein, and micronutrients to meet the nutritional needs of infants, they must be hygienically prepared and stored, and fed with kempt hands using clean feeding utensils including feeding bottles.

2.3 Complementary food consistency, frequency, and energy density

Generally, the majority of infants after 6 months should be able to eat pureed, mashed, and semi-solid foods [4, 13]. The consistency and different varieties of complementary foods must be increased gradually for infants as they get older [13]. At eight months, most infants have to be able to eat snacks (including finger foods) alone and by 12 months, many infants can eat the same kinds of foods as the rest of the family [4]. Foods such as nuts, grapes, or raw carrots should not be fed to infants younger than 12 months because they could result in the choking of the trachea [14]. Moreover, the number of times infants are fed complementary foods must be gradually increased as they get older. The energy density and nutrient content of the complementary food must determine the frequency at which infants are fed, as well as the amounts infants, can consume at each feeding [14]. To begin complementary feeding, it is recommended to start feeding infants with semi-solid and solid foods at least 2–3 times per day between 6 and 8 months and moderately increase the frequency to 3–4 times daily after 8 months [4, 13]. It is important to feed infants with complementary foods that are nutrient dense like whole grains, meat, poultry, fish, eggs, and dairy products [12]. Frequent feeding may be required if the energy density and the nutrient content of complementary foods per meal are low to meet nutrient needs for growth and development [14].

2.4 Hygienic and safe practices during complementary feeding

Complementary foods that are prepared under unhygienic conditions can make foods microbiologically unsafe to feed to the infant [15, 52]. Foods that are contaminated with microorganisms are harmful to feeding infants, especially when they are <2 years old because infants who are within these ages tend to have immature immune systems and are highly vulnerable to microbial infections [52, 53]. Poor food hygiene practice is one of the main causes of childhood diarrhea and studies have shown that about 88% of infant deaths are due to poor sanitation, poor personal hygiene, and unsafe water supplies in developing countries [52, 54]. More so, inadequate cleaning of eating utensils, improper storage of complementary foods after preparation, lack of knowledge about safe food handling, and poor environmental sanitation are major contributory factors to foodborne illnesses among infants [2, 4, 52, 55, 56]. Nonetheless, honey and honey-related foods are potential sources of the pathogenic bacteria (*Clostridium botulinum*) that cause botulism [57]. Therefore, these foods must not be introduced to infants until they are over 2 years old because the immune system of infants may not be fully developed to fight pathogenic bacteria [57]. Lastly, the following food safety and sanitary guidelines must be followed about handling complementary foods to prevent the risk of foodborne illnesses [2, 4, 56]:

- Before feeding infants, mothers and caregivers must properly wash their hands and that of their infants with soap and water
- Eating utensils must thoroughly be cleaned with soap and water before use during the preparation of complementary foods for infants
- Bottles that are difficult to clean must not be used to feed infants because they could harbor dirt/microbes that might be a potential source of contamination
- Complementary foods to be fed to infants later must be stored in either a refrigerator or freezer immediately after preparation
- Refrigerated or frozen complementary foods should be thawed and properly warmed/cooked to the right temperature before feeding to infants
- Leftover meals from eating episodes should be discarded and must not be kept to feed infants at a later time

2.5 Food allergy and complementary feeding

According to the American Academy of Pediatrics Committee on Nutrition guidelines for the introduction of complementary foods, mothers with a family history of food allergies from eggs, milk, peanuts, soy, and shellfish must delay the introduction of any of these foods to their infants [50, 58]. For infants at risk of milk allergy, dairy products must only be given after the first year of life [58]. For allergies to eggs, peanuts, soy, and shellfish, these foods must not be given to infants until they are two years of age [50]. In addition, to be able to identify potential food allergies, it is recommended that single-ingredient foods be given to infants first in the early stages of complementary feeding [13].

2.6 Expression of breast milk

In the past few decades, breast milk expression was used mainly as a means to feed preterm and sick babies [59]. However, breast milk expression has become more of a norm in many societies for mothers because of convenience and the need for mothers to return to work after delivery [59]. Currently, breast milk expression forms an essential part of breastfeeding behavior among mothers, especially in developed countries [60]. In addition, the expression of breast milk has become a useful alternative for mothers to feed their babies with breast milk when direct breastfeeding is not possible, thereby allowing mothers to continue feeding their infants with breast milk [59]. Breast milk can be expressed in two main ways, either by hand expression or by the use of pumps [61]. In the first few days after birth, hand expression may be used to initiate milk production by the stimulation of the breast with the bare hand [61].

Studies have shown that breast milk expression by hand is more effective at enhancing milk production and increasing the duration of breastfeeding [61]. Breast pump plays an important role in breast milk expression and the continuation of breastfeeding among working mothers [62]. There are three main types of breast pumps and these are manual, battery, and electric pumps [63]. A manual breast pump requires the use of the hand to manually operate a pump to remove milk from the breast into a receptacle, but the battery and electric operated pumps respectively require battery and electricity as sources of power to extract breast milk from the breast. The selection of a particular type of pump for breast milk expression is dependent on factors such as time, cost, the volume of milk required and accessibility to power [63]. The battery and electric pumps work faster than the manual pump and are more suitable for mothers who have busy work schedules. A manual pump is also cheaper and easier to operate although it is not as efficient as an electric pump [63]. The following recommended guidelines for the expression of breast milk and storage are intended to maintain the safety and quality of breast milk after expression [60, 63, 64]:

- Properly wash hands with soap and water before expressing milk. Hand sanitizers may be used if soaps and water are unavailable

- Clean breast pumps thoroughly with soap and water before use for milk expression. If expressing by hand, the receptacle to collect the breast milk must be well cleaned

- Ensure that the contact surfaces of the areas where the milk expression is to be carried out are cleaned

- Clean all utensils and breast pumps with soap and water immediately after use

- Store breast milk at the appropriate refrigerator or freezer temperature as soon as milk expression is completed

2.7 Methods of breast milk expression

2.7.1 Hand expression

Hand expression of breast milk is a technique where the hands are used instead of infants or breast pumps to extract milk out of the breasts into a container. Expressing breast milk by hand is an essential skill that lactating mothers must learn because it has the following benefits [61, 65]:

- It can be used to get colostrum out of the breast quickly to feed newborns who may be unable to suckle the breast in the early days after delivery or those who are not able to have effective latch.

- Hand expression stimulates milk production and studies have shown that expression of breast milk by hand is more effective at helping to establish milk supply within the 24 hours after birth than expression by breast pumps.

- Expression of breast milk by hand facilitates easy emptying of the breasts and this aids the prevention of engorgement and mastitis.

- Mothers who practice hand expression are more comfortable and confident about breastfeeding their infants.
- Hand expression requires no special device; it is cheaper, convenient, and easier to express breast milk by hand.

2.7.1.1 Procedure for hand expression

- The right thumb should be positioned above the left nipple with the four fingers below the nipple at about 1 to 2 inches behind the nipple. The thumb and the fingers must make a C – shape at this point.
- The thumb and fingers must be pressed and gently squeezed together back towards the chest.
- The procedure ought to be repeated in a rhythmic pattern by pressing, gently squeezing, and releasing the thumb and fingers until the milk flow stops.
- The same procedure should be repeated for the right breast by using the left thumb and fingers [66].

2.7.2 Breast pumps

Breast pumps are considered as medical devices that are used to facilitate the suction of breast milk in order to maintain or increase milk supply [16]. A typical breast pump is made up of a breast shield, pump, and milk receptacle [16]. The **breast shield is the** cone-shaped cup that fits over the nipple and the area around the areola. The pump creates a vacuum that pulls milk out of the breast. The milk receptacle is a detachable container that fits beneath the breast shield and receives breast milk simultaneously as it is being pumped.

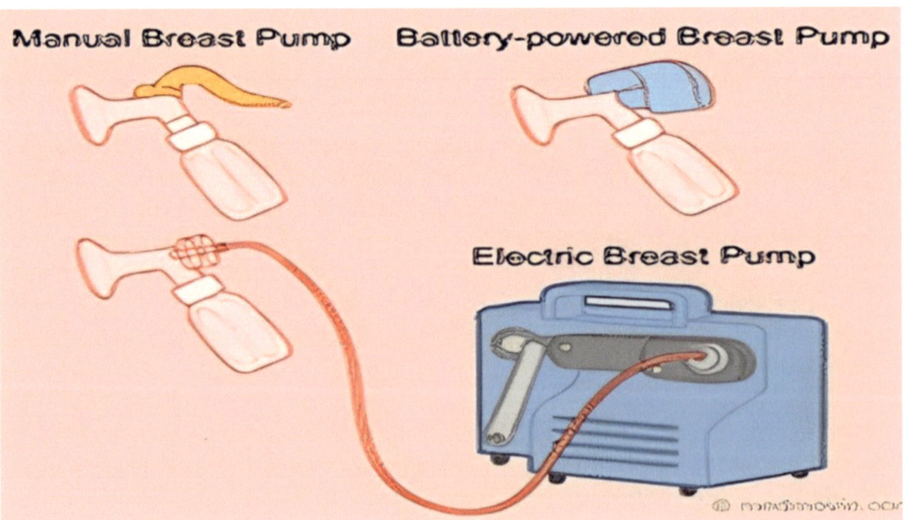

Adapted from: https://www.fda.gov/medical-devices/breast-pumps/types-breast-pumps

2.7.2.1 Manual breast pumps

These pumps are operated by hand and require the user to manually squeeze a lever consistently to create a vacuum on the breast to express milk [16]. Manual breast pumps are cheaper and can be used without electricity or battery [16]. The choice to use a manual breast pump has the following downside to it [63]. First, the use of manual pump is time-consuming and requires a lot of manual work. Manual pump is not as efficient as an electric or battery-operated breast pump due to its limited suction capability. The creation of a regular pumping rhythm is difficult when using a manual pump [16, 61].

2.7.2.2 Battery breast pumps

These pumps operate on battery for milk expression from the breast and there are two models of these pumps: single and double models [61]. The single model is used to express milk from one breast at a time and the double model is used to express milk from both breasts synchronously. Also, there are wireless breast pumps that allow for hands-free pumping [16]. Battery pumps are ideal for traveling mothers who may not have access to an electrical outlet [16]. The following downsides are associated with the use of battery-operated pumps. Battery pumps are relatively expensive compared to manual pumps. Although they are efficient at suction, their capacity may be limited depending on the amount of milk to be expressed. The intermittent charging of batteries may be inconvenient, and some batteries may not last for longer hours [16, 61].

2.7.2.3 Electric breast pumps

Electric breast pumps are motorized pumps that create suction to draw milk from the breasts and they are the most efficient breast pumps with the most output of milk expression [67]. They also come in different models that can either express milk from one breast or both breasts at the same time [67]. The choice to use an electric breast pump has the following downsides to it. Electric pumps are comparatively more expensive than manual and battery-operated pumps. The use of electric pumps may be accompanied with discomfort, pain, and soreness if the suction intensity is not regulated properly [65, 67].

2.8 Conclusion

The practice of giving prelacteal feeds such as honey, sugar water, dates, herbal tea, and fruit juice to newborn babies within 1 to 3 days after birth is more common among many cultures in developing countries than in developed countries. This practice is inappropriate because it could be a potential source of infection in newborns, and it could also lead to poor feeding of infants accompanied with many health consequences. The human breast milk is the best food for infants because it is safe, sterile, contains antibodies that protect babies against many childhood illnesses, and has all the nutrients infants need for their growth and development in the first six months of life. Breastfeeding is beneficial for both mothers and their infants. Also, breastfeeding helps to build strong emotional bond between mothers and their infants. Although breast milk continues to be an important source of nutrition for growing infants, at six months and beyond breast milk alone becomes inadequate to provide all the nutrient needs of infants. Therefore, infants must be introduced to complementary foods in addition to breast milk. Complementary foods must provide sufficient energy, protein, essential fats, and particularly, micronutrients to meet the nutritional needs of infants. During the introduction of complementary foods, mothers with a family history of food allergies must delay the introduction of any potential allergenic food to their infants until they are two years of age. One of the reasons why some mothers discontinue breastfeeding is because of busy work schedules. Therefore, the expression of breast milk has become a useful alternative for mothers to feed their infants breast milk when direct breastfeeding is not possible. Breast milk can be expressed in two main ways, either by hand expression or by the use of breast pumps.

Author details

Prince Kwabena Osei* and Alex Kojo Anderson
Department of Nutritional Sciences, College of Family and Consumer Sciences, University of Georgia, Athens, USA

*Address all correspondence to: prince.osei@uga.edu

References

[1] McAndrew F et al. Infant Feeding Survey. Leeds: Health and Social Care Information Centre; 2010, 2012

[2] Stuebe A, Schwarz E. The risks and benefits of infant feeding practices for women and their children. Journal of Perinatology. 2010;**30**(3):155-162

[3] World Health Organization. Global Nutrition Policy Review 2016-2017: Country Progress in Creating Enabling Policy Environments for Promoting Healthy Diets and Nutrition. WHO IRIS, Geneva, ID: who-275990; 2018. pp. 111-114

[4] World Health Organization. Infant and Young Child Feeding: Model Chapter for Textbooks for Medical Students and Allied Health Professionals. Geneva: WHO Press; 2009. pp. 10-26

[5] Nguyen P et al. Prelacteal and early formula feeding increase risk of infant hospitalisation: A prospective cohort study. Archives of Disease in Childhood. 2020;**105**(2):122-126

[6] Temesgen H et al. Prelacteal feeding and associated factors in Ethiopia: Systematic review and meta-analysis. International Breastfeeding Journal. 2018;**13**(1):1-12

[7] Berde AS et al. Determinants of pre-lacteal feeding practices in urban and rural Nigeria; a population-based cross-sectional study using the 2013 Nigeria demographic and health survey data. African Health Sciences. 2017;**17**(3):690-699

[8] Camps G et al. Gastric emptying and Intragastric behavior of breast Milk and infant formula in lactating mothers. The Journal of Nutrition. 2021;**151**(12):3718-3724

[9] Victora CG et al. Breastfeeding in the 21st century: Epidemiology, mechanisms, and lifelong effect. The Lancet. 2016;**387**(10017):475-490

[10] Packard V. Human Milk and Infant Formula. New York: Elsevier, Academic Press INC.; 2012. pp. 140-198

[11] Schultz ST et al. Breastfeeding, infant formula supplementation, and autistic disorder: The results of a parent survey. International Breastfeeding Journal. 2006;**1**(1):1-7

[12] Agostoni C, Przyrembel H. The timing of introduction of complementary foods and later health. Evidence-Based Research in Pediatric Nutrition. 2013;**108**:63-70

[13] West C. Introduction of complementary foods to infants. Annals of Nutrition and Metabolism. 2017;**70**(Suppl. 2):47-54

[14] Chiang KV et al. Timing of introduction of complementary foods—United States, 2016-2018. Morbidity and Mortality Weekly Report. 2020;**69**(47):1787

[15] Samady W et al. Recommendations on complementary food introduction among pediatric practitioners. JAMA Network Open. 2020;**3**(8):e2013070-e2013070

[16] Eglash A, Malloy ML. Breastmilk expression and breast pump technology. Clinical Obstetrics and Gynecology. 2015;**58**(4):855-867

[17] Tariku A et al. Factors associated with prelacteal feeding in the rural population of Northwest Ethiopia: A community cross-sectional study.

International Breastfeeding Journal. 2016;**11**(1):1-7

[18] Pirzada S et al. Use of PRELACTEAL feeds-study IN tradition. Pakistan Armed Forces Medical Journal (PAFMJ). 2021;**71**(5):1718-1721

[19] Ogundele T, Ogundele OA, Adegoke AI. Determinants of prelacteal feeding practices among mothers of children aged less than 24 months in Ile-Ife Southwest Nigeria: A community cross-sectional study. The Pan African Medical Journal. 2019;**34**:1-6. DOI: 10.116 04%2Fpamj.2019.34.172.17642

[20] Sako S. Prelacteal feeding practice and associated factors among mothers of children less than two years of age in Ethiopia: A multilevel analysis. Heliyon. 2022;**8**(4):e09339

[21] Кісельова M et al. Breastfeeding is the-"Gold Standard" old experience and new scientifically proven benefits. Неонатологія, хірургія та перинатальна медицина. 2022;**12**(2):53

[22] Shamir R. The benefits of breast feeding. Protein in Neonatal and Infant Nutrition: Recent Updates. 2016;**86**:67-76

[23] Lawrence RA. 3-Physiology of lactation. In: Breastfeeding 9th edition, A Guide for the Medical Profession. Elsevier INC; 2022. pp. 58-92

[24] Boquien C-Y. Human milk: An ideal food for nutrition of preterm newborn. Frontiers in Pediatrics. 2018;**6**:295

[25] Ríos J, Valero-Jara V, Thomas-V aldés S. Phytochemicals in breast milk and their benefits for infants. Critical Reviews in Food Science and Nutrition. 2022;**62**(25):6821-6836

[26] Nembongwe G et al. Beliefs, attitudes and practices of mothers towards breastfeeding colostrum and factors associated: Case of the Yaounde Gynaeco-obstetric and Pediatric hospital. Journal of Food Science Nutrition. 2022;**8**(130):2

[27] Andreas NJ, Kampmann B, Le-Doare KM. Human breast milk: A review on its composition and bioactivity. Early Human Development. 2015;**91**(11):629-635

[28] Breastfeeding, S.o et al. Breastfeeding and the use of human milk. Pediatrics. 2012;**129**(3):e827-e841

[29] Kordus A. The Benefits of Breastfeeding. 2014

[30] Riordan J, Wambach K. Breastfeeding and Human Lactation. 4th ed. Massachusetts: Jones & Bartlett Publishers; 2010. pp. 215-296

[31] Robbins ST, Beker LT. Infant Feedings: Guidelines for Preparation of Formula and Breastmilk in Health Care Facilities. American Dietetic Association. Pediatrics Nutrition Practice group Publishers; 2004. pp. 37-42

[32] Hester SN et al. Is the macronutrient intake of formula-fed infants greater than breast-fed infants in early infancy? Journal of Nutrition and Metabolism. 2012;**2012**:1-13. Article ID 891201. DOI: 10.1155/2012/891201

[33] Salm Ward TC, Kanu FA, Anderson AK. Trends and factors associated with breastfeeding and infant sleep practices in Georgia. Journal of Community Health. 2018;**43**(3):496-507

[34] Busch DW, Logan K, Wilkinson A. Clinical practice breastfeeding recommendations for primary care: Applying a tri-core breastfeeding conceptual model. Journal of Pediatric Health Care. 2014;**28**(6):486-496

[35] Hatsu IE, McDougald DM, Anderson AK. Effect of infant feeding on maternal body composition. International Breastfeeding Journal. 2008;**3**(1):1-8

[36] Tengku Alina TI, Wan Manan WM, Mohd Isa B. Factors predicting early discontinuation of exclusive breastfeeding among women in Kelantan, Malaysia. Health and the Environment Journal. 2013;**4**(1):42-54

[37] Yaqub A, Gul S. Reasons for failure of exclusive breastfeeding in children less than six months of age. Journal of Ayub Medical College Abbottabad. 2013;**25**(1-2):165-167

[38] Tomori C. Overcoming barriers to breastfeeding. Best Practice & Research Clinical Obstetrics & Gynaecology. 2022;**83**:60-71. DOI: 10.1016/j.bpobgyn.2022.01.010

[39] Powell R, Davis M, Anderson AK. A qualitative look into mother's breastfeeding experiences. Journal of Neonatal Nursing. 2014;**20**(6):259-265

[40] Scadden J. Breastfeeding and Lactation Consulting. Fay W. Whitney School of Nursing, University of Wyoming, Honors Capstone Project. 2022. pp. 9-15

[41] Çaka SY, Topal S, Altınkaynak S. Anne sütü ile beslenmede karşılaşılan sorunlar. Journal of Pediatric Nursing-Special Topics. 2017;**3**(2):120-128

[42] Özhüner Y, Özerdoğan N. Breast problems related to breastfeeding and alternative approaches to the solutions. 1st ed. No: 47083. Current Research in Health Sciences, Gece Publishing; 2022. pp. 220-226

[43] Berens PD. Breast pain: Engorgement, nipple pain, and mastitis. Clinical Obstetrics and Gynecology. 2015;**58**(4):902-914

[44] Kuhn L, Reitz C, Abrams EJ. Breastfeeding and AIDS in the developing world. Current Opinion in Pediatrics. 2009;**21**(1):83-93

[45] Martin CR, Ling P-R, Blackburn GL. Review of infant feeding: Key features of breast milk and infant formula. Nutrients. 2016;**8**(5):279

[46] Koletzko B et al. Global standard for the composition of infant formula: Recommendations of an ESPGHAN coordinated international expert group. Journal of Pediatric Gastroenterology and Nutrition. 2005;**41**(5):584-599

[47] Hochwallner H et al. Cow's milk allergy: From allergens to new forms of diagnosis, therapy and prevention. Methods. 2014;**66**(1):22-33

[48] Grummer-Strawn LM, Scanlon KS, Fein SB. Infant feeding and feeding transitions during the first year of life. Pediatrics. 2008;**122**(Supplement_2):S36-S42

[49] Krebs NF. Food choices to meet nutritional needs of breast-fed infants and toddlers on mixed diets. The Journal of Nutrition. 2007;**137**(2):511S-517S

[50] Kemp AS et al. Guidelines for the use of infant formulas to treat cows milk protein allergy: An Australian consensus panel opinion. Medical Journal of Australia. 2008;**188**(2):109-112

[51] Yalew BM. Prevalence of malnutrition and associated factors among children age 6-59 months at lalibela town administration, north WolloZone, Anrs, Northern Ethiopia. Journal of Nutrition Disorders Therapy. 2014;**4**(132):2161-0509

[52] Demmelash AA et al. Hygienic practice during complementary feeding and associated factors among mothers of children aged 6-24 months in Bahir Dar Zuria District, Northwest Ethiopia, 2019. Journal of Environmental and Public Health. 2020;**2020**:1-7. Article ID 2075351. DOI: 10.1155/2020/2075351

[53] Parvez SM et al. Escherichia coli contamination of child complementary foods and association with domestic hygiene in rural Bangladesh. Tropical Medicine & International Health. 2017;**22**(5):547-557

[54] Usfar AA et al. Food and personal hygiene perceptions and practices among caregivers whose children have diarrhea: A qualitative study of urban mothers in Tangerang, Indonesia. Journal of Nutrition Education and Behavior. 2010;**42**(1):33-40

[55] Redmond EC, Griffith CJ. The importance of hygiene in the domestic kitchen: Implications for preparation and storage of food and infant formula. Perspectives in Public Health. 2009;**129**(2):69-76

[56] Msuya J. Food Safety of Homemade Complementary Foods in Morogoro Municipality-Tanzania. The Ohio State University and OhioLINK Publishers; 2016. pp. 32-69

[57] Borriello PS. Infant botulism. In: Clostridia in Gastrointestinal Disease. CRC Press Publishers; 2018. pp. 39-54

[58] Briefel RR et al. Feeding infants and toddlers study: Improvements needed in meeting infant feeding recommendations. Journal of the American Dietetic Association. 2004;**104**:31-37

[59] Daniels S et al. Donor human milk for the high-risk infant: Preparation, safety, and usage options in the United States. Pediatrics. 2017;**139**(1):1-3

[60] Jiang B et al. Evaluation of the impact of breast milk expression in early postpartum period on breastfeeding duration: A prospective cohort study. BMC Pregnancy and Childbirth. 2015;**15**(1):1-13

[61] Becker GE, Smith HA, Cooney F. Methods of milk expression for lactating women. Cochrane Database of Systematic Reviews. 2016;**9**

[62] Bass JL, Gartley T, Kleinman R. Outcomes from the Centers for Disease Control and Prevention 2018 breastfeeding report card: Public policy implications. The Journal of Pediatrics. 2020;**218**:16-21

[63] Lawrence RA. Storage of human milk and the influence of procedures on immunological components of human milk. Acta Paediatrica. 1999;**88**:14-18

[64] Peters MDJ, McArthur A, Munn Z. Safe management of expressed breast milk: A systematic review. Women and Birth. 2016;**29**(6):473-481

[65] Meier PP et al. Which breast pump for which mother: An evidence-based approach to individualizing breast pump technology. Journal of Perinatology. 2016;**36**(7):493-499

[66] Meek JY, Noble L. Breastfeeding and the use of human milk. Pediatrics. 2022

[67] Leiter V et al. Pay at the pump?: Problems with electric breast pumps. Social Science & Medicine. 2022;**292**:114625

Chapter 7

Infant Feeding Practices: A Global Perspective

Aryal Laxmi, Lucas Amanda, Haseeb Yumna B, Dhaliwal Dolly and Gill Rubina

Abstract

Infant nutrition is a primary determinant of growth and development, with long-term impacts on health. The World Health Organization (WHO) offers guidelines for infant feeding, however practices vary by geographical location, culture, and biopsychosocial factors. This chapter provides a comprehensive overview of peer-reviewed and gray literature on the current infant feeding guidelines and cultural practices across the globe. The findings draw attention to the multiple drivers and barriers to exclusive breastfeeding in various regions. This chapter can serve as a building block to inform future public health initiatives and research. By addressing these barriers, we can improve maternal and infant health and reduce the burden of malnutrition and associated health consequences for infants globally.

Keywords: infant feeding policies, cultural patterns, breastfeeding, social influences, global, breastfeeding support, nutrition, guidelines, cultural practice, culture

1. Introduction

According to the World Health Organization (WHO), undernutrition is associated with the deaths of 2.7 million children annually, which is 45% of all child deaths [1]. WHO recommends early initiation of breastfeeding within 1 h of birth, exclusive breastfeed (EBF) for the first 6 months of life, and introduction of nutritionally adequate, safe complementary foods at 6 months with continued breastfeeding up to 2 years of age [1]. Breastfeed of infants is associated with higher cognitive development, reduced risk of infections in both childhood and adulthood, reduced risk of obesity in adulthood, reduced serum cholesterol levels in adulthood, and a small reduction in systolic blood pressure in adulthood [2]. Breastfeeding also significantly reduces the risk of developing type 2 diabetes mellitus [2]. However, only 44% of infants under 6 months of age are exclusively breastfed, indicating that significant barriers exist to providing nutrition to infants [1]. Identifying and reducing these barriers is critical to improving infant nutrition globally, thus improving health outcomes in all populations.

Adequate nutrition is necessary in maintaining overall health for all populations, but is especially important in the infant population. Infant malnutrition is associated with growth stunting, developmental delays, and increased mortality, especially from diarrheal and respiratory illness [3]. Poor nutrition in infancy, particularly in the first year of life, is associated with negative health outcomes across the full lifespan. Malnutrition in the first year of life is associated with significantly elevated incidence of impaired IQ in adulthood, causing a nine-fold increase in adults with disability-range IQ relative to those with sufficient nutrition in the first year of life [4]. Furthermore, adult offspring of parents who were malnourished in the first year of life also demonstrate reduced IQ, even accounting for socioeconomic status (SES) and parental IQ [5].

Significant barriers to meeting infant nutrition guidelines exist globally. Economic factors such as poverty can limit access to healthcare, food, and other resources which are critical to both maternal and infant health. Similarly, geographic isolation reduces access to critical resources. Social factors such as a mother's need to work outside the home, availability of family support networks, availability of community healthcare workers, and maternal autonomy are also influential on infant nutrition. Additionally, many cultural factors influence perceptions of breastfeeding and introduction of other foods. Family systems are essential in promoting maternal and child nutrition; all family and close community members play a role in the care of infants, particularly grandmothers and nuclear household members [6]. The dyadic relationship between mother and infant is particularly important, as it is well understood that infant health thrives where mothers are well-supported and healthy; infants also take nutritional cues from mothers, including maternal diet during pregnancy [7]. Education about infant nutrition and maternal-infant health is also of critical importance, because lack of maternal knowledge about infant feeding guidelines is associated with earlier cessation of breastfeeding and early introduction of solids [8]. Across the globe, infant nutrition faces significant challenges, which vary in nature by region and community. In this chapter, we explore infant feeding practices across different regions of the globe and specific barriers in different communities to better understand what progress must be made to improve global infant nutrition.

2. North America

Infant nutrition guidelines in North America recommend EBF for the first 6 months of life, followed by continued breastfeeding alongside complementary foods until 12 months of age. However, adherence to these guidelines is not always consistent due to various cultural and societal influences within countries. Unfortunately, early weaning can lead to a range of issues including increased risk of infections, malnutrition, allergens, and chronic diseases later in life [1, 9].

A mother's close network, such as her spouse, grandmother, and close friends, play a critical role in infant feeding decisions and is associated with an increased likelihood of following medical guidelines for longer durations [10]. Interestingly, a mother's distant network, including neighbors and relatives, have been found to encourage earlier introduction of family foods than recommended by medical professionals [11]. In Mexico, the Mexican Social Security Institute (IMSS) recommends the integration of family diet reflecting cultural practices between six and 12 months [12]. Despite high initial breastfeeding rates among Mexican mothers at 86%, 92% of infants are fed complementary food before reaching the recommended weaning age [13]. Factors such as maternal employment, maternal education, and maternal age all affect the recommended timeframe for introducing complementary foods [14]. Interestingly, Indigenous Mexican mothers are found to be more compliant with IMSS and WHO infant feeding recommendations than non-Indigenous Mexican mothers [13].

Cultural perspectives play a crucial role in infant feeding within North America. In some African American communities, the decision to breastfeed can be rooted in generational trauma of wet nursing during slavery and, for some, a preference for formula feeding [15]. Unfortunately, negative connotations of wet nursing (woman who breastfeeds and cares for another's child) and slavery create a cultural barrier that denies African American women and infants the many benefits of breastfeeding [15]. Conversely, in many indigenous communities, the act of breastfeeding is highly valued and an essential cultural practice [16]. The rate of breastfeeding among Chinese Canadian mothers was 68%, lower than the overall rate of breastfeeding in British Columbia, Canada, which is 85–87% [17]. This difference in rates may be attributed to Chinese beliefs of yin-yang theory and a focus on protecting the mother's body from illness postpartum, while Western medicine places emphasis on the baby's body [17]. Chinese immigrant populations in Canada report mothers following the traditional postpartum practice of *zuo yuezi*, which involves new mothers staying at home, avoiding contact with cold items, and increasing the consumption of hot food [17]. This highlights the importance of understanding how cultural context can impact infant feeding practices and deviate from the guidelines provided within the region.

Furthermore, obesity's impact on North American society is a critical factor that contributes to infant feeding practices. Approximately 30% of children in the United States are overweight or obese, with this trend consistently increasing for the past 20 years [18]. During an infant's first 6 months of life, rapid weight gain has been associated with later obesity and related comorbidities [19]. Interestingly, mothers who had not previously breastfed or those who experienced higher stress levels tended to feed their infants more out of concerns about hunger [20]. One element of increased stress may be attributed to the timing of a mother's return to employment. In the United States, employment has little to no impact on breastfeeding initiation. The literature suggests that in the United States, employment has little to no impact of breastfeeding initiation, however, the return to employment is a central factor influencing breastfeeding duration [21]. Therefore, the development of institutional and fiscal policies that offer employed mothers, especially in low-income groups, the support related to breastfeeding is vital for infant health.

3. Australia

Australia has similar breastfeeding guidelines are also in agreement with WHO recommendations and breastfeeding initiation rates however, at 3 and 6 months of age, breastfeeding rates fall below global standards [22]. For instance, in New South Wales, only 17.5% of infants are being exclusively breastfed until 6 months of age and there is a trend towards earlier introduction to complementary feeding [22]. This difference is more extensive in rural communities where 96% of Australian infants were breastfed at birth, 39% exclusively breast to 4 months, and 15% were breastfed for the recommended 6 months [23]. Although there are numerous factors impacting infant feeding decisions, maternal breastfeeding intention is a significant predictor of exclusivity and duration [24].

A particular concern in Australia from a recent study, highlights the exposure to breastmilk substitutes while in hospital. It is reported that 29% of infants were given breastmilk substitutes while in hospital [25]. This is in part due to the lack of antenatal education at the time of birth and the need for more support for breastfeeding continuing on in the early neonatal period. Almost one third of infants lose their

EBF status as a result of the early introduction of breastfeeding substitutes, therefore changing the landscape of infant feeding practices in Australian neonates [26].

4. South America

The South American region faces many challenges to achieving WHO recommendations for infant feeding practices, including social, economic, and cultural barriers. Both urban and rural communities face specific difficulties, in both cases associated with low income and education levels [27]. Low access to nutritionally high-quality food is a common theme across the region, which is associated with nutritional inadequacies in infants and children, as well as higher intake of ultraprocessed foods [28]. Additionally, many communities hold cultural beliefs surrounding breastfeeding which decrease both the length of time infants are breastfed and the period of EBF [29]. Many studies show that women in South American low-income communities report having access to community healthcare workers and pediatricians who they have positive relationships with, while others report cultural barriers between healthcare workers and mothers [29, 30]. Mothers generally report a positive opinion of breastfeeding, but report struggle to meet WHO guidelines and the recommendations of local healthcare workers, indicating a strong need to address existing barriers to improving both maternal and infant health [30].

In Latin America, 75% of people live in urban settings, in contrast to 47% of the global population; this is associated with a rise in the number of people living in urban poverty, which has significant consequences for infant nutrition [27]. Childhood malnutrition in Latin America has declined in recent years, but the burden of malnutrition has shifted toward the urban setting, particularly where women must work outside of the home for income [27]. The need to return to work reduces maternal ability to maintain EBF, thus encouraging the use of infant formula and other complementary food products prior to the end of the recommended 6-month exclusivity window. In urban settings, more than 90% of infants are initially breastfed, but are much less likely to be exclusively breastfed, as milk-based complement foods are much more prevalent in urban communities [27]. While urban mothers are more likely to need to return to work outside the home, rural mothers are more likely to lack access to a variety of nutrient-rich supplementary foods, leading to an overall lower nutritional status for rural infants [27]. Thus, both urban and rural mothers in Latin America face geographic challenges to meeting WHO recommendations.

Access to high-quality nutrition is an ongoing struggle described across the South American region, which impacts both mothers and infants. In a Brazilian cohort study on infant feeding practices in 9- to 24-month-old infants, the percentage of children who met minimum standards for diet was significantly increased relative to past studies, but this improvement appears to be mediated by the use of ultraprocessed, high-sugar foods [28]. At 24 months of age, 76.1% of infants had met the minimum acceptable diet, and 80.1% met minimum dietary diversity, compared to approximately 50% in previous studies [28]. However, 99.4% of infants were consuming ultraprocessed foods at 24 months of age, while 30.5% were consuming no fruits or vegetables; by 15 months of age, all participants were consuming sweetened beverages [28]. Additionally, only 45.1% of infants were still breastfeeding at 24 months [28]. There was a reduction in breastfeeding alongside earlier consumption of sugar and lower consumption of eggs and pulses than previous studies, suggesting that women in Brazil are relying on ultraprocessed and sugar-rich foods to fill in existing nutritional gaps, rather than a closure of food disparities.

One of the significant cultural beliefs impacting breastfeeding practices in South America is the belief that breast milk is a cause of diarrheal illness in children [29]. Diarrhea is a leading cause of morbidity in children under 5 years of age, and is a significant aspect of health risk in small children, which in many communities in South America is at least partially attributed to breast milk [29]. In a study of cultural factors surrounding breastfeeding conducted in rural Peru, 85% of women reported ceasing breastfeeding before their infants reached the age of 2 years, citing four main factors: low breast milk supply, need to return to work and chores, belief that breast milk lacks nutritional value after 6 months, and belief that breast milk causes diarrheal illness [29]. Specifically, women reported the belief that breast milk can cause illness if exposed to heat or sun, if produced during a time of maternal physical or emotional unwellness, or if a subsequent pregnancy took place before the first child was weaned [29]. The same cohort also reported a poor relationship with local healthcare workers on a background of inappropriate understanding of these cultural beliefs and practices, likely causing distrust of advice given by healthcare workers [29]. This study describes how cultural beliefs can disrupt successful breastfeeding and create barriers between healthcare workers and local communities, worsening these communities access to reliable healthcare information.

Culturally aware advocacy from community health teams could improve understanding of the role of breastfeeding in infant health and nutrition. Many studies across South America have shown that women who have positive relationships with their local healthcare workers continue to seek advice, and report having positive perceptions of breastfeeding [30]. One study of Brazilian mothers' perceptions of breastfeeding and complementary foods reported common beliefs that breastfeeding benefits both mother and child, improves mother-child bonding, and is economically beneficial and practical [30]. This population of women cited both their mothers and healthcare workers as supports for continued breastfeeding, and the majority of women continued to breastfeed exclusively until 6 months of age, before introducing complementary foods such as rice flour, milk, fruit juices, and banana [30]. Mothers who began complementary feeding before the recommended 6-month window cited the infant "looking too skinny" or being "unsatisfied" with breast milk alone, while mothers who delayed introduction of foods beyond 6 months cited financial burdens; women who were unable to follow healthcare workers' recommendations reported frustration with being unable to comply, suggesting that having a well-received healthcare body does improve education and health literacy, but is potentially insufficient in addressing barriers to meeting WHO recommendations such as low income and inaccessibility of food [30].

Grandmothers of infants in South American communities are an important source of stability and advice, especially where mothers are adolescents [31]. In a Colombian study on the role of grandmothers in infant feeding practices, grandmothers were household decision makers in most households, and regularly advocated for breastfeeding and high-quality maternal diet, such as advocating for culturally significant, healthier meals over sugar-rich, ultraprocessed foods [31]. Mothers reported that this role is "essential to [the infant's] upbringing", and relied on grandmothers for guidance, advice, and support during times of illness or stress [30]. This suggests that by encouraging strong family support systems, the security and stability of mother-infant dyads can be improved, especially where adolescent mothers are involved.

Another study in Colombia examined modifiable risk factors in failure to initiate early breastfeeding and failure to exclusively breastfeed among a group of mother-infant dyads, and found that C-sections, lack of skilled attendant at birth, prelacteal feeding, and maternal overweight or obesity were all factors in non-adherence to recommendations [32]. Prelacteal feed refers to food given to newborns prior to initiation of breastfeeding, and includes provisions such as sugar and sugar juices, as well as honey, ghee (refined butter), and water or milk-based supplements [33, 34]. Improvements to patient education, pre- and perinatal healthcare, and postnatal follow-up are important to reduce the impact of these factors on mothers and their ability to successfully follow WHO guidelines regarding infant feeding practices.

In summary, the South American region faces a number of cultural, social, and economic challenges to the promotion of WHO-recommended infant feeding practices, but research suggests that this has improved in recent years. Continued improvement of healthcare advocacy and culturally aware community healthcare work, alongside a reduction in community poverty levels, are goals which will continue to improve maternal and infant health and nutrition.

5. Europe

A widespread phenomenon-emerging in many European countries is the effect of what is considered high health literacy on the impact of infant feeding practices. Many mothers from European countries have the education and accessibility to cultivate what they deem acceptable timelines and food group introductions for infant weaning.

The diet introduced to infants and children can greatly impact the overall health of the child, thus creating a window of time in which parents have the opportunity to influence their child's future eating behaviors [35]. In many countries where the literacy level is high such as France, this creates a strain for the mother who can experience increased levels of stress in order to try to implement the best habits in her child [36]. Information in many European countries such as France, Germany, Spain, and Hungary comes in the form of the internet, social media, healthcare professionals, friends, and family. Studies have shown however, the various avenues of information are not especially significant without understanding the parent's financial situation and education level [37]. French parents predominantly utilize healthcare professionals as their primary source of advice on childcare feeding due to the fact that consultations for children between the age of 0 and 16 are free and mandatory [38]. This is in contrast to mothers in England and Finland who were not as influenced by doctors in their infant feeding practices due to the disparity in the role of the health care professional. Mothers from Sweden in particular, are the most active in looking up information on the internet and thus are able to comprehend that information in a way that is safe and effective in child rearing [39]. Previous studies have found many correlations between the use of written sources and the number of years of formal education and higher incomes for mothers. Mothers in Sweden who have experienced more years of formal education may choose the written source as this involves searching and reading in contrast to mothers from Spain who rely on passive and informal methods such as family and friends for infant feeding information [40].

France is a model for the effect of immigrant-dominant cultural practices on the effect of breastfeeding as well. In Paris and its surrounding suburbs, women who were born in foreign countries have higher breastfeeding rates compared to other French regions. This is in part due to the fact that many of these women represent first-generation mothers who despite moving to a new country still identify with their traditional values, many of which are from middle eastern or African countries that place a greater value on breastfeeding [41]. This favorable attitude toward breastfeeding can be observed intergenerationally as well between first and second-generation mothers, many of whom are greatly influenced by the cultural practices of their foreign-born mothers before them [41].

A study that focused on Italy reports that women are more likely to breastfeed longer if they are more educated, a trend seen in central to northern Italy where literacy rates are higher [42]. Higher levels of education correlate to more demanding jobs and the subsequent effect of maternity leave then plays an important role in breastfeeding for Italian mothers. Studies conducted in northern Italy have found the longer the leave, the longer mothers breastfed their children [43]. These results are consistent with studies conducted in Norway as well, where such societies have many women employed in various professional jobs that therefore shape the workforce in developed nations to accommodate mothers and infant feeding [43]. Maternity leave is an important construct that shapes the first few months of both the infant's and the mother's life, and even after resumption of employment, Italian mothers still reported high motivation to continue breastfeeding [43]. Women in professional jobs have more control over their work and schedule and this allows them to develop a positive relationship between balancing employment and infant feeding.

Developed countries have guidelines for infant feeding practices that influence the parent's decision on what foods to provide and at what times. These guidelines, however, do not necessarily guarantee optimal health for a newborn, as seen in Sweden in the 1990s. National recommendations during this time for Sweden caused many infants to be introduced to disproportionately large amounts of gluten without ongoing breastfeeding and thus a coeliac disease epidemic emerged [44]. The food content at this time also changed, with many infant cereals manufactured with almost double the amount of gluten and the usage of less protein-rich flour [44]. This provides an example of how the national guidelines can shift from unfavorable to favorable currently based on public health research and the ability of nations like Sweden to rectify infant feeding practices in a political manner.

In Greece, a national breastfeeding promotion program named 'Alkyoni' introduced breastfeeding awareness and educational activities for parents and healthcare professionals [45]. Along with this program, a baby-friendly initiative was introduced which created baby-friendly hospitals, and businesses including restaurants, shops, and pharmacies [45]. This provides an example of a nation taking proactive steps to ensure that the stigma surrounding breastfeeding is removed and that mothers are encouraged to breastfeed their babies longer. As numerous other local initiatives continue to become baby-friendly in Greece, higher rates of breastfeeding contribute to the overall health of babies and the shift of the national ideologies to become more cognisant of infant feeding practices [45].

6. Asia

Breastfeeding is a crucial tenant of infant nutrition in Asia. While the importance of this practice is well recognized, rates of EBF for up to 6 months, prior to the introduction of supplements, have steadily declined [46]. In South Asia, the early introduction of milk supplements have been attributed to a rise in inadequate nutrition for infants aged 6–24 months [46]. The premature use of such supplements reduces suckling, and thus milk volume, a negative cascade which promotes early cessation of breastfeeding [46].

There are several factors that impact breastfeeding trends. In Bangladesh and Iraq, maternal education and high familial SES were inversely associated with duration of breastfeeding [33, 46]. These trends are consistent with those in North America and Australia but were not found to impact the duration of breastfeeding in Japan [47]. Contrary to common belief, access to health and nutrition care was also linked to a shorter time span of breastfeeding in several states across India [46]. This highlights the need for appropriate education for not only the mother, but also for the post-natal healthcare team. Furthermore, returning to work was not found to be a detriment to the continuation of breastfeeding in Japan. However, the reason for this relationship is an area for further study [47].

Early initiation of breastfeeding, specifically within 1 h postbirth, is linked to a significant decrease in infection-specific infant mortality [34]. This may be attributed to the high protein and nutrient rich colostrum that is often produced soon after birth and substantially contributes to an infant's immune system.

However, despite the well-established benefits of early Breastfeeding, in 2013, only 23.4% of infants in India were reportedly breastfed within 1 h of birth [34]. Preventing infants from consuming colostrum is a widespread practice in parts of Asia often prompted by a lack of education regarding the benefits offered by colostrum, in addition to a misconception that colostrum is unhygienic [34]. In West Bengal, India, villages often delay breastfeeding based on the misbelief that post parturition breast milk requires a few days to be ready for consumption [34]. Research also indicates that familial dynamics, specifically in South Asia the lack of decision-making power provided to the mother can hinder prompt initiation of breastfeeding [48].

Furthermore, early breastfeeding is also found to be 9 times lower in caesarean section versus vaginal delivery, a finding that is consistent across multiple research studies [33]. During caesarean section, the use of anaesthesia, as well as the post-operational recovery often results in a third-party providing care for the infants in the hours following birth [33]. Thus, alternative feeding is commonly used until the mother is well enough to explore breastfeeding [33].

Delaying breastfeeding is strongly associated with prelacteal feeding [34]. This practice has been linked to lower rates of literacy, and out of hospital deliveries [34]. Additionally, prelacteal feeding is also influenced by religion. In Islam, infants are often introduced to sweet provisions prior to breastfeeding [34]. Furthermore, misinformation such as familial beliefs that prelacteal feeding would prevent the development of neonatal illnesses (i.e., jaundice) or provide energy when there is insufficient lactation, also underlie the use of this practice [33].

Unfortunately, the use of prelacteal feed acts as a barrier to the EBF [33]. The use of water or milk-based pre lacteal feeds has been associated with a delay in lactation [34].

A potential mitigator of delayed breastfeeding is maternal education which targets cultural beliefs underlined by false information, as well as the taboos surrounding breastfeeding and colostrum [33]. Further improvements can be made through the inclusion of counselling alongside regular antenatal visits. Such support helps prepare pregnant mothers for breastfeeding prior to birth [34]. The use of counselling to improve early breastfeeding has been a proven model in areas such as Bolivia and Madagascar [34]. It is also important to note that early initiation of breastfeeding is less likely in mother's who experienced obstetric problems. Therefore, research supports the early identification and support to such high-risk mothers [34].

7. Africa

Despite the global advocacy by the World Health Organization (WHO) for EBF, a significant number of African countries are still experiencing remarkably low rates of EBF that begin as low as 10% [48–50]. Infant nutrition guidelines in African countries recommend EBF for the first 6 months of life, followed by continued breastfeeding alongside complementary foods until 12 months of age [50–54]. Breastfeeding is widely acknowledged as the typical and optimal method of feeding infants, and most mothers support the recommendation to exclusively breastfeed their babies for around 6 months [50, 54]. However, in Africa, poor comprehension and cultural attitudes towards EBF, as well as conflicts between traditional beliefs and the promotion of EBF, are the primary impediments to the sustainability of this practice [51–53].

7.1 Socioeconomic factors

Research results in regards to the association between EBF and the mother's education and SES has been inconsistent with multiple studies showcasing opposing results. In a Morrocan SES, researchers found a strong association between maternal employment and EBF [55]. Many mothers were aware of the benefits of EBF, with higher levels of awareness among those with higher education and SES [55]. Nonetheless, a study in West Africa found that almost half of the participants believed that formula-feeding was more convenient than breastfeeding, which was especially important for working mothers [50]. Additionally, a study conducted in Congo did not find an association between EBF up to 6 months and the mother's family income [56]. The researchers suggested this may have been due to a variety of reasons, including limited access to complementary foods and breast-milk substitutes due to a lower income. As a result, EBF may have been the sole choice they had for feeding their babies.

Furthermore, researchers in Cameroon found that women of higher SES preferred the use of infant formula against WHO recommendations [54]. Study participants also admitted that they and their affluent, educated peers sometimes chose formula instead to display their wealth and social status [54]. The contradictory results of the above-mentioned studies suggests that socioeconomic factors may contribute to the low rates of EBF in African countries.

7.2 Social support

Access to healthcare services across the continent have also been found to account for low EBF rates [57–59]. Although access to a health facility provides an opportunity to receive and respond to health promotion messages, relevant messages about breastfeeding may not have been effectively communicated to mothers during antenatal care. A research study carried out in Tanzania discovered that despite 91% of mothers receiving medical attention during the antenatal period, only 39% of pregnant women and 25% of postpartum mothers received counselling on breastfeeding [59]. Previous studies from Ghana and Nigeria reported that mothers who used traditional healthcare services were more likely to practice optimal breastfeeding; however, a more recent study discovered that mothers who frequently attend antenatal visits (ANC) were more likely to bottle-feed their babies than those who did not attend ANC visits [57, 60, 61]. This is also a critical issue in regards to mothers with HIV whose fear of HIV transmission and status disclosure are among reasons for the low prevalence of EBF in South Africa [62, 63].

In rural areas of Egypt, mothers were found to be more likely to initiate breastfeeding within the first hour after delivery compared to Egyptian urban mothers [58]. Additionally, mothers with no education were found to be more likely to initiate breastfeeding within the first hour after delivery compared to educated mothers [58, 64]. However, the results of the 2008 EDHS indicate that health providers did not provide proper advice to pregnant women about breastfeeding [58]. Surprisingly, similar to findings mentioned previously, mothers who received regular antenatal care or delivered with the assistance of a trained health provider were less likely to initiate breastfeeding within the first hour after delivery than those who received no medical or antenatal care [58]. In fact, 52% of mothers who received regular antenatal care initiated breastfeeding within the first hour of delivery, while the percentage was 67% for mothers who did not receive any antenatal care [58].

The impact of marketing and unethical marketing tactics used in the baby formula industry also plays a role in infant feeding in North Africa [65]. A study by WHO found that 38% of Moroccan mothers were offered recommendations for specific milk brands by health professionals [65]. Additionally, 19% of mothers were offered free milk samples inside the hospital, 20% were offered samples outside the hospital, and 26% were offered samples both inside and outside of the hospitals [65]. The promotion of baby formula decreases the likelihood of adherence to EBF.

7.3 Sociocultural factors

There is a common belief in numerous cultures that breastfeeding alone is insufficient for nourishing a child, and that it is necessary to provide complementary solid foods or liquids in order to address thirst and promote healthy growth and development. This is prelacteal feeding and it is one of the most significant practices that hinder proper infant nutrition in African culture [66]. It can lead to lactation failure, insufficient milk production, infection, diarrhea, and short duration of breastfeeding [66–68]. Moreover, there is a vicious cycle between prelacteal feeding and delayed breastfeeding initiation, which may delay the production of breast milk and further encourage the use of prelacteal feeds [66, 69]. A study conducted in Egypt which included 647 mother-infant dyads found that about 58% of newborns receive prelacteal feeds [66]. The primary reasons for giving prelacteal feeds were tradition (61.0%) and mother's/mother in law's advice (58.3%) [66]. A study conducted in Kenya reported that the belief that prelacteal feeds protect the baby from stomach problems was common not only among breastfeeding mothers but also among community health or social workers [70]. Some communities believe that prelacteal feeds are necessary to clean the baby's bowels, keep the mouth and throat moist, keep the baby warm, soothe the baby, relief pain, and allow stool to be passed [66, 67]. In East African countries, some cultures believe that a male infant needs solid foods immediately after birth in order to be strong and healthy and that if practicing EBF, the bones will weaken [50, 71]. Other various explanations for prelacteal feeding can be explained by a study conducted in rural areas of Cameroon [59]. Firstly, breastfeeding mothers experienced societal pressure from their elders to follow this customary practice and were hesitant to cause any disagreements [59]. Secondly, the women believed that all members of the family should benefit from the highly treasured farm produce, including infants [59]. Lastly, they were prohibited from engaging in sexual activity while breastfeeding [59]. More recently, East Africa and various non-governmental organizations have collaborated and formed groups to tackle the shortcomings in EBF and come up with solutions to enhance its positive health effects [50].

This includes efforts to improve EBF at healthcare centers and in the community, while also partnering with the media as a primary tool to raise awareness [50].

EBF practices can be influenced by a mother's perception of her own breast milk production. Multiple studies conducted in Tanzania and Kenya have found that the main reason for introducing complementary food early was the belief that the amount of breast milk produced by the mother is insufficient for the child's growth [59, 72, 73]. As a result, these mothers perceived their child to be thirsty, leading them to introduce herbal medicine for cultural reasons, which was identified as one of the key factors for early mixed feeding [59]. Additionally, Indigenous African people commonly use herbal and medicinal preparations, which are believed to protect infants from evil spirits and improve their chances of survival [56, 59]. As a result of this belief system, EBF is often considered not only an impractical idea but also a "harmful practice" that endangers the lives of infants [56]. In Cameron, a study found that participants with low education and low occupations believed that one should wait to breastfeed only after the colostrum has passed [54]. Other studies found that participants of various religions discarded the colostrum because it was regarded as impure, unhealthy, or harmful and subsequently, they delayed the first breastfeeding for a few hours or even days [59, 66].

Additional research has highlighted the cultural expectations and social norms that encourage women to breastfeed. Qualitative research conducted in Benin showed that mothers perceived breastfeeding as a daily and on-demand activity, often initiated by the infant's cries [74]. In Nigeria, some women regarded breastfeeding as a religious privilege because breastmilk was considered a natural gift from God [70, 74]. Researchers from Nigeria explained how breastfeeding is a crucial part of African women's maternal identity and is deeply ingrained in their psyche [74, 75]. In other studies from DRC and Mali, breastfeeding was considered a child's right and a necessary aspect of a mother's duty [76, 77]. Deviating from this norm could lead to sanctions; resistance to breastfeeding in Ghana and Nigeria has been found to result in negative reactions, such as family disapproval, anger, or stigmatizing allegations that the mother or child was HIV-positive or illegitimate [75, 78, 79].

Another study in Nigeria found that awareness (95.3%) and knowledge (82.0%) of EBF was high among surveyed mother but the practice of EBF (33.5%) was very low [62]. Socio-cultural beliefs in Nigeria, such as the perception babies continued to be hungry after breastfeeding, the fear of babies becoming addicted to breast milk, lack of family support and the need to return to work were found to influence the mothers' decision to breastfeed or bottle-feed [60, 63, 80]. In Nigerian communities, new mothers typically do not have the autonomy to make infant feeding decisions, as these decisions are often made by the father or grandmother [60, 63]. Grandmothers, who usually provide significant support to nursing mothers, are knowledgeable in infant feeding practices, but their skills are often based on traditional belief systems [60, 63]. Based on their role, grandmothers can influence a mother's decision to breastfeed or bottle-feed, which may be an additional reason for suboptimal feeding practices among mothers in Nigeria [60, 63, 81].

8. Conclusions

In conclusion, infant feeding practices are crucial for ensuring the health and well-being of infants globally, but adherence to recommended guidelines for EBF and complementary feeding is influenced by a variety of cultural, societal, and environmental factors. These factors vary across regions, with each region facing unique challenges and barriers to achieving optimal infant feeding practices.

High-income countries like those found in North America, Europe, and Australia face similar challenges in adhering to guidelines for EBF and complementary feeding, including cultural and societal influences. However, in Australia, breastfeeding rates fall below global standards, and the exposure to breastmilk substitutes in hospitals is a particular concern. In Europe, high health literacy among mothers influences their infant feeding practices, creating a need for more support for mothers in implementing the best practices for their children.

South America faces numerous challenges in achieving the WHO recommendations for infant feeding practices, including social, economic, and cultural barriers. Both urban and rural communities face specific difficulties, with low access to nutritionally high-quality food being a common theme across the region, leading to nutritional inadequacies in infants and children. Breastfeeding rates have been declining in Asia, with early introduction of milk supplements being attributed to inadequate nutrition for infants. Various factors influence breastfeeding trends, including maternal education, familial SES, access to health and nutrition care, and returning to work. In Africa, poor comprehension, and cultural attitudes towards EBF, conflicts between traditional beliefs and promotion of EBF, and inadequate communication and understanding about breastfeeding are the primary impediments to the sustainability of this practice. Socioeconomic factors, social support, and sociocultural factors also play a role in the low rates of EBF.

Overall, there is a need for increased support for mothers, especially in low-income groups, to ensure that all infants have access to the health benefits of EBF and appropriate complementary feeding practices. This support should be tailored to the unique challenges faced by each region and should involve advocacy from community health teams, maternal education, counseling, and early identification and support for high-risk mothers. By addressing these barriers, we can improve maternal and infant health and reduce the burden of malnutrition and associated health consequences for infants globally.

Conflict of interest

The authors declare no conflict of interest.

Author details

Aryal Laxmi[1*], Lucas Amanda[2], Haseeb Yumna B[1], Dhaliwal Dolly[1] and Gill Rubina[1]

1 Faculty of Medicine, The University of Queensland, Brisbane, Queensland, Australia

2 Faculty of Medicine, The University of Queensland-Ochsner Clinical School, Brisbane, Australia, New Orleans, USA

*Address all correspondence to: l.aryal@uq.net.au

References

[1] World Health Organization, UNICEF. Global Strategy for Infant and Young Child Feeding. Vol. 53(3). WHO; 2017

[2] Robinson S, Fall C. Infant nutrition and later health: A review of current evidence. Nutrients. 2012;**4**:859-874. DOI: 10.3390/nu4080859

[3] Djoumessi YF. The impact of malnutrition on infant mortality and life expectancy in Africa. Nutrition. 2022;**103-104**:111760. DOI: 10.1016/J.NUT.2022.111760

[4] Waber DP, Bryce CP, Girard JM, Zichlin M, Fitzmaurice GM, Galler JR. Impaired IQ and academic skills in adults who experienced moderate to severe infantile malnutrition: A 40-year study. Nutritional Neuroscience. 2014;**17**(2):58-64. DOI: 10.1179/1476830513Y.0000000061

[5] Waber DP, Bryce CP, Girard JM, Fischer LK, Fitzmaurice GM, Galler JR. Parental history of moderate to severe infantile malnutrition is associated with cognitive deficits in their adult offspring. Nutritional Neuroscience. 2016;**21**(3):195-201. DOI: 10.1080/1028415X.2016.1258379

[6] Aubel J, Martin SL, Cunningham K. Introduction: A family systems approach to promote maternal, child and adolescent nutrition. Maternal & Child Nutrition. 2021;**17**(S1):e13228. DOI: 10.1111/MCN.13228

[7] Monterrosa EC, Pelto GH. The mother-child food relationship in the study of infant and young child feeding practices. Sight and Life. 2017;**31**(1):46-51

[8] Hart CN, Drotar D. Maternal knowledge of nutrition, problem-solving abilities and the introduction of complementary foods into infants' diets. Early Child Development and Care. 2006;**176**(7). DOI: 10.1080/03004430500207005

[9] Lanigan JA, Bishop JA, Kimber AC, Morgan J. Review systematic review concerning the age of introduction of complementary foods to the healthy full-term infant. European Journal of Clinical Nutrition. 2001;55:309-320. Available from: https://www. nature.com/ejcn

[10] Kaufman KJ, Hall LA. Influences of the social network on choice and duration of breast-feeding in mothers of preterm infants. Research in Nursing & Health. 1989;**12**:149-159. DOI: 10.1002/nur.4770120305

[11] Attree P. Low-income mothers, nutrition and health: A systematic review of qualitative evidence. Maternal & Child Nutrition. 2005;**1**:227-240. DOI: 10.1111/j.1740-8709.2005.00022.x

[12] el Área de Nutrición y Desarrollo Infantil, Instituto Mexicano del Seguro Social. Guía para una alimentación SANA, VARIADA y SUFICIENTE [pdf]. 2020 [cited 2023 Apr 14]. Available from: https://www.imss.gob.mx/sites/all/statics/pdf/guarderias/Menu-0-12-meses.pdf

[13] Gonzá Lez-Cossío T, Rivera-Dommarco J, Moreno-Macías H, Monterrubio E, Sepú Lveda J. Poor Compliance with appropriate feeding practices in children under 2 y in Mexico 1. The Journal of Nutrition Community and International Nutrition. 2006;**136**:2928-2933. Available from: https://academic.oup.com/jn/article/136/11/2928/4664269

[14] Gonzalez-Perez GJ, Vega-Lopez MG, Cabrera-Pivaral C, Romero-Valle S.

Sociodemographic factors associated with early cessation of breastfeeding in Guadalajara, Mexico. Ecology of Food and Nutrition. 2001;**40**(1):67-84. DOI: 10.1080/03670244.2001.9991638

[15] Green VL, Killings NL, Clare CA. The historical, psychosocial, and cultural context of breastfeeding in the African American community. Breastfeeding Medicine. 2021;**16**(2). DOI: 10.1089/bfm.2020.0316

[16] Blue V, Jernigan B, D'amico EJ, Duran B, Buchwald D. Multilevel and community-level interventions with Native Americans: Challenges and opportunities. Prevention Science. 2018. DOI: 10.1007/s11121-018-0916-3

[17] Chen WL. Understanding the cultural context of Chinese mothers' perceptions of breastfeeding and infant health in Canada. Journal of Clinical Nursing. 2010;**19**(7-8):1021-1029. DOI: 10.1111/J.1365-2702.2009.02956.X

[18] Fryar CD, Carroll MD, Ogden CL. Prevalence of Overweight, Obesity, and Severe Obesity among Children and Adolescents aged 2-19 years: United States, 1963-1965 Through 2015-2016. 2018. Available from: https://stacks.cdc.gov/view/cdc/58669

[19] Gillman MW, Ludwig DS. How early should obesity prevention start? New England Journal of Medicine. 2013;**369**(23). DOI: 10.1056/nejmp1310577

[20] Bushaw A, Lutenbacher M, Karp S, Dietrich M, Graf M. Infant feeding beliefs and practices: Effects of maternal personal characteristics. Journal for Specialists in Pediatric Nursing. 2020;**25**(3):e12294. DOI: 10.1111/JSPN.12294

[21] Galtry J. The impact on breastfeeding of labour market policy and practice in Ireland, Sweden, and the USA. Social Science and Medicine. 2003;**57**(1):167-177. DOI: 10.1016/S0277-9536(02)00372-6

[22] Reid J, Schmied V, Beale B. 'I only give advice if I am asked': Examining the grandmother's potential to influence infant feeding decisions and parenting practices of new mothers. Women and Birth. 2010;**23**(2):74-80. DOI: 10.1016/J.WOMBI.2009.12.001

[23] Helps C, Barclay L. Aboriginal women in rural Australia; a small study of infant feeding behaviour. Women and Birth: Journal of the Australian College of Midwives. 2015;**28**(2):129-136. DOI: 10.1016/J.WOMBI.2014.12.004

[24] Matriano MG, Ivers R, Meedya S. Factors that influence women's decision on infant feeding: An integrative review. Women and Birth. 2022;**35**(5):430-439. DOI: 10.1016/J.WOMBI.2021.10.005

[25] Hunt RW, Ryan-Atwood TE, Davey M-A, Gaston J, Wallace E, Anil S. Victorian Perinatal Services Performance Indicators. 2018. Available from: https://bettersafercare.vic.gov.au

[26] Netting MJ, Moumin NA, Knight EJ, Golley RK, Makrides M, Green TJ. The Australian Feeding Infants and Toddler Study (OzFITS 2021): Breastfeeding and early feeding practices. Nutrients. 2022;**14**(1). DOI: 10.3390/nu14010206

[27] Ruel MT. Urbanization in Latin America: Constraints and opportunities for child feeding and care. Food and Nutrition Bulletin. 2000;**21**(1). DOI: 10.1177/156482650002100103

[28] de Andrade EDO, de Rebouças AS, Filho JQ, Ambikapathi R, Caulfield LE, Lima AÂM, et al. Evolution of infant feeding practices in children from 9 to 24 months, considering complementary feeding indicators and food processing:

Results from the Brazilian cohort of the MAL-ED study. Maternal & Child Nutrition. 2022;**18**(4). DOI: 10.1111/MCN.13413

[29] Nuño Martínez N, Wallenborn J, Mäusezahl D, Hartinger SM, Muela Ribera J. Socio-cultural factors for breastfeeding cessation and their relationship with child diarrhoea in the rural high-altitude Peruvian Andes—A qualitative study. International Journal for Equity in Health. 2021;**20**(1). DOI: 10.1186/s12939-021-01505-3

[30] Lindsay AC, Machado MT, Sussner KM, Hardwick CK, Peterson KE. Infant-feeding practices and beliefs about complementary feeding among low-income Brazilian mothers: A qualitative study. Food and Nutrition Bulletin. 2008;**29**(1). DOI: 10.1177/156482650802900102

[31] Concha N, Jovchelovitch S. Grandmothers: Central scaffolding sources impacting maternal and infant feeding practices in Colombia. Maternal & Child Nutrition. 2021;**17**(S1):e13162. DOI: 10.1111/MCN.13162

[32] Finnie S, Peréz-Escamilla R, Buccini G. Determinants of early breastfeeding initiation and exclusive breastfeeding in Colombia. Public Health Nutrition. 2020;**23**(3):496-505. DOI: 10.1017/S1368980019002180

[33] Al-Marzoki JM, Abdulkareem AH. Sociocultural influences in feeding pattern in children below two years in Babylon Iraq. Journal of Advanced Medical Research. 2015;**25**:7-13

[34] Patel A, Banerjee A, Kaletwad A. Factors associated with prelacteal feeding and timely initiation of breastfeeding in hospital-delivered infants in India. Journal of Human Lactation. 2013;**29**(4). DOI: 10.1177/0890334412474718

[35] Blake-Lamb TL, Locks LM, Perkins ME, et al. Interventions for childhood obesity in the first 1000 d: A systematic review. American Journal of Preventive Medicine. 2016;**50**

[36] Loudon K, Buchanan S, Ruthven I. The everyday life information seeking behaviours of first-time mothers. Journal of Documentation. 2016;**72**:24-46

[37] De Rosso S, Nicklaus S, Ducrot P, Schwartz C. Information seeking of French parents regarding infant and young child feeding: Practices, needs and determinants. Public Health Nutrition. 2022;**25**(4):879-892. DOI: 10.1017/S1368980021003086

[38] Service-public.fr. Suivi médical de l'enfant: examens médicaux obligatoires ("Medical Follow-Up of the Child: Compulsory Medical Examinations"). République française. 2020. Available from: https://www.service-public.fr/particuliers/vosdroits/F967

[39] Plantin L, Daneback K. Parenthood, information and support on the internet. A literature review of research on parents and professionals online. BMC Family Practice. 2009;**10**:34

[40] Gage, H., Williams, P., Von Rosen-Von Hoewel, J. et al. Influences on infant feeding decisions of first-time mothers in five European countries. European Journal of Clinical Nutrition 66, 914-919 (2012). DOI: 10.1038/ejcn.2012.56

[41] Hawkins SS, Lamb K, Cole TJ, et al. Influence of moving to the UK on maternal health behaviours: Prospective cohort study. BMJ. 2008;**336**:1052-1055

[42] Lauria L, Spinelli A, Grandolfo M. Prevalence of breastfeeding in Italy: A population based follow-up study. Annali dell'Istituto Superiore di Sanità. 2016;**52**:457-461. DOI: 10.4415/ANN_16_03_18

[43] Liamputtong P. Infant feeding beliefs and practices across cultures: An introduction. In: Liamputtong P, editor. Infant Feeding Practices. New York, NY.: Springer; 2011. DOI: 10.1007/978-1-4419-6873-9_1

[44] Ivarsson A. The Swedish epidemic of coeliac disease explored using an epidemiological approach—Some lessons to be learnt. Best Practice & Research Clinical Gastroenterology. 2005;**19**(3):425-440

[45] Iliodromiti Z, Zografaki I, Papamichail D, Stavrou T, Gaki E, Ekizoglou C, et al. Increase of breast-feeding in the past decade in Greece, but still low uptake: Cross-sectional studies in 2007 and 2017. Public Health Nutrition. 2020;**23**(6):961-970. DOI: 10.1017/S1368980019003719

[46] Ramachandran P. Breast-feeding practices in South Asia. Indian Journal of Medical Research. Jun 2004;**119**(6):13-15. PMID: 15243170

[47] Inoue M, Binns CW, Otsuka K, Jimba M, Matsubara M. Infant feeding practices and breastfeeding duration in Japan: A review. International Breastfeeding Journal. 2012;7). DOI: 10.1186/1746-4358-7-15

[48] Tylleskär T, Jackson D, Meda N, Engebretsen IM, Chopra M, Diallo AH, et al. Exclusive breastfeeding promotion by peer counsellors in sub-Saharan Africa (PROMISE-EBF): A cluster-randomised trial. The Lancet. 2011;**378**(9789):420-427

[49] Vitalis D, Vilar-Compte M, Nyhan K, Pérez-Escamilla R. Breastfeeding inequities in South Africa: Can enforcement of the WHO Code help address them?—A systematic scoping review. International Journal for Equity in Health. 2021;**20**:1-7

[50] Dukuzumuremyi JP, Acheampong K, Abesig J, Luo J. Knowledge, attitude, and practice of exclusive breastfeeding among mothers in East Africa: A systematic review. International Breastfeeding Journal. 2020 Dec;**15**:1-7

[51] Asfaw MM, Argaw MD, Kefene ZK. Factors associated with exclusive breastfeeding practices in Debre Berhan District, Central Ethiopia: A cross sectional community based study. International Breastfeeding Journal. 2015;**10**(1):1-9

[52] Bhattacharjee NV, Schaeffer LE, Marczak LB, Ross JM, Swartz SJ, Albright J, et al. Mapping exclusive breastfeeding in Africa between 2000 and 2017. Nature Medicine. 2019;**25**(8):1205-1212

[53] Chakona G. Social circumstances and cultural beliefs influence maternal nutrition, breastfeeding and child feeding practices in South Africa. Nutrition Journal. 2020;**19**(1):1-15

[54] Dapi LN, Tambe AB, Axberg F, Lundström L, Hörnell A. After giving birth to a baby, breastfeeding becomes your responsibility: Infant feeding perceptions and practices among women in Yaoundé, Bamenda and Bandja, Cameroon, Africa. International Research Journal of Public and Environmental Health. 2018;**5**(3):38-45

[55] Habibi M, Laamiri FZ, Aguenaou H, Doukkali L, Mrabet M, Barkat A. The impact of maternal socio-demographic characteristics on breastfeeding knowledge and practices: An experience from Casablanca, Morocco. International Journal of Pediatrics and Adolescent Medicine. 2018;**5**(2):39-48

[56] Babakazo P, Donnen P, Akilimali P, Ali NM, Okitolonda E. Predictors of discontinuing exclusive breastfeeding before six months among mothers in Kinshasa: A prospective study.

International Breastfeeding Journal. 2015;**10**:1-9

[57] Aidam BA, Perez-Escamilla R, Lartey A, Aidam J. Factors associated with exclusive breastfeeding in Accra, Ghana. European Journal of Clinical Nutrition. 2005;**59**:789-796

[58] El-Zanaty F, Way A. Egypt Demographic and Health Survey 2008. Cairo, Egypt: Ministry of Health/Egypt, El-Zanaty and Associates/Egypt, and Macro International; 2009

[59] Maonga AR, Mahande MJ, Damian JD, Msuya SE. Factors affecting exclusive breastfeeding among women in Muheza district Tanga northeastern Tanzania: A mixed method community based study. Maternal and Child Health Journal. 2016;**20**:77-87

[60] Ogbo FA, Agho KE, Page A. Determinants of suboptimal breastfeeding practices in Nigeria: Evidence from the 2008 demographic and health survey. BMC Public Health. 2015;**15**(1):1-2

[61] Ogunlesi T, Dedeke O, Okeniyi J, Oyedeji G. Infant and toddler feeding practices in the Baby Friendly Initiative (BFI) era in Ilesa, Nigeria. The Internet Journal of Nutrition and Wellness. 2004;**1**:2

[62] Onah S, Osuorah DI, Ebenebe J, Ezechukwu C, Ekwochi U, Ndukwu I. Infant feeding practices and maternal socio-demographic factors that influence practice of exclusive breastfeeding among mothers in Nnewi South-East Nigeria: A cross-sectional and analytical study. International Breastfeeding Journal. 2014;**9**(1):1

[63] Agunbiade OM, Ogunleye OV. Constraints to exclusive breastfeeding practice among breastfeeding mothers in Southwest Nigeria: Implications for scaling up. International Breastfeeding Journal. 2012;7:1

[64] Mohammed ES, Ghazawy ER, Hassan EE. Knowledge, attitude, and practices of breastfeeding and weaning among mothers of children up to 2 years old in a rural area in El-Minia Governorate, Egypt. Journal of Family Medicine and Primary Care. 2014;**3**(2):136

[65] M&C Saatchi World Services. Multi-country study examining the impact of breast-milk substitutes marketing on infant feeding decisions and practices: commissioned report [pdf]. World Health Organization and the United Nations Children's Fund (UNICEF). 2022 (WHO/UHL/MCA/22.01). Available from: https://apps.who.int/iris/bitstream/handle/10665/354094/WHO-UHL-MCA-22.01-eng.pdf

[66] El-Gilany AH, Abdel-Hady DM. Newborn First Feed and Prelacteal Feeds in Mansoura, Egypt. BioMed Research International. 2014;**2014**:7. DOI: 10.1155/2014/258470

[67] Moshaddeque Hossain M, Radwan MM, Arafa SA, Habib M, DuPont HL. Prelacteal infant feeding practices in rural Egypt. Journal of Tropical Pediatrics. 1992;**38**(6):317-322

[68] Jagzape T, Lohkare A, Vagha J, Lakhkar BB. Prevalence of prelacteal feeding practice in Wardha and the effect of antenatal education on it. Pediatric Oncall. 2009;**6**. Art# 56

[69] Athavale AV, Athavale SA, Deshpande SG, Zodpey SP, Sangole S. Initiation of breast-feeding by urban women. Health and Population: Perspectives and Issues. 2004;**27**(2):117-125

[70] Coetzee B, Tomlinson M, Osawe S, Amibiku AL, Kagee A, INFANT Study Team, et al. Barriers to and facilitators of adherence to exclusive breastfeeding practices among HIV infected and

non-infected women in Jos, Nigeria. Maternal and Child Health Journal. 2017;**21**:953-960

[71] Arts M, Geelhoed D, Schacht C, Prosser W, Alons C, Pedro A. Knowledge, beliefs, and practices regarding exclusive breastfeeding of infants younger than 6 months in Mozambique: A qualitative study. Journal of Human Lactation. 2011;**27**(1):25-32

[72] Kimani-Murage EW, Madise NJ, Fotso JC, Kyobutungi C, Mutua MK, Gitau TM, et al. Patterns and determinants of breastfeeding and complementary feeding practices in urban informal settlements, Nairobi, Kenya. BMC Public Health. 2011;**11**(1):396

[73] Matsuyama A, Karama M, Tanaka J, Kaneko S. Perceptions of caregivers about health and nutritional problems and feeding practices of infants: A qualitative study on exclusive breastfeeding in Kwale, Kenya. BMC Public Health. 2013;**13**(1):525

[74] Alive & Thrive and UNICEF. Factors Influencing the Practice of Exclusive Breastfeeding and Other Infant Feeding Practices in the First Six Months of Life in West and Central Africa [pdf]. Alive & Thrive and UNICEF. 2022. Available from: https://www.aliveandthrive.org/sites/default/files/literature_review_-_breastfeeding_in_west_africa_-_feb2022.pdf

[75] Ogbonna M, Williamson IR, Mitchell H. It was never an option not to breastfeed: Exploring breastfeeding experiences and intentions of multigravidae in Southern Nigeria. African Journal for the Psychological Study of Social Issues. 2018;**21**:51-65

[76] Burns J, Emerson JA, Amundson K, Doocy S, Caulfield LE, Klemm RD. A qualitative analysis of barriers and facilitators to optimal breastfeeding and complementary feeding practices in South Kivu, Democratic Republic of Congo. Food and Nutrition Bulletin. 2016;**37**(2):119-131

[77] Dettwyler KA. More than nutrition: Breastfeeding in urban Mali. Medical Anthropology Quarterly. 1988;**2**(2):172-183

[78] Iddrisu S. Exclusive Breastfeeding and Family Influences in Rural Ghana: A Qualitative Study [Internet] [Dissertation]. Malmö högskola/Hälsa och samhälle; 2013. Available from: http://urn.kb.se/resolve?urn=urn:nbn:se:mau:diva-27075

[79] Afaya A, Fuseini K, Anaman-Torgbor J, Salia S, Adatara P, Afaya R. Family belief systems and practices that influence exclusive breastfeeding in Sagu. Ghana: Numid Horizon; 2017;**12017**:23-32

[80] Agbo HA, Envuladu EA, Adams HS, Inalegwu E, Okoh E, Agba A, et al. Barriers and facilitators to the practice of exclusive breast feeding among working class mothers: A study of female resident doctors in tertiary health institutions in Plateau State. Journal of Medical Research. 2013;**2**(1):112-116

[81] Grassley J, Eschiti V. Grandmother breastfeeding support: what do mothers need and want? Birth. 2008;**35**(4):329-335

Chapter 8

Compliance to Infant and Young Child Feeding (IYCF) Indicators amongst Infants of Rural Saharanpur, India

Monika Jain and Vandana

Abstract

Optimal Infant and Young Child Feeding (IYCF) practices hold paramount importance for child survival, health, growth, and development. This study was done to assess the IYCF practices followed by the rural dwellers of Saharanpur, Uttar Pradesh, India. A cross-sectional survey was carried out in 18 randomly selected Anganwadi Centres of Behat Tehsil in Saharanpur district. The data were collected from 800 mothers whose children aged 1–3 years were registered in these anganwadis. Information was gathered using questionnaires and interviews. Results showed that 99.5% mothers initiated breastfeeding their infants with in first hour of birth. Minimum dietary diversity, minimum meal frequency as well as minimum acceptable diet were the three IYCF core indicators that were not followed by about 95% of mothers. Infant and young child feeding practices in the selected rural area are not satisfactory and there is not 100% compliance to something as important as exclusive breastfeeding for 6 months. There should be a more focused approach towards awareness generation, and sincere efforts should be made to improve infant feeding practices so as to make a positive impact on eradication of malnutrition amongst rural children.

Keywords: breastfeeding, complementary feeding, IYCF, infant nutrition, malnutrition

1. Introduction

Nutrition of young children is an essential component of ensuring their growth and Infant and young child feeding (IYCF) practices have a direct effect on the health, development, and nutritional status of all children who are below 2 years of age. This, ultimately, has an impact on child survival. Improving IYCF practices in children 0–23 months of age is, therefore, crucial to improved development, nutrition, and health. World Health Organization (WHO) and UNICEF adopted the Global Strategy for infant and young child feeding in the year 2002. With the objective of reinvigorating the attention of the world to the influence that feeding practices have on the nutritional status, growth, and development, health, and survival of the vulnerable segment of infants and young children, the strategy was formulated [1].

WHO guiding principles related to complementary feeding of the breastfed child [2] along with guiding principles for feeding non-breastfed children between 6 and 24 months of age [3] provide significant evidence-based literature as well as guidance on optimal feeding practices for supporting growth, health, and behavioral development for infants and young children (IYC) aged <2 years, that can be accepted globally. The indicators that support programmatic action and contribute to monitoring progress on IYCF at both national and global levels were published in the year 2008. These indicators serve as an important tool in assessing infant and young child feeding practices. A set of eight core and seven optional indicators were recommended through this guidance document. These indicators have served as the standard for data collection and reporting on IYCF practices at a global level [3]. Below is the brief explanation of these indicators.

1.1 Breastfeeding indicators

1.1.1 Ever breastfed (EvBF)

Indicator: Percentage of children born in the last 24 months who were ever breastfed.

1.1.2 Early initiation of breastfeeding (EIBF)

Indicator: Percentage of children born in the last 24 months who were put to the breast within 1 hour of birth.

1.1.3 Exclusively breastfed for the first 2 days after birth (EBF2D)

Indicator: Percentage of children born in the last 24 months who were fed exclusively with breast milk for the first 2 days after birth.

1.1.4 Exclusive breastfeeding under 6 months (EBF)

Indicator: Percentage of infants 0–5 months of age who were fed exclusively with breast milk during the previous day.

1.1.5 Mixed milk feeding under 6 months (MixMF)

Indicator: Percentage of infants 0–5 months of age who were fed formula and/or animal milk in addition to breast milk during the previous day.

1.1.6 Continued breastfeeding 12–23 months (CBF)

Indicator: Percentage of children 12–23 months of age who were fed breast milk during the previous day.

1.2 Complementary feeding indicators

1.2.1 Introduction of solid, semi-solid, or soft foods 6–8 months (ISSSF)

Indicator: Percentage of infants 6–8 months of age who consumed solid, semi-solid, or soft foods during the previous day.

1.2.2 Minimum dietary diversity 6–23 months (MDD)

Indicator: Percentage of children 6–23 months of age who consumed foods and beverages from at least five out of eight defined food groups during the previous day.

1.2.3 Minimum meal frequency 6–23 months (MMF)

Indicator: Percentage of children 6–23 months of age who consumed solid, semi-solid, or soft foods (but also including milk feeds for non-breastfed children) at least the minimum number of times during the previous day.

1.2.4 Minimum milk feeding frequency for non-breastfed children 6–23 months (MMFF)

Indicator: Percentage of non-breastfed children 6–23 months of age who consumed at least two milk feeds during the previous day.

1.2.5 Minimum acceptable diet 6–23 months (MAD)

Indicator: Percentage of children 6–23 months of age who consumed a minimum acceptable diet during the previous day.

1.2.6 Egg and/or flesh food consumption 6–23 months (EFF)

Indicator: Percentage of children 6–23 months of age who consumed egg and/or flesh food during the previous day.

1.2.7 Sweet beverages consumption 6–23 months

Indicator: Percentage of children 6–23 months of age who consumed a sweet beverage during the previous day.

1.2.8 Unhealthy food consumption 6–23 months (UFC)

Indicator: Percentage of children 6–23 months of age who consumed selected sentinel unhealthy foods during the previous day.

1.2.9 Zero vegetables or fruits consumption 6–23 months (ZVF)

Indicator: Percentage of children 6–23 months of age who did not consume any vegetables or fruits during the previous day.

1.3 Other indicators

1.3.1 Bottle feeding 0–23 months (BF)

Indicator: Percentage of children 0–23 months of age who were fed from a bottle with a nipple during the previous day.

1.3.2 Infant feeding area graphs (AGs)

Whilst the indicators recommended above are useful for comparing population groups, targeting programmes, and evaluating progress over time, they provide a limited understanding of how population-level feeding patterns change with the age of the infant. In addition to calculating numerical indicators, presenting graphic displays of how IYC are fed is also recommended.

1.4 Importance of infant and young child feeding

Progression related to enhancement of the "Infant and Young Child Feeding" (IYCF) practices mainly in developing countries is very slow because of various factors such as poverty and poor hygienic conditions [4]. Proper breastfeeding and practices related to complementary feeding play an essential role in both child survival and child development. Physical growth can be counted amongst the best indicator of the wellbeing of child and it is massively affected by the feeding practices. But, in spite of the theories available and work done it is hard to establish the relation between quality of feeding and the effect of feed factors on the nutritional status of children. It can vary to a great extent per se depending on the kind of living conditions and the context [5]. Adequate nutrition during infancy and early childhood is essential to ensure the growth, health, and development of children to the potential they hold [6, 7]. The chances of getting ill are high in infants when the nutrition is poor. Moreover, research suggests that childhood obesity, a burgeoning public health problem, may also be a consequence of inappropriate nutrition [8, 9]. Early nutritional deficits have a long-term effect on growth as well as the overall health. Malnutrition during the first 2 years of life results in stunting. Therefore, as an adult such infants will not be able to attain their potential height and will remain shorter relatively. There is now enough research concluding that early childhood malnutrition impairs the child's intellectual performance [10, 11]. Another impairment is also seen in their physical work capacity. The consequences of girl child malnutrition are graver because their reproductive capacity gets negatively affected when they grow up into adult women. Such women have higher probability to bear infants with low birth weight and they tend to suffer from more obstetric complications. In a country where many children are malnourished, it has negative implications for its national development [12–14]. Thus, the significance of investing resources as well as time in IYCF cannot be ignored, if we aspire to have a healthy society, healthy nation, and a healthy world.

2. Review of literature

As per the 2020 report of WHO, around 144 million children below 5 years were stunted, 47 million children, and 14.3 million children were wasted and severely wasted respectively. On the other hand, 38.3 million children below 5 years were overweight or obese [15]. Even after the continuous developments made, dietary quality still remains to be suboptimal amongst the infants and young children all over the world and the improvements are not much observed since the past decade. Merely around 39% children of urban areas and 23% children of rural areas belonging to less than 5 years of age are reported of receiving a minimally diversified diet [16].

The children that were ever breastfed were approximately 91.6%. About 79.0% children were put to the breast within the time of an hour after giving birth and they (79.6%) were reported of having colostrum. From the data of children belonging to 6–8 months of age, not even half (41.5%) reported receiving semi-solid, solid, or soft foods in the previous day. Greater percentage of children continued to be breastfed during 1 year (81.7%) and 2 years (68.9%). Merely 13.6% were fed with iron-rich or iron-fortified foods developed for infants and young children. Most of the children (89.2%) belonging to 6–23 months of age had breastfeeding considered adequate as per their age [17]. It was observed that fewer mothers practiced early initiation of breastfeeding. The increase in early initiation of breastfeeding can be attributed to two primary facts. Firstly, it is a result of the sensitization and training provided to peripheral health workers and public health staff regarding various aspects of breastfeeding and secondly, the fact that most of the deliveries take place in public health facilities also contributes to the higher rates of early breastfeeding initiation [18]. This study reported very poor IYCF practices with merely 15.0% of moms who began breastfeeding within an hour of giving birth, whereas more than a third (38.3%) said they would breastfeed exclusively until their baby was 6 months old, although with pre-lacteal meals. Merely 21 (5.3%) infants were breastfed exclusively for 6 months without any pre-lacteal meals. Only 29.8% of babies started supplementary feeding at 6 months, according to the main indicator [18]. The breast milk and animal milk (cow/buffalo) were used by nearly 40.2% of women to feed their children, followed by solely breastmilk for the first 6 months (38.3%), breast milk and formula milk (10.7%), breast milk and water (4.0%), and breast milk and solid food (1.3%). Approximately 5.5% of women did not feed their children with breast milk at all [19].

Approximately 45% of children of less than 5 years of age globally have been reported of dying because of undernutrition. Undernutrition is considered to be a vital causable factor increasing susceptibility towards malaria, diarrhea, and pneumonia [20]. Poor infant and young child feeding (IYCF) practices, specifically at the time of initial thousand days, i.e., from birth till 2 years, lead to malnutrition, deprived psychosocial development, reduced school performance, and decreased productivity in later years of life, thus setting up a vicious cycle [20].

Amongst the core indicators for assessing IYCF practices, it was observed that only 65.0% of mothers started breastfeeding within 1 hour of birth [21]. The infant feeding methods, which include both breastfeeding and supplemental feeding, have a significant impact in defining a child's nutritional health. Adequate nutrition in infancy and early childhood is precious in supporting children's growth, development, and health to fullest. Merely 34.8% of infants worldwide are exclusively breastfed for the initial 6 months of life, with the remainder receiving additional foods or liquids in the interim. The initial 2 years of life are a key time for ensuring children's proper growth and development through adequate eating. Optimal breastfeeding could result in the prevention of 13% deaths amongst children below the age of 5 years, globally, whilst proper supplemental eating could reduce under-5 mortality by another 6% [22]. Breastfeeding is beneficial not only to a young child's survival, health, nutrition, and the developing baby's trust and sense of security, but it also helps with brain development and learning preparation. Breastfed babies have an IQ that is about 8 points greater than non-breastfed babies. The connection between starvation and baby feeding has long been known. According to current scientific research, malnutrition results in 60% of all deaths in children below 5 years, either directly or indirectly. Over two-thirds of these overall deaths occur within the 1 year of life and are generally linked to improper feeding practices. Only 35% of infants globally are nursed exclusively for the initial 4 months of their lives [23].

An evaluation depicted that proper breastfeeding and complementary feeding related practices could solely lead to prevention of deaths by 19% in under five children [24]. Every year, above 9 million children below 5 years die around the world. Malnutrition is the foremost cause of death in children below the age of five, with 70% of deaths occurring in the initial 1 year of life. Feeding strategies for infants and young children have a direct impact on their nutritional health and, ultimately, their survival [25]. Optimal infant feeding practices include the initiation of breastfeeding within an hour of birth, exclusive breastfeeding during the initial 6 months of life, and continuous breastfeeding for 2 years accompanied by appropriate complementary feeding.

As per the data from India, only 46% of children in the age group of 6–9 months in Uttar Pradesh are consuming semi-solid or solid foods along with breastmilk [26]. In India, child feeding appears to be prejudiced by traditional and economic structures. Poor beliefs and fads towards child feeding practices have been recognized to be amongst the chief reasons for health amongst the children, mostly in developing nations. Insufficient nutrition knowledge and adherence to social practices lead to low-quality feeding practices. Social variables and taboos strongly influence the feeding practices and eating patterns.

With this backdrop, a need to observe the compliance to IYCF was felt and an attempt was made to study the adherence to IYCF core indicators amongst 1–3 years old children registered in anganwadis (an anganwadi centre is set up by the central or state government in India to implement the Integrated Child Development Scheme. The main purpose of anganwadis is to enhance the capability of the mother to look after the normal health and nutritional needs of the child through proper nutrition and health education) at rural Saharanpur in India. The study presented below is a part of a comprehensive project undertaken to assess the nutritional status and dietary diversity of rural children from Saharanpur, India.

3. Materials and methods

3.1 Research design and locale

This study was a cross-sectional descriptive study without any intervention. The setting of the study was Muzaffarabad block of Behat Tehsil of Saharanpur, a district in the north Indian state of Uttar Pradesh which is also the most populated state of the country.

The 3410 anganwadi centres in Saharanpur district (Uttar Pradesh) cater to the nutritional needs of infant and school going children in the age group of 6 months to 6 years. Muzaffarabad block is located under the Behat Tehsil of Saharanpur. As of the 2011 India census, the Muzaffarabad block of Saharanpur district had a population of 303,055. Out of this, 162,641 are males, and the female count was 146,414 [27]. This block has 50,478 children in the age bracket of 0–6 years. Amongst them, 26,484 are boys, and 23,994 are girls. The total number of anganwadis present in the Muzaffarabad block is 111. The anganwadis of Muzaffarabad block were selected for this study. In the Muzaffarabad block there are 164 villages. Nine villages were selected through the simple random sampling technique. The names of the selected villages were as follows: Khushalipur, Satpura, Badshapur, Mirzapur-Grant,

Kaluwala-Jahanpur, Jayantipur, Hamirpur, Raheempur, and Ahmadpura. Out of the 9 selected villages 3 villages, namely, Kaluwala-Jahanpur, Khushalipur, and Ahmadpura villages had four anganwadi centres each. The remaining six villages have one anganwadi centre each. Thus, the total number of anganwadis which became a part of the study were 18. The total number of registered children varied from 40 to 60 in each of these anganwadis.

3.1.1 Ethical considerations

In accordance with the guidelines given in Handbook on National Ethical Guidelines for Biomedical and Health Research Involving Human Participants [28], written informed consent for participation of children in the study was obtained from the mother/father of the children. Only non-invasive data was collected from the subjects with utmost care.

3.2 Sampling

To select eligible children of age group 1 to 3 years, multi-stage random sampling was used in which, first we selected Tehsil (T) randomly from Saharanpur district, then at second stage Block (B) was selected randomly amongst the available blocks within Tehsil. Now, within a selected block, 34 anganwadi centres available in the villages of that block were selected.

3.2.1 Sample size calculation

A random sampling technique using Slovin's formula [29] was used to calculate the sample size for the present study which was computed to be 793.17. It was rounded off to 800.

3.2.2 Participant recruitment

Amongst the selected anganwadis, the beneficiaries in the age group of 1–3 years were listed and data was collected after seeking requisite permission of Data Protection Officer (D.P.O) from Vikas Bhawan. The officer certified the data collection after due vigilance and conformity to ethical and other guidelines. The purpose and details of the study were explained and written informed consent was obtained from the guardian of the children who were a part of the study.

3.3 Data collection procedure

The data collection was conducted from January 2019 to October 2020. A majority of data were collected using questionnaires. The questionnaires for present study were designed in Hindi language, so that native people can understand the questions. Face-to-face interviews were conducted with mothers at their homes in Hindi/local dialect. All the relevant information about infants was collected with the support of Asha Sahyoginis (grass root functionaries associated with anganwadis) which were present at specified anganwadis along with mothers. Interview took 30–40 minutes for each subject. Data collection was usually done between 10:00 am and 5:00 pm every day barring Sunday.

3.4 Background information and socioeconomic status (SES)

A self-designed and semi-structured questionnaire was used to collect the socio-demographic information from the mothers or caregivers of the subjects through the personal interview method. The data included information regarding background information of subjects and parents/caregivers. Information included name, age, gender, family type, occupation, family income, education of parents, and the like. Questionnaire was prepared in Hindi. Information was collected by the interview technique.

3.5 Infant and young child feeding practices (IYCF)

A well-structured and pretested questionnaire based on IYCF practices was used for data collection. These questions provide the information needed to calculate the key indicators given by WHO about IYCF, outlining exclusive breastfeeding and complementary feeding [30]. This questionnaire was adapted from the standardized questionnaire of World Health Organization and UNICEF [31]. There are eight feeding indicators which are closed-ended questions with two options of "Yes" and "No". The indicators are the initiation of breastfeeding within 1 hour of birth, exclusive breastfeeding for 6 months, continued breastfeeding for 1 year, initiation of complementary feeds after six to 8 months, minimum meal frequency, minimum meal diversity, minimum acceptable diet, and consumption of iron-rich foods. The questions related to these indicators were included in the questionnaire for IYCF indicators, a scoring system was established. Indicator with the appropriate response was given a score of 1 and if inappropriate it was marked as 0. A score of 7–8 was considered as excellent, 4–6 as good, and < 4 as poor.

3.6 Statistical analysis

All the data were recorded in the software Statistical Package for Social Sciences (SPSS) Version 20. To describe the data, descriptive statistics mainly frequency analysis, percentage analysis, mean, and SD were used. Chi-square was used to find the associations of age and gender with different IYCF indicators and $p < 0.05$ was considered as significant.

4. Results

The mean age of the children was 24.0 ± 6.97 months. Out of 800 children whose data were collected 53.5% were boys and 46.5% were girls. About two-thirds (67.2%) of the children came from nuclear families, 24.1% from joint, and remaining 8.6% from extended families. With respect to education of parents, 65.5% mothers and 35.7% fathers were illiterate. Family income of 81.1% families was less than Rupees 1865 per month. Most of the fathers were poor, marginal farmers whilst mothers were housewives spending much time working in their fields. More than half of the children were following non-vegetarian food habits (53.7%), 37.5% were lacto-vegetarians, and 8.7% were lacto-ovo vegetarian.

Retrospective data collection was done to get an insight into adherence to IYCF practices, the results of which are presented in **Table 1**. The early initiation of breastfeeding, exclusive breastfeeding till 6 months, and consumption of iron-rich or

s. no	Core of indicators	"Yes", as response N (%)
1	Early initiation of breastfeeding	796 (99.5)
2	Exclusive breastfeeding till 6 months	755 (94.3)
3	Continued breastfeeding at 1 year	699 (87.3)
4	Introduction of solid, semi-solid, or soft foods	70 (8.7)
5	Minimum dietary diversity	41 (5.5)
6	Minimum meal frequency	40 (5.0)
7	Minimum acceptable diet	44 (5.5)

Table 1.
Number of affirmative (Yes) responses to infant and young child feeding practices (IYCF) core indicators.

iron-fortified food was practiced by nearly 90% of the mothers, the optimal feeding practices related to minimum dietary diversity, minimum meal frequency, and minimum acceptable diet were followed by nearly 5% mothers only.

Table 2 reveals the core indicators of age-wise association of children (1–3 years aged) with infant and young child feeding practices. Results showed that there was no significant association of age and early initiation of breastfeeding, exclusive breastfeeding under 6 months, minimum diversity, and consumption of iron-rich foods.

Core indicators	Status	All children	1–2	2–3	Chi-square	p-value
Early initiation of breastfeeding	Yes	796 (99.5)	447 (99.1)	349 (100.0)	χ^2 = 3.11	0.07^{NS}
	No	4 (0.5)	4 (0.8)	0 (00.0)		
Exclusive breastfeeding under 6 months	Yes	755 (94.3)	430 (95.3)	325 (93.1)	χ^2 = 1.82	0.17^{NS}
	No	45 (5.6)	21 (4.6)	24 (6.8)		
Continued breastfeeding at 1 year	Yes	699 (87.4)	411 (91.1)	288 (82.5)	χ^2 = 13.22	0.00*
	No	101 (12.6)	40 (8.8)	61 (17.4)		
Introduction of solid, semi-solid, or soft foods	Yes	70 (8.7)	28 (6.2)	42 (12.0)	χ^2 = 8.36	0.00*
	No	730 (91.2)	423 (93.7)	307 (87.9)		
Minimum dietary diversity	Yes	41 (5.1)	21 (4.6)	20 (5.7)	χ^2 = 0.46	0.49^{NS}
	No	759 (94.8)	430 (95.3)	329 (94.2)		
Minimum meal frequency	Yes	44 (5.5)	15 (3.3)	25 (7.1)	χ^2 = 6.09	0.01*
	No	756 (94.5)	436 (96.6)	324 (92.8)		
Minimum acceptable diet	Yes	44 (5.5)	21 (4.7)	23 (6.5)	χ^2 = 1.41	0.02*
	No	86 (10.7)	430 (95.3)	44 (12.6)		
Consumption of iron-rich or iron-fortified foods	Yes	714 (89.2)	409 (90.6)	305 (87.3)	χ^2 = 2.22	0.13^{NS}

*Statistically significant ($p < 0.05$).
^{NS}Non-significant.

Table 2.
Age-wise association of children with infant and young child feeding practices (IYCF) core indicators.

However, the continued breastfeeding at 1 year, the introduction of solid, semi-solid food, minimum meal frequency, and minimum acceptable diet were significantly associated with age.

Table 3 shows the gender-wise association of children with infant and young child feeding practices core indicators. The results demonstrated that there was no association of gender with any of the IYCF core indicators.

Table 4 presents the mean of infant young and child feeding practices (IYCF) scores of age and gender-wise categorized children. Based on the results, the characteristics of IYCF are classified in three ways, excellent, good, and poor. Only one boy had a mean score of 7.0 ± 0.0 and two girls also had a mean score of 7.0 ± 0.0 who belonged to the 1–2 year age group and had an excellent level of IYCF. Similarly, 48.42% (n = 200) and 43.82% (n = 181) were boys and girls having mean intake values of 4.06 ± 0.27 and 4.04 ± 0.26, respectively of 1–2 year age groups who had the good level of IYCF, whilst 5.08% (n = 21) boys exhibiting mean intake of 2.33 ± 0.47 and 1.93% (n = 8) girls exhibiting mean intake of 2.38 ± 0.51 demonstrated poor level of IYCF under same age groups children. The children from 2 to 3 year age groups were 0.51% (n = 2) boys demonstrating a mean intake 7.0 ± 0.0 and 0.77% (n = 3) girls demonstrating the mean intake 7.0 ± 0.0, which showed the excellent practices of IYCF, whereas 48.57% (n = 188) boys presenting mean intake 4.06 ± 0.26 and 40.31% (n = 156) girls presenting mean intake 4.08 ± 0.38 demonstrated the good level of

Core indicators (IYCF)	Status	All children	Boys	Girls	Chi-square	p-value
				N (%)		
Early initiation of breastfeeding	Yes	796 (99.5)	425 (99.2)	371 (99.7)	$\chi^2 = 0.747$	0.387^{NS}
	No	4 (0.5)	3 (0.7)	1 (0.2)		
Exclusive breastfeeding under 6 months	Yes	755 (94.3)	403 (94.1)	352 (94.6)	$\chi^2 = 0.081$	0.776^{NS}
	No	45 (5.6)	25 (5.8)	20 (5.3)		
Continued breastfeeding at 1 year	Yes	699 (87.3)	373 (87.1)	326 (87.6)	$\chi^2 = 0.042$	0.837^{NS}
	No	101 (12.6)	55 (12.8)	46 (12.3)		
Introduction of solid, semi-solid, or soft foods	Yes	70 (8.7)	37 (8.6)	33 (8.8)	$\chi^2 = 0.013$	0.910^{NS}
	No	730 (91.2)	391 (91.3)	339 (91.1)		
Minimum dietary diversity	Yes	41 (5.1)	23 (5.3)	18 (4.8)	$\chi^2 = 0.117$	0.732^{NS}
	No	759 (94.8)	405 (94.6)	354 (95.1)		
Minimum meal frequency	Yes	40 (5.0)	21 (4.9)	19 (5.1)	$\chi^2 = 0.017$	0.896^{NS}
	No	756 (94.5)	407 (95.0)	353 (94.8)		
Minimum acceptable diet	Yes	44 (5.5)	23 (5.3)	21 (5.6)	$\chi^2 = 0.028$	0.867^{NS}
	No	756 (94.5)	405 (94.6)	351 (94.3)		
Consumption of iron-rich or iron-fortified foods	Yes	714 (89.2)	379 (88.5)	335 (90.0)	$\chi^2 = 0.468$	0.494^{NS}
	No	86 (10.7)	49 (11.4)	37 (9.9)		

**Statistically significant ($p < 0.05$).*
^{NS}*Non-significant.*

Table 3.
Gender-wise association of children with infant and young child feeding practices (IYCF) core indicators.

Characteristics	Age (years)	N	Mean ± SD		
			All children	Boys	Girls
Excellent (7–8)	1–2	428	7.00 ± 0.00	7.00 ± 0.00	7.00 ± 0.00
Good (4–6)			4.05 ± 0.24	4.06 ± 0.27	4.04 ± 0.26
Poor (<4)			2.34 ± 0.48	2.33 ± 0.47	2.38 ± 0.51
Excellent (7–8)	2–3	372	7.00 ± 0.00	7.00 ± 0.00	7.00 ± 0.00
Good (4–6)			4.07 ± 0.28	4.06 ± 0.26	4.08 ± 0.30
Poor (<4)			2.45 ± 0.50	2.44 ± 0.51	2.45 ± 0.51
Excellent (7–8)	All children	800	7.00 ± 0.00	7.00 ± 0.00	7.00 ± 0.00
Good (4–6)			4.06 ± 0.26	4.06 ± 0.26	4.06 ± 0.25
Poor (<4)			2.40 ± 0.49	2.38 ± 0.49	2.43 ± 0.50

Table 4.
Age- and gender-wise mean infant and young child feeding practices (IYCF) scores of children.

Parameters	Variables	All children	Yes	No	Chi square	p-value
			N (%)			
Religion	Hindu	377 (47.1)	339 (42.3)	38 (4.7)	$\chi^2 = 0.74$	0.10[NS]
	Muslim	421 (52.6)	358 (44.7)	63 (7.8)		
	Sikh	2 (0.2)	2 (0.2)	00 (0.0)		
Type of family	Nuclear	538 (67.2)	488 (61.0)	70 (8.7)	$\chi^2 = 1.05$	0.58[NS]
	Joint	193 (24.1)	168 (21.0)	25 (3.1)		
	Extended	69 (8.6)	63 (7.8)	6 (0.7)		
Place of delivery	House	104 (13.0)	95 (11.8)	9 (1.1)	$\chi^2 = 1.70$	0.19[NS]
	Govt. hospital	696 (87.0)	604 (75.5)	92 (11.5)		
Birth order	First	150 (18.7)	133 (16.6)	17 (2.1)	$\chi^2 = 8.75$	0.03*
	Second	376 (47.0)	317 (39.6)	59 (7.3)		
	Third	188 (23.5)	167 (20.8)	21 (2.6)		
	Above third	86 (10.7)	82 (10.2)	4 (0.5)		
Education of mother	Illiterate	516 (64.5)	442 (55.2)	74 (9.2)	$\chi^2 = 4.38$	0.35[NS]
	Primary	216 (27.0)	197 (24.6)	19 (2.3)		
	Intermediate	29 (3.6)	26 (3.2)	3 (0.3)		
	High school	16 (2.0)	14 (1.7)	2 (0.2)		
	College	23 (2.8)	20 (2.5)	3 (0.3)		
Occupation of mother	Housewife	714 (89.2)	649 (81.1)	95 (11.8)	$\chi^2 = 4.72$	0.19[NS]
	Informal work	23 (2.8)	23 (2.8)	0 (00.0)		
	Own work	20 (2.5)	17 (2.1)	3 (0.3)		
	Formal	13 (1.6)	10 (1.2)	3 (0.3)		

*Statistically significant ($p < 0.05$).
[NS]Non-significant.

Table 5.
Background information of children associated with factors influencing continuation of breastfeeding up to 1 year.

IYCF. Further, amongst the children who were aged 2–3 years, 4.13% (n = 16) were boys and had a mean 2.44 ± 0.51 and 5.68% (n = 22) were girls who had a mean of 2.45 ± 0.51 reflecting the poor level of IYCF. Moreover, overall, 1.0% (n = 8) children exhibiting a mean intake 7.00 ± 0.0 showed an excellent level of IYCF and 90.62% (n = 725) exhibiting a mean of 4.06 ± 0.26 had a good level, whilst 8.37% (n = 67) showing mean 2.40 ± 0.49 had poor level of IYCF.

Table 5 shows the association of children's background information with factors influencing the continuation of breastfeeding for up to 1 year. From the results, no significant association was found amongst religion, type of family, place of delivery, education of mother, and occupation of the mother with factors influencing the continuation of breastfeeding for up to 1 year. Whereas, the birth order of the children was significantly found associated with factors, which were influencing the continuation of breastfeeding for up to 1 year.

5. Discussion

In the present study, primary breastfeeding introduction (within 60 minutes of birth) has been observed in 99.5% of children that is much greater than found in a report of the NFHS-5 [32] for India (42%) and Uttar Pradesh (23.9%). Another study revealed that the breastfeeding introduction by 85% mothers has been observed within 60 minutes or just after the birth. The intense increment in the number of mothers whose delivery was done at a health central is mainly caused by the persistent promotion of the free delivery services in the country resulting in a great chance for the health specialists to stimulate the breastfeeding introduction within 60 minutes of birth [33].

According to a study conducted by Gaurav et al. [34] on the children of less than 2 years of age in Uttar Pradesh, 65% of the subjects had initiated breastfeeding within an hour. The increment in the number of mothers adopting early breastfeeding could be because of the awareness and training of health workers related to health facilities and of public health workers related to several aspects of breastfeeding. Furthermore, it could also be because of greater number of births taking place in public health facilities. Another study by Patel et al. [35] showed that introduction of breastfeeding was primarily done by 57.5% of mothers in Gujarat.

About 94.3% of mothers who have children under the age of 6-months exclusively breastfed their infants. This practice is much higher compared to that reported by NFHS-5 [32] for Uttar Pradesh being 59.7%. This variation could be owing to the cultural and socioeconomic differences amongst the studied subjects.

In this study, most of the participants were housewives that can enhance the probability of breastfeeding to their child as it is less expensive when they have poor level of economic status. The proportion of the children was found 72.5%, which were absolutely breastfed; it has been confirmed by a report of NFHS-4 [36]. The prevalence of exclusive breastfeeding was found to be 75.0% [37]. The major cause for this observation could be the usual perception of mothers related to breast milk not being enough and needs to be supplemented with other milk sources such as animal or formula milk. Additionally, some of the mothers do not have proper knowledge about the accurate positioning and attachment to the breast that also results in hindering the practice of exclusive breastfeeding. Amongst the children of 6–12 months of age, 87.3% had continued breastfeeding up to 1 year. The percentage (72.1%) is nearly similar to a study conducted in Delhi [38] but lesser than the study of West Bengal in which 91.1% of the children of 12–23 months of age were breastfed till 1 year of age [39]. Another study conducted by Gupta et al. [40] reported that 71.5% of mothers continued breastfeeding for 1 year or more. The widely prevalent practices of extended breastfeeding in rural part of India must be protected. Only 8.7% mothers had knowledge about the complementary feeding of food such as liquid, semi-solid, and solid food must be started with breastfeeding after the age of 6-months. The children will vomit all after feeding, which was the common cause of the postponed complementary feeding. The ignorance has been found as another significant reason for the same. The enhancement in feeding practices was probable via appropriate utilization of current health facilities facilitating the mothers to appreciate the rationale of the practices so that worthy feeding practices could be continued [41].

Amongst the seven food groups utilized for assessing the minimum diversity, 5.5% of the children consumed foods from 4 or more groups in the present study. As observed in some other studies, a smaller number of children were receiving foods from four or more groups like 32.6% by Khan et al. [42], 30.0% by Das et al. [43], 15.7% by Chaudhary et al. [18], and 37.7% by Arzu et al. [44] respectively. Contrary to these studies, 79.6% children belonging to urban Meerut were having a diverse diet to desirable level [11]. Lower dietary diversity could be due to lack of knowledge and awareness related to appropriate complementary feeding habits in rural areas. Additionally, the lower socioeconomic status, excessive indulgence of mother in daily work activities, and lower birth gap may also be the causes of inadequate complementary feeding-related practices.

The minimum meal frequency observed in the present study was in 5% of children. This proportion was lesser in comparison to other studies such as 89.3% reported by Satija et al. [45]; 70.0% by Das et al. [43]; and 72.5% by Arzu et al. [44] respectively. The lowest meal frequency reported was 43.4% in a study conducted in urban Meerut by Singhal et al. [19]. The reason behind the lower percentage of minimum meal frequency in the present study could be because of the predominant consumption of animal milk as the major feed for the infants after the age of 6 months.

In the present study, minimum acceptable diet was given to 5.5% of children which was lesser than the report of the NFHS-5 [32] for India (11.1%) and Uttar Pardesh (6.1%). Another study [46] in West Bengal has shown that minimum acceptable diet was given to 7.5% of children due to the lack of postnatal counseling by the health workers as well as infrequent antenatal health clinics and maternal illiteracy. Contrary to these, two more findings were also reported by Das et al. [35] and Singhal et al. (19) who showed that 36.8% and 37.7% respectively of children received minimum acceptable diet which was much higher than the data of present study as well as data of NFHS-5 [32].

The prevalence related to good intake of iron-rich or iron-fortified foods in the present study is greater than the prevalence shown in other studies like 33.1% in Zambia, [47] 21.4% in Ethiopia [48], and 19.6% in Madagascar (19.6%) [49]. The difference in the results could be because of the variation seen in socioeconomic status, norms, beliefs, and cultural practices related to the feeding of children. Animal sources of foods are usually consumed only at the time of holidays in Ethiopia because of the reason that they are included as luxury foods in the diet and not to fulfill the daily requirements [50]. In this study done in rural Saharanpur, large proportion of subjects were non-vegetarians and, in these families, meat is cooked at least once in a week.

6. Conclusion

It could be concluded from the study that minimum dietary diversity, minimum meal frequency, and minimum acceptable diet are the core IYCF indicators that are least complied with. Most of the mothers adhered to early initiation of breastfeeding. This promising finding could be attributed to large number of deliveries taking place at hospitals/health centres against home deliveries which has long been a trend in rural India. Exclusive breastfeeding for 6 months was also practiced by the major part of the study population. It has been observed in India that in poor families, infants usually live on breastfeeding only. This practice, a boon for 6 months, becomes a detriment to infant growth and development as nearly one-thirds of the mothers comprising study group failed to initiate complementary feeding at 6 months of age. Poverty alleviation programmes, adult education programmes, and a more focused behavior change communication approach by Anganwadi workers hold the potential to enhancing the compliance to IYCF indicators.

Acknowledgements

We acknowledge the cooperation received from study participants, anganwadi workers, and the authorities of Uttar Pradesh who permitted to undertake the data collection.

Conflict of interest

None.

Author details

Monika Jain* and Vandana
Food Science and Nutrition Division, Banasthali Vidyapith, India

*Address all correspondence to: drmonikajain2000@gmail.com

References

[1] World Health Organization and UNICEF. Global Strategy for Infant and Young Child Feeding. Geneva: World Health Organization; 2003. Available from: http://apps.who.int/gb/archive/pdf files/WHASS/eassis.pdf

[2] Pan American Health Organization and World Health Organization. Guiding Principles for Complementary Feeding of the Breastfed Child. Washington, DC: Division of Health Promotion and Protection; 2003. Available from: http://www.who.int/nutrition/publications/guiding_principles_compfeeding_breastfed.pdf

[3] WHO. Guiding Principles for Feeding Non-breastfed Children 6-24 Months of Age. Geneva: World Health Organization; 2005. p. 40. Available from: https://www.who.int/maternal_child_adolesent/documents/9241593431/en/

[4] Park K. Park's Textbook of Preventive and Social Medicine. 21st ed. Jabalpur, India: M/S Banarsidas Bhanot; 2011

[5] Moore ER, Bergman N, Anderson GC, Medley N. Early skin-to-skin contact for mothers and their healthy newborn infants. Cochrane Database of Systematic Reviews. 2016;**11**:CD003519. DOI: 10.1002/14651858

[6] Martorell R, Kettel Khan L, Schroeder DG. Reversibility of stunting: Epidemiological findings in children from developing countries. European Journal of Clinical Nutrition. 1994;**58**(Suppl.1):45-57

[7] Black RE, Allen LH, Bhutta ZA, Caulfield LE, de Onis M, Ezzati M, et al. Maternal and child undernutrition: Global and regional exposures and health consequences. Lancet. 2008;**371**(9608):243-260. DOI: 10.1016/S0140-6736(07)61690-0

[8] Martorell R, Khan LK, Schroeder DG. Reversibility of stunting: Epidemiological findings in children from developing countries. European Journal of Clinical Nutrition. 1994;**48**(Suppl 1):S45-S57

[9] Pollitt E, Gorman KS, Engle PL, Rivera JA, Martorell R. Nutrition in early life and the fulfillment of intellectual potential. The Journal of Nutrition. 1995;**125**(4 Suppl):1111S-1118S. DOI: 10.1093/jn/125

[10] Grantham-McGregor SM, Cumper G. Jamaican studies in nutrition and child development, and their implications for national development. The Proceedings of the Nutrition Society. 1992;**51**(1):71-79. DOI: 10.1079/pns19920012

[11] Haas JD, Murdoch S, Rivera J, Martorell R. Early nutrition and later physical work capacity. Nutrition Reviews. 1996;**54**(2):41-48. DOI: 10.1111/j.1753-4887.1996.tb03869.x

[12] Bahl R, Frost C, Kirkwood BR, Edmond K, Martines J, Bhandari N, et al. Infant feeding patterns and risks of death and hospitalization in the first half of infancy: Multicentre cohort study. Bull World Health Organization. 2005;**83**(6):418-426

[13] Victora CG, Horta BL, Loret de Mola C, Quevedo L, Pinheiro RT, Gigante DP, et al. Association between breastfeeding and intelligence, educational attainment, and income at 30 years of age: A prospective birth cohort study from Brazil. Lancet Glob Health. 2015;**3**(4):e199-e205

[14] Baker EJ, Sanei LC, Franklin N. Early initiation of and exclusive breastfeeding

in large-scale community based programmes in Bolivia and Madagascar. Journal of Health, Population, and Nutrition. 2006;**24**(4):530-539

[15] Clark AB, Reijnierse EM, Lim WK, Maier AB. Prevalence of malnutrition comparing the GLIM criteria, ESPEN definition and MST malnutrition risk in geriatric rehabilitation patients: RESORT. Clinical Nutrition. 2020;**39**(11):3504-3511. DOI: 10.1016/j.clnu.2020.03.015

[16] Khandelwal S, Kondal D, Chakravarti AR, Dutta S, Banerjee B, Chaudhry M, et al. Infant and young child feeding practices in an Indian maternal-child birth cohort in Belagavi, Karnataka. International Journal of Environmental Research and Public Health. 2022;**19**(9):1-12. DOI: 10.3390/ijerph19095088

[17] Dafursa K, Gebremedhin S. Dietary diversity among children aged 6-23 months in Aleta Wondo District, Southern Ethiopia. Journal of Nutrition and Metabolism. Nov 2019;**13**:2869424. DOI: 10.1155/2019/2869424

[18] Chaudhary SR, Govil S, Lala MK, Yagnik HB. Infant and young child feeding index and its association with nutritional status: A cross-sectional study of urban slums of Ahmedabad. Journal of Family and Community Medicine. 2018;**25**(2):88-94. DOI: 10.4103/jfcm.JFCM_82_17

[19] Singhal P, Garg SK, Chopra H, Jain S, Bajpai SK, Kumar A. Status of infant and young child feeding practices with special emphasis on breastfeeding in an urban area of Meerut. Journal of Dental and Medical Sciences. 2013;7(4):7-11. DOI: 10.3126/ajms.v6i6.12067

[20] Black RE, Victora CG, Walker SP, Bhutta ZA, Christian P, De Onis M, et al. Maternal and child undernutrition and overweight in low-income and middle-income countries. The Lancet. 2013;**382**(9890):427-451. DOI: 10.1016/S0140-6736(13)60937-X

[21] Gupta V, Mohapatra D, Kumar V. Nutritional assessment among children (under five years of age) using various anthropometric indices in an urban area of district Rohtak, Haryana. India. International Journal of Business Research. 2015;**6**(9):629-633. DOI: 10.4103/IJCFM.IJCFM_14_19

[22] WHO. Infant and young child feeding: Model chapter for textbooks for medical students and allied health professionals. World Health Organization. 2009:1-4. Available from: http://www.who.int/iris/handle/10665/44117

[23] MHRD. Department of women and child development. Food and Nutrition Board. Government of India. National Guidelines on Infant and Young Child Feeding. 2006:7-8. Available from: https://wcd.nic.in/sites/default/files/nationalguidelines.pdf

[24] Jones RN. Global epidemiology of antimicrobial resistance among community-acquired and nosocomial pathogens: A five-year summary from the SENTARY antimicrobial surveillance program (1997-2001). Seminars in Respiratory and Critical Care Medicine. 2003;**24**(1):121-134. DOI: 10.1086/653053

[25] WHO. Global Strategy for Infant and Young Feeding. Geneva, Switzerland: World Health Organization; 2003. p. 133. Available from: http://apps.who.int/iris/bitstream/10665/42590/1/9241562218.pdf

[26] Sapra D, Ray S, Jindal AK, Patrikar S. Infant and young child feeding practices amongst children referred to the paediatric outpatient department.

Medical Journal, Armed Forces India. 2015;**71**(4):359-362. DOI: 10.1016/j.mjafi.2014.04.002

[27] Census 2011. Saharanpur District: Census 2011 Data. Available from: https://www.census2011.co.in/census/district/503-saharanpur.html [Accessed: December 5, 2017]

[28] ICMR. Indian Council of Medical Research. Handbook on National Ethical Guidelines for Biomedical and Health Research Involving Human Participants. New Delhi: Indian Council of Medical Research; 2018. pp. 1-170

[29] George PS, Murthy MN. Prevalence of undernutrition among preschool children (3-6 years) attending anganwadi centers in urban Mysuru. Indian Journal of Medical Specialities. 2021;**12**(3):127-131. DOI: 10.4103/injms.injms_11_21

[30] Nakel MP, Naval SS, Mahajan SM, Salve SB. Study of infant and young child feeding (IYCF) practices with reference to IYCF indicators among mothers attending immunization clinic at a tertiary care hospital, Aurangabad (MS). Indian Journal of Nutrition. 2018;**5**(2):188.1-188.5

[31] World Health Organization and UNICEF. Indicators for Assessing Infant and Young Child Feeding Practices: Part 1: Definitions: Conclusions of a Consensus Meeting held 6-8 November 2007 in Washington D.C; USA. USA: World Health Organization; 2008. Available form: https://apps.who.int/iris/handle/10665/43895

[32] NFHS-5. National Family Health Survey. India Fact Sheet [Internet]. Ministry of Health and Family Welfare. Mumbai, India: International Institute for Population Science; 2019-2021. Available from: http://rchiips.org/nfhs/factsheet_NFHS-5.shtml [Accessed: October 19, 2021]

[33] Demilew YM, Tafere TE, Abitew DB. Infant and young child feeding practice among mothers with 0-24 months old children in Slum areas of Bahir Dar city, Ethiopia. International Breastfeeding Journal. 2017;**12**(1):1-9. DOI: 10.1186/s13006-017-0117-x

[34] Gaurav GK, Kumar A, Garg SK, Singh G, Mittal C. Infant and young child feeding practices in rural Meerut U.P. Journal of Dental and Medical Sciences (IOSR-JDMS). 2019;**18**(5):32-40. DOI: 10.9790/0853-1805083240

[35] Patil CL, Turab A, Ambikapathi R, Nesamvni C, Chandyo RK, Bose A, et al. Early interruption of exclusive breastfeeding: Results from the eight-country MAL-ED study. Journal of Health, Population and Nutrition. 2015;**34**(10):1-10. DOI: 10.1186/s41043-015-0004-2

[36] NFHS-4. National Family Health Survey. India Fact Sheet. Ministry of Health and Family Welfare. Mumbai, India: International Institute for population Science; 2015-16. Available from: http://rchips.org./NFHS/nfhs3.html. [Accessed: December 20, 2017]

[37] Mahmood SE, Srivastava A, Shrotriya VP, Mishra PJ. Infant feeding practices in the rural population of north India. Family Community Medicine. 2012;**19**(2):130-135. DOI: 10.4103/2230-8229.9830

[38] Aggarwal A, Verma S, Faridi M, Dayachand. Complementary feeding-reasons for inappropriateness in timing, quantity and consistency. Indian Journal of Pediatrics. 2008;**75**(1):49-53. DOI: 10.1007/s12098-008-0006-9

[39] Sinhababu A, Mukhopadhyay DK, Panja TK, Saren AB, Mandal NK, Biswas AB. Infant-and young child-feeding practices in Bankura district,

West Bengal, India. Journal of Health, Population, and Nutrition. 2010;**28**(3):294-299. DOI: 10.3329/jhpn.v28i3.5559

[40] Gupta A, Sobti J, Rohde JE. Infant feeding practices among patients of pediatricians and general practitioners. Indian Journal of Pediatrics. 1992;**59**(2): 193-196. DOI: 10.1007/BF02759981

[41] Sethi V, Kashyap S, Seth V. Effect of nutrition education of mothers on infant feeding practices. Indian Journal of Pediatrics. 2003;**70**(6):463-466. DOI: 10.1007/BF02723133

[42] Khan AM, Kayina P, Agrawal P, Gupta A, Kannan AT. A study on infant and young child feeding practices among mothers attending an urban health center in East Delhi. Indian Journal of Public Health. 2012;**56**(4):300-304. DOI: 10.4103/0019-557X.106420

[43] Das N, Chattopadhyay D, Chakraborty S, Dasgupta A. Infant and young child feeding perceptions and practices among mothers in a rural area of West Bengal, India. Annals of Medical and Health Sciences Research. 2013;**3**(3):370-375. DOI: 10.4103/2141-9248.117955

[44] Arzu T, Sujan AK, Juliana FM, Hossain S. Study of IYCF indicators on practices and knowledge of mothers in rural areas. American Journal of Public Health Research. 2018;**6**(3):130-133. DOI: 10.12691/ajphr-6-3-1

[45] Satija M, Sharma S, Chaudhary A, Kaushal P, Girdhar S. Infant and young child feeding practices in a rural area of North India. Asian Journal of Medical Sciences. 2015;**6**(6):60-65. DOI: 10.3126/ajms. v6i6.12067

[46] Chakraborty S, Gupta SB, Chaturvedi B, Chakraborty SK. A study of protein energy malnutrition (PEM) in children (0 to 6 years) in a rural population of Jhansi district (U.P.). Indian Journal of Community Medicine. 2006;**31**(4):291-292

[47] Marinda PA, Genschick S, Khayeka-Wandabwa C, Kiwanuka-Lubinda R, Thilsted SH. Dietary diversity determinants and contribution of fish to maternal and under-five nutritional status in Zambia. PLoS One. 2018;**13**(9):1-18. DOI: 10.1371/journal.pone.020400

[48] Tiruneh DT, Weldeslassie AG, Kassa A, Tefera Z, De Cock M, Elen J. Systematic design of a learning environment for domain-specific and domain-general critical thinking skills. Educational Technology Research and Development. 2016;**64**(3):481-405. DOI: 10.1007/s11423-015-9417-2

[49] Rakotomanana H, Gates GE, Hildebrand D, Stoecker BJ. Situation and determinants of the infant and young child feeding (IYCF) indicators in Madagascar: Analysis of the 2009 demographic and health survey. BMC Public Health. 2017;**17**(1):812-821. DOI: 10.1186/s12889-017-4835-1

[50] Haileselassie M, Redae G, Berhe G, Henry CJ, Nickerson MT, Tyler B, et al. Why are animal source foods rarely consumed by 6-23 months old children in rural communities of Northern Ethiopia? A qualitative study. PLoS One. 2020;**15**(1):1-21. DOI: 10.1371/journal.pone.0225707

Chapter 9

Suboptimal Child Feeding and Its Determinants

Nega Degefa

Abstract

Inappropriate feeding during the early childhood period plays a detrimental role in the child's growth, development, and overall health. Some of these are suboptimal feeding practices, which have a negative impact on a child's nutritional status and well-being. Suboptimal child feeding is a common problem in developing countries, despite the efforts that have been made to address it. This book chapter explores the determinants of suboptimal child feeding and identifies the various factors that contribute to it among caregivers. By reviewing existing literature and the author's prior work, the chapter provides comprehensive insights into suboptimal feeding during childhood and its contributing factors. The book chapter reviews recent research on suboptimal child feeding practices and contributing factors. It also presents the findings and interprets the researcher's own work on the topic. The chapter highlights the importance of the research findings in enriching the existing body of knowledge and informing future research in the field. It also concludes that a multidimensional approach is needed to address the socioeconomic, maternal, family, and environmental factors that contribute to suboptimal child-feeding practices. This approach will help to ensure better health outcomes for children.

Keywords: suboptimal child feeding, child feeding practices, determinants, breastfeeding, complementary feeding

1. Introduction

In this book chapter, the author summarizes their own research findings, as well as the findings of other studies, on the topic of suboptimal child feeding practices and their determinants. A detailed explanation of suboptimal child feeding practices and their contributing factors is provided.

Suboptimal child feeding practices are becoming increasingly important because they can significantly impact a child's health and well-being. In the early years of life, children's brains and bodies are rapidly developing, and they need the right nutrients to support this growth and development. Suboptimal feeding practices can lead to nutrient deficiencies, which can have long-lasting consequences for a child's health [1, 2].

Suboptimal child feeding is a serious problem that can have several negative consequences for children's health and development. The determinants of suboptimal child feeding can be categorized into three main groups: maternal factors, socio-economic factors, and environmental factors [3]. Suboptimal child feeding can lead to several health problems, including undernutrition, overweight and obesity, iron deficiency anemia, and vitamin A deficiency [2]. The topic of suboptimal child feeding is relevant, important, and timely because it has a significant impact on children's health and development.

In this book chapter, suboptimal child feeding is defined as any deviation from the World Health Organization's (WHO) optimal feeding recommendations, which include early initiation of breastfeeding within one hour of birth, appropriate complementary feeding at 6 months of age, and continuation of breastfeeding for up to 2 years or beyond. However, many infants and children do not receive optimal feeding. For example, only about 44% of infants aged 0–6 months worldwide were exclusively breastfed over the period of 2015–2020 [4].

The main issues and challenges related to suboptimal child feeding include lack of awareness, limited access to healthy foods, and cultural beliefs. There are several approaches that can be considered to address the issue of suboptimal child feeding, including educating parents about the importance of good nutrition, providing families with access to healthy foods, and challenging cultural beliefs about breastfeeding and complementary feeding [2].

The purpose of this chapter is to provide an overview of suboptimal child feeding practices and their determinants by exploring the author's own work as well as the work of others on the topic. This will help to depict the scope of the problem, the attempts that have been made to resolve it, and the future direction of research and interventions to improve child feeding and well-being.

The chapter begins by defining suboptimal child feeding and discussing the different factors that can contribute to it. The chapter then discusses the significance of suboptimal child feeding, highlighting the fact that it can lead to several health problems, including undernutrition, overweight and obesity, iron deficiency anemia, and vitamin A deficiency. The chapter then discusses the key challenges associated with improving child-feeding practices. The chapter then discusses some interventions that can be used to improve child-feeding practices.

The chapter concludes by noting that suboptimal child feeding is a complex problem with no easy solutions. However, by understanding the determinants of the problem and the key challenges associated with it, we can develop effective interventions to improve child-feeding practices and improve the health and development of children.

The chapter does not attempt to cover all aspects of the topic of suboptimal child feeding thoroughly. However, it provides a comprehensive overview of the topic and offers insights that can be used to improve child-feeding practices.

2. Definition of optimal breastfeeding

WHO and UNICEF recommend that optimal breastfeeding includes:

- Early initiation of breastfeeding within 1 hour of birth.
- Exclusive breastfeeding for the first 6 months of life, meaning no other foods or liquids are provided, including water.
- Introduction of nutritionally adequate and safe complementary (solid) foods at 6 months together with continued breastfeeding up to 2 years of age or beyond [4].

Below are listed some of the benefits of optimal breastfeeding.

- Protects babies from infections.
- Provides babies with all the nutrients they need for their first 6 months of life.
- Helps babies develop a healthy gut microbiome.
- Reduces the risk of obesity and chronic diseases later in life.
- Promotes bonding between mothers and babies.

Not all mothers can exclusively breastfeed for 6 months. However, they can still provide their babies with many of the benefits of breastfeeding by breastfeeding as often as possible and for as long as they are able.

2.1 Definition of suboptimal child feeding

Suboptimal child feeding refers to any feeding practices that deviate from the World Health Organization's (WHO) recommendations for children aged 0–2 years. These practices include delaying the initiation of breastfeeding, introducing formula or other liquids before 6 months of age, stopping breastfeeding before 2 years of age, and inadequate feeding. Suboptimal child feeding is considered when these practices occur [4].

Suboptimal breastfeeding is when infants do not receive the recommended amount of breast milk. There are two main risk factors for suboptimal breastfeeding: not breastfeeding exclusively for the first 6 months of life, and stopping breastfeeding before the age of two [5].

2.2 Types of suboptimal child feeding

Based on how the feeding approach deviates from the World Health Organization's (WHO) recommendations for optimal child feeding, suboptimal child feeding can be classified into the following:

A. Delayed initiation of breastfeeding is a condition in which a baby is not put to the breast within the first hour of birth. This is contrary to the World Health Organization's (WHO) recommendation, which states that all babies should be breastfed within the first hour of life. Delayed initiation of breastfeeding is critical because it can deprive the baby of the essential colostrum, which is the first milk produced by the mother. Colostrum is high in antibodies and nutrients, and it provides the baby with important protection against infection. Delayed initiation of breastfeeding can also make it more difficult for the mother and baby to establish a good breastfeeding pattern [6, 7].

B. Non-exclusive breastfeeding before 6 months refers to the introduction of any foods or fluids before the age of 6 months. The World Health Organization (WHO) recommends exclusive breastfeeding for the first 6 months of a child's life, meaning that the infant receives only breast milk without any additional food or liquids (except for oral rehydration salts, drops, or syrups of vitamins, minerals, or medicines as needed).

C. Early cessation of breastfeeding is the discontinuation of breastfeeding before the child reaches the age of 2 years. The World Health Organization (WHO) recommends that mothers continue to breastfeed their children until at least 2 years of age or beyond, along with the introduction of nutritionally adequate and safe complementary foods.

There are many benefits to breastfeeding for both the mother and the child. Breastfeeding helps to protect the child from infection, allergies, and obesity. It also helps to promote the development of the child's brain and immune system. For mothers, breastfeeding can help to reduce the risk of postpartum depression and cancer.

D. Inadequate breastfeeding is a condition in which a child does not receive enough breast milk. This can happen for a variety of reasons, including poor latch, insufficient milk supply, incorrect breastfeeding techniques, or maternal issues. Inadequate breastfeeding can lead to poor infant nutrition and growth. Inadequate breastfeeding can lead to poor infant nutrition and growth. A child who is not getting enough breast milk may be more likely to experience weight loss, growth delays, and other health problems. Our study supports this finding, showing that poor latch can lead to inadequate feeding of the child. This is because a poor latch can make it difficult for the baby to suck effectively, which can lead to them not getting enough milk [8].

E. Inappropriate breastfeeding practices: These include feeding infants with bottles, teats, or pacifiers, which can interfere with proper breastfeeding techniques and reduce milk supply. Study have also suggested that exposure of infants to artificial nipples (bottle feeding) has been strongly associated with breastfeeding problems [9]. This is because artificial nipples are easier for infants to suck on than the breast. As a result, infants may prefer the bottle and may not be as motivated to breastfeed.

Our work on the introduction of Prelacteal feeding, a form of suboptimal feeding, has shown that a significant number of mothers (16.8%) introduced Prelacteal feeds within the first 3 days after birth [10]. This means that one in every six newborns receives some form of Prelacteal food or fluid. This can lead to improper establishment of breastfeeding and a decreased likelihood of achieving effective suckling, which can result in poor disease protection and frequent infection.

Another study on breastfeeding practices that assessed the positioning and attachment of mothers during breastfeeding found that poor attachment and positioning were observed among a notable proportion of mother [8]. This is the single most important cause of inadequate breastfeeding. This has a significant impact on the health of the child, and it raises the need to reconsider the approach to enhancing maternal counseling during the postnatal period to improve effective feeding and prevent the child from illness.

A study by the authors found that even among caregivers of sick children, inappropriate feeding practices were observed. This is even though there are well-established recommendations to increase feeding during and after common childhood illnesses [11]. This finding suggests how deeply rooted the problem of suboptimal feeding practices is. The study's findings highlight the importance of interventions that address the underlying determinants of feeding practices during illness to ultimately improve children's well-being.

3. Determinants of suboptimal child feeding

Determinants of suboptimal breastfeeding can vary across different populations and contexts. Several factors have been identified through research and evidence that contribute to suboptimal breastfeeding rates.

Our study on Prelacteal feeding found that mothers' knowledge of breastfeeding, exposure to counseling on optimal breastfeeding during antenatal care (ANC) follow-up, and receipt of immediate postnatal care were predictors of suboptimal feeding in the form of Prelacteal feeding. These findings emphasize the importance of considering a wide range of participants, including mothers with poor knowledge about breastfeeding, who have no exposure to counseling on breastfeeding, and those without immediate postnatal care [10].

Studies have shown that mothers who lack accurate information about breastfeeding may face difficulties in establishing and maintaining breastfeeding. This is because they may not know how to deal with challenges such as not knowing the benefits of breastfeeding, not knowing how to properly latch their babies, and not knowing how to manage common breastfeeding challenges. This lack of knowledge can lead to mothers giving up on breastfeeding early. Therefore, it is important for mothers to have access to accurate information about breastfeeding. This information can help them to overcome challenges and breastfeeding successfully [12, 13].

Accurate information and support are essential for mothers to make informed decisions about breastfeeding and breastfeed successfully. Societal and cultural norms, beliefs, and practices can influence breastfeeding rates, and negative attitudes and practices can hinder optimal breastfeeding practices. In short, mothers need the right information and support to breastfeed successfully, and society should foster a supportive environment for breastfeeding [14].

The support and practices within the healthcare system can significantly impact breastfeeding outcomes. Factors such as limited access to skilled lactation support, inconsistent advice from healthcare professionals, and inadequate postpartum care can contribute to suboptimal breastfeeding [15].

Maternal employment status also affects breastfeeding. Returning to work shortly after childbirth without supportive policies, such as paid maternity leave, flexible work arrangements, and dedicated breastfeeding spaces, can create challenges for mothers who wish to continue breastfeeding [16].

Marketing and availability of formula milk: Aggressive marketing of infant formula and the easy availability of formula milk products can influence maternal decisions and undermine exclusive breastfeeding.

Studies have shown that social support is a critical factor that affects breastfeeding. Lack of support from family members, partners, and the broader community can make breastfeeding more challenging for mothers. Lack of understanding, unsupportive attitudes, and limited assistance with household chores and childcare can worsen breastfeeding rates [17, 18].

Maternal physical and mental health are important factors that can interfere with successful child feeding practices. Issues such as difficulties with breastfeeding due to pain or insufficient milk supply, postpartum depression, or stress can negatively affect the initiation and maintenance of breastfeeding [19, 20].

Inappropriate use of complementary foods is the most common determinant of suboptimal breastfeeding. For example, introducing complementary foods too early, before the recommended age of 6 months, can reduce breastfeeding duration as well as exclusivity.

4. The impact of suboptimal child feeding

The global prevalence of suboptimal child feeding is high. According to the World Health Organization (WHO), about 44% of infants under 6 months are exclusively breastfed. Additionally, many children are fed unhealthy diets that are high in processed foods and low in nutrient-rich foods. Few children receive nutritionally adequate and safe complementary foods; in many countries less than a fourth of infants 6–23 months of age meet the criteria of dietary diversity and feeding frequency that are appropriate for their age [4].

In Africa, about 37% of infants under 6 months of age were exclusively breastfed in 2017 [21]. In Ethiopia, only 59% of infants under 6 months are exclusively breastfed. Contrary to the WHO recommendation that children under age 6 months should be exclusively breastfed, 14% of infants 0–5 months also consume plain water, 1% of them consume non-milk liquids, 8% consume other milk, and 13% consume complementary foods in addition to breast milk (**Figure 1**). Notably, 6% of infants under age 6 months are not breastfed at all [22].

Suboptimal breastfeeding can have various negative impacts on child health. Breast milk is the optimal source of nutrition for infants and provides a wide range of essential nutrients and antibodies that support their growth and development. When breastfeeding is suboptimal or not practiced at all, it can lead to the following consequences for child health.

In 2019, suboptimal breastfeeding was associated with 2.8% (95% uncertainty interval (UI) 2.1–3.5) of disability-adjusted life years (DALYs) among children under

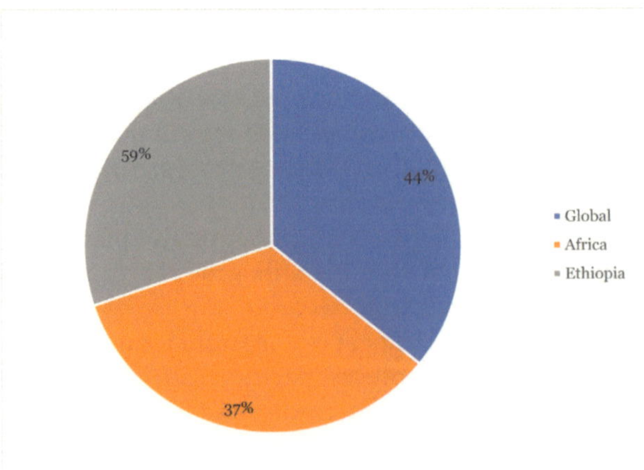

Figure 1.
Proportion of infants under 6 months who are exclusively breastfed.

5 years of age. This means that suboptimal breastfeeding was responsible for 2.8% of the total burden of disease in children under 5 years of age.

Suboptimal breastfeeding was also associated with 146,000 under-5 deaths (95% UI 104,000–197,000) in 2019. This means that suboptimal breastfeeding was responsible for 146,000 deaths of children under 5 years of age in 2019.

The burden of suboptimal breastfeeding is significant, and it is important to take steps to improve breastfeeding practices in order to reduce the number of deaths and DALYs associated with this problem [5].

Evidence shows that suboptimal breastfeeding increases the risk of infections in infants [23–25]. This is because breast milk contains high levels of antibodies and immune-boosting substances that help protect infants against various infections, including respiratory and gastrointestinal infections. Suboptimal breastfeeding, on the other hand, impedes these protective substances, leaving infants more susceptible to illnesses and with a higher risk of developing infections.

Suboptimal breastfeeding unquestionably leads to nutritional deficiencies among infants. Breast milk is the main and initial source of nutrients for infants, and it is uniquely tailored to meet their nutritional needs. It provides an ideal balance of proteins, fats, carbohydrates, vitamins, and minerals. When infants are not fed optimally, they may not acquire all the necessary nutrients for their growth and development, leading to nutritional deficiencies and associated health problems [1, 26].

Increased risk of chronic diseases: Studies have shown that suboptimal breastfeeding is associated with a higher risk of developing chronic diseases later in life. These include conditions such as obesity, type 2 diabetes, asthma, allergies, and certain types of cancers. Breastfeeding provides long-term health benefits that can help reduce the incidence of these diseases [27].

Impaired cognitive development: Breast milk contains essential fatty acids, such as docosahexaenoic acid (DHA), which are critical for brain development. Infants who are not breastfed or receive suboptimal breastfeeding may have a higher risk of impaired cognitive development, including lower intelligence quotient (IQ) scores and decreased academic performance.

Increased risk of obesity: Breastfeeding has been shown to play a role in preventing childhood obesity. Suboptimal breastfeeding, particularly when combined with early introduction of solid foods or the use of formula, may increase the risk of obesity in childhood and later in life [28, 29].

Emotional and psychological impacts: Breastfeeding promotes a strong emotional bond between mother and child. It provides comfort, security, and a sense of closeness, which contributes to the child's emotional well-being. Lack of breastfeeding or suboptimal breastfeeding practices may affect the mother-child bonding and emotional development of the child [30].

It is important to note that while breastfeeding is highly beneficial, some mothers may face challenges or circumstances that prevent them from breastfeeding exclusively. In such cases, alternative feeding methods should be adopted to ensure the infant receives adequate nutrition. Consulting with healthcare professionals and lactation specialists can provide guidance and support to address any breastfeeding difficulties and ensure the best possible outcomes for the child health.

Protecting, promoting, and supporting breastfeeding will save more lives of babies and children than any other single preventive intervention. Globally, exclusive and continued breastfeeding could help prevent 13% of deaths among children under 5 years old. Breastfed children have fewer childhood infections, fewer chronic diseases,

3–5 extra points of IQ, higher earning potential, more opportunities to prioritize education, and healthier mothers. Breastfeeding reduces burdens on society in terms of health spending, hospitalizations, and absenteeism. It also saves families money because it obviates the need for commercial substitutes [31].

5. Interventions and strategies

Suboptimal child feeding practices can have long-term consequences on a child's health and development. To address these issues, various interventions and strategies can be implemented. Here are some approaches that can help reduce suboptimal child-feeding practices:

Nutrition education: Providing parents, caregivers, and communities with accurate and practical information on infant and child nutrition is crucial. This education can focus on topics such as breastfeeding, introducing complementary foods, nutrient requirements, portion sizes, and the importance of a balanced diet [32].

Breastfeeding support: Promote and support exclusive breastfeeding for the first 6 months of a child's life, as recommended by the World Health Organization (WHO). This can involve training healthcare providers and establishing lactation support programs to assist mothers with breastfeeding challenges [4].

Complementary feeding guidance: Educate caregivers on the appropriate timing and methods for introducing complementary foods to infants around 6 months of age. Emphasize the importance of nutrient-rich and diverse foods, proper food preparation, and responsive feeding practices.

Peer support and counseling: Establish support groups, mother-to-mother networks, or community health workers to provide guidance, encouragement, and practical advice on optimal child feeding practices. Peer support can be particularly effective in promoting behavior change [15].

Food affordability and accessibility: Addressing economic barriers to accessing nutritious foods is essential. Implement strategies such as social protection programs, agricultural development initiatives, and market interventions to improve affordability and availability of nutrient-rich foods for families [33, 34].

Parenting programs: Incorporate child feeding and nutrition education into existing parenting programs. These programs can provide comprehensive support on various aspects of childcare, including feeding practices, responsive feeding, meal planning, and portion control [35].

Quality healthcare services: Strengthen healthcare systems to provide quality services related to child nutrition and feeding practices. Ensure that healthcare providers are trained in evidence-based guidelines, and that they offer consistent and accurate counseling to parents and caregivers [36].

Policy and advocacy: Advocate for policy changes that support optimal child feeding practices. This can include regulations on marketing of unhealthy foods, mandatory labeling of nutritional information, and workplace policies that support breastfeeding and parental leave [37].

Monitoring and evaluation: Establish mechanisms to monitor and evaluate the effectiveness of interventions and strategies aimed at reducing suboptimal child feeding practices. Regular assessments and data collection can help identify gaps and refine approaches for better outcomes [38].

6. Gaps in knowledge and future directions

Despite progress, there are still gaps in knowledge and areas that require further attention in addressing suboptimal child feeding practices. These gaps include:

Cultural influences: A deeper understanding of cultural influences on feeding behaviors is needed to develop culturally appropriate interventions.

Behavior change strategies: Effective behavior change strategies that can be implemented at the individual, family, and community levels need to be identified.

Critical periods and long-term effects: Critical periods during early childhood when specific feeding practices have the greatest impact on long-term health outcomes need to be investigated. Longitudinal studies are needed to understand the long-term effects of suboptimal feeding practices.

Socioeconomic determinants: Complex relationships between socioeconomic status, food security, and feeding behaviors need to be understood to inform targeted interventions.

Technology-based interventions: The potential of technology in delivering child-feeding interventions needs to be explored.

Male involvement: Fathers and male caregivers need to be engaged to promote their active involvement in child feeding decisions and practices.

Policy interventions and environmental factors: The impact of policy interventions needs to be assessed, and environmental factors such as the availability of healthy foods need to be explored to inform strategies to create supportive environments for optimal child feeding.

International partnerships: Collaboration among researchers, practitioners, policymakers, and communities worldwide needs to be promoted to facilitate knowledge sharing, exchange of best practices, and scaling up effective interventions.

7. Conclusion

Suboptimal child feeding is a widespread problem with serious consequences for children's health and development. However, there are effective interventions that can help parents and caregivers provide their children with nutritious and balanced diets. These interventions include nutrition education, breastfeeding support, complementary feeding guidance, peer support, and parenting programs. Comprehensive interventions must address food affordability and accessibility, healthcare services, and supportive policies. It is also important to recognize the cultural context of different communities, conduct further research, and address gaps in knowledge to tailor interventions to the specific needs and challenges of each community.

Future efforts should focus on understanding the cultural influences on child feeding practices, identifying effective ways to change feeding behaviors, investigating the long-term effects of different feeding practices, addressing socioeconomic factors that affect feeding practices, exploring the use of technology to improve feeding practices, promoting male involvement in feeding practices, and implementing policy and environmental changes to improve feeding practices. Collaboration, knowledge sharing, and international partnerships will be essential for developing evidence-based interventions and scaling them up globally.

Acknowledgements

I am grateful to Intech Open, an open-access publisher of books and journals, for inviting me to contribute to this chapter. I would also like to thank Mr. Kristian Josic, the publishing process manager, for his unwavering support and guidance throughout the development of this chapter.

Conflict of interest

The author declares no conflict of interest.

Accronyms and abbrevaition

WHO	World health organization
IQ	intelligence quotient
DALY	disability-adjusted life years

Author details

Nega Degefa
Arba Minch University, Arba Minch, Ethiopia

*Address all correspondence to: nega.degefu@amu.edu.et

References

[1] Ersino G, Henry CJ, Zello GA. Suboptimal feeding practices and high levels of undernutrition among infants and young children in the rural communities of Halaba and Zeway, Ethiopia. Food and Nutrition Bulletin. 2016;**37**(3):409-424

[2] UNICEF. Early childhood nutrition: Preventing malnutrition in infants and young children. 2023. Available from: https://www.unicef.org/nutrition/early-childhood-nutrition#:~:text=Poor%20diets%20in%20early%20childhood%20can%20lead%20toto%20death%20from%20common%20childhood%20diseases%20like%20diarrhoea

[3] Geda NR, Feng CX, Janzen B, Lepnurm R, Henry CJ, Whiting SJ. Infant and young child feeding practices in Ethiopia: Analysis of socioeconomic disparities based on nationally representative data. Archives of Public Health. 2021;**79**:1-10

[4] World Health Organization. Infant and young child feeding. 2021. Available from: https://www.who.int/news-room/fact-sheets/detail/infant-and-young-child-feeding#:~:text=WHO%20and%20UNICEF%20recommend%3A%201%20early%20initiation%20ofup%20to%202%20years%20of%20age%20or%20beyond

[5] Global Burden of Disease. Suboptimal breastfeeding. 2019. Available from: https://www.healthdata.org/results/gbd_summaries/2019/suboptimal-breastfeeding-level-3-risk

[6] Sundaram ME, Labrique AB, Mehra S, Ali H, Shamim AA, Klemm RD, et al. Early neonatal feeding is common and associated with subsequent breastfeeding behavior in rural Bangladesh. The Journal of Nutrition. 2013;**143**(7):1161-1167

[7] Patil CL, Turab A, Ambikapathi R, Nesamvuni C, Chandyo RK, Bose A, et al. Early interruption of exclusive breastfeeding: Results from the eight-country MAL-ED study. Journal of Health Population and Nutrition. 2015;**34**(1):1-10

[8] Degefa N, Tariku B, Bancha T, Amana G, Hajo A, Kusse Y, et al. Breast Feeding Practice: Positioning and Attachment during Breast Feeding among Lactating Mothers Visiting Health Facility in Areka Town, Southern Ethiopia. Iran: Mashhad University of Medical Science; 2019

[9] Kebebe T, Assaye H. Intention, magnitude and factors associated with bottle feeding among mothers of 0-23 months old children in Holeta town, Central Ethiopia: A cross sectional study. BMC Nutrition. 2017;**3**(1):53

[10] Megersa N, Tariku EZ, Yesera G, Gutema BJSAJoCH. Prevalence of prelacteal feeding and its associated factors among mothers of under-24-month-old children at Arba Minch Zuria District, Ethiopia: A cross-sectional study. South African Journal of Child Health. 2021;**15**(2):112-117

[11] Degefa N, Tadesse H, Aga F, Yeheyis T. Sick Child Feeding Practice and Associated Factors among Mothers of Children Less than 24 months Old, Burayu Town, Ethiopia. Iran: Mashhad University of Medical Science; 2019

[12] Hoche S, Meshesha B, Wakgari N. Sub-optimal breastfeeding and its associated factors in rural

communities of Hula District, southern Ethiopia: A cross-sectional study. Ethiopian Journal of Health Sciences. 2018;**28**(1):49-62

[13] Tamiru D, Belachew T, Loha E, Mohammed S. Sub-optimal breastfeeding of infants during the first six months and associated factors in rural communities of Jimma Arjo Woreda, Southwest Ethiopia. BMC Public Health. 2012;**12**(1):363

[14] Chakona G. Social circumstances and cultural beliefs influence maternal nutrition, breastfeeding and child feeding practices in South Africa. Nutrition Journal. 2020;**19**(1):47

[15] Center for Disease Control and Prevention. Supporting evidence: Maternity care practices. 2021. Available from: https://www.cdc.gov/breastfeeding/data/mpinc/supporting-evidence.html

[16] Chen J, Xin T, Gaoshan J, Li Q, Zou K, Tan S, et al. The association between work related factors and breastfeeding practices among Chinese working mothers: A mixed-method approach. International Breastfeeding Journal. 2019;**14**(1):1-13

[17] Raj VK, Plichta SB. The role of social support in breastfeeding promotion: A literature review. Journal of Human Lactation. 1998;**14**(1):41-45

[18] Baño-Piñero I, Martínez-Roche ME, Canteras-Jordana M, Carrillo-García C, Orenes-Piñero E. Impact of support networks for breastfeeding: A multicentre study. Women and Birth. 2018;**31**(4):e239-ee44

[19] Chee Din MA, Mohd Fahmi Teng NI, Abdul MZ. Maternal depression and child feeding practices: Determinants to malnutrition among young children in Malaysian rural area. Women's Health. 2023;**19**:17455

[20] Woldetensay YK, Belachew T, Ghosh S, Kantelhardt EJ, Biesalski HK, Scherbaum V. The effect of maternal depressive symptoms on infant feeding practices in rural Ethiopia: Community based birth cohort study. International Breastfeeding Journal. 2021;**16**(1):27

[21] Mekebo GG, Argawu AS, Likassa HT, Ayele W, Wake SK, Bedada D, et al. Factors influencing exclusive breastfeeding practice among under-six months infants in Ethiopia. BMC Pregnancy and Childbirth. 2022;**22**(1):630

[22] Federal Democratic Republic of Ethiopia-Ministry of Health. The Ethiopia mini demographic and health survey. 2019. Available from: https://www.unicef.org/ethiopia/reports/2019-ethiopia-mini-demographic-and-health-survey

[23] Hajeebhoy N, Nguyen PH, Mannava P, Nguyen TT, Mai LT. Suboptimal breastfeeding practices are associated with infant illness in Vietnam. International Breastfeeding Journal. 2014;**9**(1):12

[24] Abdulla F, Hossain MM, Karimuzzaman M, Ali M, Rahman AJPO. Likelihood of infectious diseases due to lack of exclusive breastfeeding among infants in Bangladesh. PLos One. 2022;**17**(2):e0263890

[25] Sharma R, Sood A, Nair PJ. Infant feeding practices and risk of occurrence of diarrheal and respiratory infections in infancy-a hospital based study. International Journal of Contemporary Pediatrics. 2017;**4**(5):1717-1720

[26] Oot L, Sethuraman K, Ross J, Sommerfelt A. The effect of suboptimal

breastfeeding on preschool overweight/obesity: A model in profiles for country-level advocacy. 2017

[27] Organization PAH, Organization WH. Breastfeeding and complementary feeding. 2019. Available from: https://www.paho.org/en/topics/breastfeeding-and-complementary-feeding#:~:text=Women%20who%20breastfeed%20compared%20with%20women%20who%20don%E2%80%99tand%20a%2037%25%20lower%20risk%20of%20ovarian%20cancer

[28] Scherbaum V, Srour ML. The role of breastfeeding in the prevention of childhood malnutrition. World Review of Nutrition and Dietetics. 2016;**115**:82-97

[29] Rito AI, Buoncristiano M, Spinelli A, Salanave B, Kunešová M, Hejgaard T, et al. Association between characteristics at birth, breastfeeding and obesity in 22 countries: The WHO European childhood obesity surveillance initiative–COSI 2015/2017. Obesity Facts. 2019;**12**(2):226-243

[30] Care BH. Breastfeeding and bonding. 2018. Available from: https://breastpumps.byramhealthcare.com/blog/2018/11/23/breastfeeding-bonding

[31] World Health Organization. Protecting, supporting and promoting breastfeeding. 2022. Available from: https://www.who.int/westernpacific/activities/protecting-supporting-and-promoting-breastfeeding

[32] Dattilo AM, Saavedra JM. Nutrition education: Application of theory and strategies during the first 1,000 days for healthy growth. In: Nutrition Education: Strategies for Improving Nutrition and Healthy Eating in Individuals and Communities. Switzerland: Karger Publishers; 2020. pp. 1-18

[33] Lee A, Mhurchu CN, Sacks G, Swinburn B, Snowdon W, Vandevijvere S, et al. Monitoring the price and affordability of foods and diets globally. Obesity Reviews. 2013;**14**(Suppl. 1):82-95

[34] Development WBCfS. Food affordability – The role of the food industry in providing affordable, nutritious foods to support healthy and sustainable diets. 2022. Available from: https://www.wbcsd.org/Programs/Food-and-Nature/Food-Land-Use/FReSH/Resources/Food-Affordability-The-role-of-the-food-industry-in-providing-affordable-nutritious-foods-to-support-healthy-and-sustainable-diets

[35] Daniels LA. Feeding practices and parenting: A pathway to child health and family happiness. Annals of Nutrition & Metabolism. 2019;**74**(Suppl. 2):29-42

[36] World Health Organization. Quality health services. 2020. Available from: https://www.who.int/news-room/fact-sheets/detail/quality-health-services

[37] Michaud-Létourneau I, Gayard M, Pelletier DL. Strengthening advocacy and policy change for infant and young child feeding. Maternal & Child Nutrition. 2019;**15**(Suppl. 2):e12749

[38] Bamberger JM, Clark M, Sartorius R. Monitoring and evaluation: Some tools, methods, and approaches: The World Bank. 2009. Available from: http://documents.worldbank.org/curated/en/829171468180901329/Monitoring-and-evaluation-some-tools-methods-and-approaches

Section 3

Infant Nutrition and Feeding for Infants with Special Problems

Chapter 10

Premature Infant Care and Feeding

Enos Mirembe Masereka, Clement Munguiko, Linda Grace Alanyo, Kenyonyozi Rubagumya, Brenda Nabawanuka, Julian Aryampa, Alex Tumusiime and Emmanuel Kimera

Abstract

The burden of premature birth is still high worldwide at 10.6% and ranges from 5 to 18% of all babies born. About 80% of these occur in Africa and South Asia. In Sub-Saharan Africa, the burden ranges from 3.4 to 49.4%. In almost all countries, premature birth rates are on increase, which poses a threat to newborn health. Premature babies usually present with complications that hinder their ability to feed. Due to this, premature babies are at risk of insufficient nutrient supply, leading to undernutrition, failure to thrive and early newborn deaths. However, improved newborn feeding can avert these deaths. In line with this noble cause, this chapter focused on care and feeding of premature babies in hospital and home settings, feeding development, feeding difficulties, and growth and development monitoring for premature babies.

Keywords: premature, infant, nutrition, care, feeding

1. Introduction

A premature baby is one who is born alive before 37 weeks of pregnancy [1, 2]. The burden of premature birth is still high worldwide at 10.6% and ranges from 5 to 18% of all babies born [2]. About 80% of these occur in Africa and South Asia [1, 3]. In Sub-Saharan Africa, the burden ranges from 3.4 to 49.4% [4] and is highest in Malawi with 18.1 premature births per 100 births, Comoros (16.7), Congo (16.7), Zimbabwe (16.6), Equatorial Guinea (16.5), Mozambique (16.4), Gabon (16.3), and Mauritania (15.4) [1]. Recent demographic and health surveys of Sub-Saharan African countries showed that Eastern Africa and Southern Africa as well were likely to register high premature births with 7.34 and 11.19%, respectively [5]. Most of the body systems of premature babies are usually not fully developed. As a result, they require support in the majority of aspects of life, including their feeding. If the support rendered is insufficient, they are more likely to have complications such as feeding difficulties, micronutrient deficiencies, and poor growth and development. Due to this, premature babies are at great risk of death compared to babies born mature. The majority of the survivors face lifelong disabilities, such as visual, hearing, and learning problems. The challenge of premature birth and death is worth to be addressed if countries are to achieve Sustainable Development Goals (SDGs), especially goal 3, subsection 3.2 that aims at ending all the preventable deaths of newborn babies and children aged under 5 years by 2030. Improved care and feeding of preterm babies can avert these deaths. This book chapter addresses the challenges associated with feeding preterm babies and is hoped to make a significant contribution toward ending deaths due to nutrition-associated comorbidities among this group of newborns.

2. Care and feeding of premature babies in hospital and at home

The body structures and systems of premature babies are usually not fully developed. As a result, premature babies usually have poor muscle tone, incomplete rooting, and weak gag reflexes. Premature babies also have incompetent lower esophageal sphincter and impaired rectal sphincter reflex. In addition, premature babies have high metabolic needs and are unable to store nutrients. Due to this, they are more likely to develop difficulties such as failure to suckle enough milk from the breast, poor gastric emptying, slowed intestinal motility, and impaired bowel emptying. All these affect feeding abilities and contribute to the development of nutritional deficiencies. The good news is that many of these babies can survive and grow especially if they are cared for and fed adequately.

The survival rates of premature infants can greatly improve if the emphasis is put on optimizing nutritional demands and appropriate feeding. The use of breast milk for premature babies as the feeding choice is highly recommended. In addition to nutritional values, breast milk provides premature babies with immunological defense, hormones, and enzymes that are essential for growth and development. Feeding should be initiated within 30 minutes to 1 hour of birth. Exclusive breastfeeding for 6 months is recommended. The mode of feeding initially will depend on whether the baby is stable or not. Stable babies may be able to breastfeed, while unstable babies may need parenteral nutrition in the first 24 hours. Premature babies weighing 1.5–2.0 kg or less are admitted to the Neonatal Intensive Care Unit (NICU) as well as those who are unstable. Premature babies below 1.5 kg are unstable so should not be fed by mouth for at least the first 24 hours. Initially, the health worker should establish an intravenous line and give intravenous fluids such as dextrose 10%, infant maintenance solution, or neonatal cocktail. Intravenous nutrition should provide glucose, amino acids, minerals, and vitamins plus fat in some preparations.

On day one, babies less than 1500 g should be given 80 mls per kg per day and for infants greater than 1500 g should be given 60 mls per kg per day. This should be divided and given every 2–3 hours. Once the baby stabilizes, oral feeds can be started through a Nasal Gastric Tube (NGT). From day two of life, it is important to introduce oral feeds mostly Expressed Breast Milk (EBM) with feed volumes estimated based on the body weight of the baby while continuing with intravenous fluids that have other electrolytes, especially potassium and sodium. If the baby has a birth weight of 1500 g or less and is stable, feeding is started with EBM of 5 mls and is increased carefully by 5 mls each day as shown in **Table 1**. Do not exceed the daily maximum volume of feeds as shown in **Table 2**. If the baby is between 1500 and 2000 g and is stable, then feeding can be started with 7.5 mls of EBM and also increased accordingly. If the premature baby has a weight of more than 2000 g, 10 mls of EBM is given and is also increased steadily as explained earlier.

The first choice of milk for feeding preterm babies is expressed breast milk from the mother of the baby. The second choice is donor breast milk. The donor breast milk

Day	IV	NGT
1	4mls per hour	0
2	3mls per hour	5mls 3 hourly
3	2mls per hour	10 mls 3 hourly
4	1 ml per hour	15mls 3 hourly
5	0 ml	18mls 3 hourly
6		21mls 3 hourly
7+		24mls 3 hourly

Table 1.
Intravenous and nasal gastric feeds.

Age	Total daily fluid/milk volume
Day 1	60 mls/kg/day
Day 2	80 mls/kg/day
Day 3	100 mls/kg/day
Day 4	120 mls/kg/day
Day 5	140 mls/kg/day
Day 6	160 mls/kg/day
Day 7	180 mls/kg/day

Table 2.
Total feeds given per kgs per day.

should be pasteurized. Donor pasteurized milk should be screened for human immunodeficiency virus, hepatitis B, hepatitis C, and venereal diseases. In cases where EBM from the mother or donor breast milk is not available, the premature babies may be fed on formula milk such as modified cow milk containing energy 80 kcal, protein 2.0 g, fat 4.5 g, calcium 77–110 mg, and phosphate 33–63 mg. However, premature babies fed on formula milk have been found to carry a high risk of developing Necrotizing Enterocolitis (NEC) compared to those fed on breast milk. There has also been an increase in NEC with fast or early EBM or formula milk compared to slow or delayed introduction of these feeds. While the baby is on these feeds, it is important to check random blood sugar. Usually, a random blood sugar of 2.8–8 mmols per dl or 49–140 mg per kg is considered to be within the normal range. The health worker should also monitor the quantity of fluids being given as well as the amount of urine passed within 24 hours. At least six wets per day are normal. This translates into about 0.5–1.0 ml per kg per hour. Also, observe signs of fluid overload such as swelling of face and difficulty in breathing.

After a lengthy stay in the hospital, premature babies are usually discharged to home and care is continued from there but still under the remote support of the health care worker. The premature baby will be discharged if he or she no longer needs intravenous fluids and can tolerate at least 8 oral feeds per day. The caretaker should be counseled on exclusive breastfeeding for the first 6 months, complementary feeding at 6 months of uncorrected chronological age and to practice appropriate weaning practices when the baby is able to eat adequately. The mother or caretaker is encouraged to bring back the baby as soon as he or she develops danger signs such as feeding poorly or getting complications such as diarrhea. The baby should be discharged on multivitamin supplements and iron syrup for about 6 months. The baby should be brought back to the clinic on day 6 for the first postnatal visit. At this visit, the baby should be weighed. The baby's weight should be monitored weekly until 2.5 kg weight is attained.

3. Supplementary feeding in premature babies

Premature babies at birth have low nutrient stores since most nutrients are transferred from the mother to the baby in the last trimester of pregnancy. For instance, babies accumulate about 60% of total iron stores during the last trimester of pregnancy. In addition, during fetal growth and development in utero, the transfer of some mineral ions, such as calcium and phosphorus, from the pregnant woman to her fetus takes place in the third trimester, mainly between 32 and 36 weeks of pregnancy. This means that premature babies miss out on this and therefore are at higher risk of suffering from iron deficiency anemia and osteopenia. For these babies to catch up with normal growth and prevent these complications, additional nutrients are required. Due to this, the fortification of the baby's feeds is necessary. Feeds for premature babies should be fortified with iron, calcium, phosphorus, and vitamin D. A baby who is on full enteral feeds, should be given Vitamin D 400–1000 units per day until 6 months, calcium 120–140 mg per kg per day for the first month of life, phosphorus 60–90 mg per kg per day. At 2 weeks of age, the baby should be given iron 2–4 mg per kg per day up to 6 months of age and folate 2.5 mg weekly up to 6 months.

4. Complementary feeding and weaning practices in premature babies

When breast milk alone is no longer sufficient to satisfy the nutritional requirements of the baby, the addition of other foods and liquids to the baby's diet is necessary. The exact timing is still a debate on whether other feeds should be introduced at 6 months of age corrected or 6 months of age uncorrected. No clear recommendations for premature babies. However, premature babies are a vulnerable group who have increased nutritional requirements, are at risk of developing gastro-esophageal reflux, respiratory problems, and have delayed gross motor development. Delayed introduction of complementary feeding may result in insufficient nutritional needs [6]. It is therefore helpful for premature babies to start receiving complementary foods at 6 months of uncorrected chronological age. The weaning process should be initiated when the infant has reached at least 5 kg of body weight, is able to eat from a spoon and the weaning diet is able to provide adequate nutrition. Weaning should be started between 5 and 8 months of uncorrected age to ensure that sensitive periods for the acceptance of solid foods are not missed and to allow the development of the appropriate feeding skills.

5. Feeding development and feeding difficulties in premature babies

Feeding difficulties are common complications experienced by premature babies hospitalized in NICU. Premature babies display significant difficulty feeding by mouth in the weeks following birth. Initially, they lack sucking skills. The overall prevalence of feeding difficulty among premature babies is as high as 42% and ranges from 6 to 84%. However, the degree of difficulty feeding entirely depends on the gestation age at birth. The problem of difficulty feeding continues to manifest among premature babies even several months after birth but reduces as the baby grows. Specific symptoms of difficulty feeding change with time as the baby grows and transits from a liquid-based diet to complementary foods. The symptoms of difficulty feeding may include behaviors such as (i) refusing to eat appropriate volumes of food or developmentally appropriate varieties of foods, (ii) symptoms of dysphagia or aspiration such as coughing, choking, gagging, or respiratory compromise while eating, (iii) difficulty feeding behaviors such as increased stress, crying, irritability, and (iv) delayed eating skills such as difficulty chewing. The contributing factors to difficulty feeding behaviors in premature babies include poor sucking skills and poor suck-swallow-breath coordination, among others [7].

The development of suckling takes two forms, that is to say, nonnutritive and nutritive sucking. Nonnutritive suckling is the type of sucking seen when an infant is not feeding. To elicit nonnutritive sucking, a finger is generally placed in the infant's mouth. In premature babies, this type of sucking is generally seen as a precursor to nutritive sucking. Some degree of nonnutritive sucking can often be elicited weeks before nutritive sucking emerges [8]. However, nonnutritive sucking generally becomes more rhythmic and stronger as the baby grows [9]. Nonnutritive sucking development among premature babies is an important milestone in the maturation process and reflects the subsequent improvement in suckling. Nutritive sucking occurs when a baby is feeding and results in the baby drawing milk into the mouth from the breast or bottle. Greater displacement of the tongue is required during nutritive sucking as compared to nonnutritive sucking [10]. Nutritive sucking is also characterized by slower, more rhythmical sucking movements, with regular breaks required for swallowing and breathing [10]. Like nonnutritive sucking, nutritive sucking skills generally improve with age and practice [11]. Once they approach mature age, it is often assumed that the nutritive feeding skills of premature babies can match those of mature babies. However, the sucking patterns of premature babies often remain significantly less coordinated and less efficient than those of mature babies at term age and beyond [12].

Swallowing and breathing utilize a common space within the pharynx, and hence, difficulties are often observed when sucking, swallowing, and breathing are not well coordinated [13]. Components of sucking, swallowing, breathing, and their coordinated activity mature at different times and rates [14]. Premature babies often swallow preferentially at different phases of respiration than those of their mature counterparts [15] and that restricts milk flow. Oral support during feeds may reduce pauses in sucking, increase rate and volume of intake during feeds. Externally paced feeding improves physiological stability during feeding [16]. For premature babies who are bottle-fed, the use of slow-flowing nipples over faster-flowing nipples improves physiological stability during feeds [17]. Babies born very premature continue to display frequent oxygen desaturation events during feeding at a mature age and spend on average 20% of their feeding time with arterial oxygen saturation levels less than 90 [18]. This may be a result of apnea events in premature babies during swallowing [19]. Apnea times have been found to reduce as babies mature [20]. Due to these issues, premature babies greatly rely on caregivers to feed them, provide adequate support and assistance during feeding, and recognize any distress cues as may occur during feeding [21].

Optimizing feeding during prematurity requires interventions aimed at directly assisting oral feeding to reduce complications that may come along. These interventions can be classified as:

a. Feeding the baby based on behavioral cues such as demand feeding, semi-demand feeding, and structured cue-based feeding. Feeding the baby *"on-demand"* simply means not worrying about the clock. *Semi-demand feeding uses infant cues and timing to determine when to offer a feed.* For example, if the baby fusses, cries, or wants to suck. The *cue-based* clinical *pathway* for oral *feeding* initiation and advancement of premature babies results in the earlier achievement of full oral *feeding*. Assessing readiness for feeding can be subjective and without *structure. Cue-based feeding* is more objective and individually tailored.

b. Strategies aimed at preparing the infant before a feed, such as oral stimulation prior to feeds, suck training, and oral tactile stimulation before feeds. *Suck training* exercises are helpful for gaining proper tongue function. Suck training increases the percentage of oral intake between 34 and 38 weeks of gestation. During suck training, the following steps should be observed; (1) the trainer should first wash hands to prevent transmitting infections to the baby. (2) the fingernails of the trainer should be short and smooth to prevent possible oral injuries, (3) the trainer should stroke the middle of the baby's lower lip with the index finger to encourage the baby to widely open his or her mouth, (4) when the baby opens the mouth, the trainer should place the finger, nail side down, into the front of the baby's mouth, (5) the baby will then suck the finger into his or her mouth, (6) if the tongue of the baby does not twist around the finger, the trainer can stroke the roof of the baby's mouth (palate), then softly press down on the back of the baby's tongue while stroking the tongue forward. This will help to pull the finger out of the baby's mouth somehow, (7) allow the baby to suck it back in, (8) then repeat this practice at least three times or until you feel the tongue come forward over the gum. Oral tactile stimulation before feeds is another strategy that can be used to prepare the premature baby to feed. It appears to improve the frequency of sucking and rate of intake during feeds and has been reported to improve the rate of breastfeeding. Oral tactile stimulation has also been reported to shorten the transition time to exclusive oral feeding.

c. Strategies aimed at supporting the infant during feeds, such as oral support during feeding and externally paced feeding. During oral support, *the jaw and cheek are supported* by placing the middle finger under the chin and the thumb and index fingers on the cheeks. It makes swallowing easier for the baby. External pacing means tipping the bottle down to slow milk flow or removing the bottle from the baby's mouth to impose a break in sucking. This *slows down the flow of milk into the nipple and the mouth,* allowing the baby to eat more slowly, and take breaks.

d. Interventions aimed at assisting respiratory support for oral feeding. Preterm babies often require noninvasive respiratory support, such as nasal continuous positive airway pressure and or high-flow nasal cannulas, to achieve full oral feeding. However, some forms of respiratory support strategies are feared by healthcare teams, as they may disrupt breath coordination if not carefully used.

6. Growth and development monitoring in premature babies

Normal growth is the progression of changes in height, weight, and head circumference that are compatible with established standards for a given population. Normal growth is a reflection of overall health and nutritional status. Premature babies are at risk for poor growth while in the Neonatal Intensive Care Unit (NICU) and after discharge. They must be closely monitored and may require interventions to promote better growth. Poor growth among preterm babies is usually an early indicator of health problems, such as nutritional and medical conditions. Parameters such as height, weight, and head circumference of a premature baby will vary depending on the gestational week of their birth and their overall health at birth as indicated in **Tables 3** and **4**. For example, a preterm baby with a gestational age of 24 weeks may attain 5 g per day while the one born at 33 weeks or later can put on as much as 30 g per day. The required weight gain in preterm babies who are born with a birth weight of more than 2 kg is 20–30 g per day. Similarly, the height of premature babies increases by about 1.1 centimeters every week until the completion of the ideal gestational age, which is about 40 weeks. A healthy premature baby is likely to first show improvement in the head circumference, followed by weight and height.

In premature babies, growth is monitored using different growth charts based on gestation age. Up to 36 weeks gestation, the Olsen and Bertino charts are the best growth charts to assess appropriateness for gestational age. For instance, small for gestational age or large for gestational age status. They perform relatively poorly in growth monitoring for premature babies beyond 36 weeks of age. Between 36 to 50 weeks of corrected age (10 weeks post-term), the Fenton chart is the best growth chart to assess longitudinal growth in premature babies over this period. After 4 to 8 weeks post-term, the World Health Organization growth charts for normal children can be used.

Developmental *monitoring* observes how the child grows and changes over time and whether the child meets the typical developmental milestones in playing, learning, speaking, behaving, and moving. Most premature babies go on to develop like babies born at term. But the earlier premature babies are born, the more likely it is that they will have development problems.

Gestational age in weeks	Weight in kilograms	Height in centimeters	Head circumference in centimeters
24	0.6	30	21.1
26	0.8	33	23
28	1	35.6	25
30	1.3	38.5	27
32	1.7	41.1	29
34	2.1	44	30.5
36	2.6	46.5	32.1
38	3.1	48.5	33.5
40	3.4	50.5	34.9

Table 3.
Weight, height, and head circumference of premature babies (girls).

Gestational age in weeks	Weight in kilograms	Height in centimeters	Head circumference in centimeters
24	0.65	31	22
26	0.83	34	23.5
28	1.1	36.5	25.8
30	1.4	39	27.5
32	1.8	42	29.5
34	2.25	44.9	31
36	2.7	47	32.8
38	3.2	49.5	34
40	3.6	51	35

Table 4.
Weight, height, and head circumference of premature babies (boys).

7. Summary and conclusion

The burden of premature labor and birth is still high worldwide at 10.6% and ranges from 5 to 18% of all babies born. About 80% of these occur in Africa and South Asia. In Sub-Saharan Africa, the burden ranges from 3.4 to 49.4%. In almost all countries, premature birth rates are on increase, which poses a threat to newborn health. Preterm babies are more likely to have feeding difficulties, suffer micronutrient deficiencies, and exhibit poor growth and developmental patterns. Due to this, premature babies are at great risk of death compared to babies born mature. The majority of the survivors face lifelong disabilities such as visual, hearing, and learning problems. However, there is still a window of opportunity to prevent these nutritional dilemmas, whereby improved care and feeding of preterm babies in the hospital and at home can avert these deaths as follows; a premature baby who is unstable should be given intravenous fluids in the first 24 hours. Once the baby stabilizes, oral feeds (mostly EBM) can be started on day two through a Nasal Gastric Tube (NGT) till day 7 or more while continuing the intravenous fluids until the baby is able to suckle. Babies who are able to suckle should be allowed to breastfeed immediately or within 1 hour after birth. It is recommended that the feeds of premature babies are fortified with iron, calcium, phosphorus, and vitamin D as these micronutrient stores are not adequately built and stored while the baby is still in utero. Appropriate and timely complementary feeds should be introduced to meet the nutritional needs of the baby and the weaning process should be initiated when the infant has reached at least 5 kg of body weight, is able to eat from a spoon and the diet is able to provide adequate nutrition. Sucking development and ability should always be assessed as this may pose a nutritional threat if the baby is unable to breastfeed adequately.

Acknowledgements

Authors extend their gratitude to Mountains of the Moon University www.mmu.ac.ug for the favorable environment and access to online resources *via* the university online library during the writing of this book chapter.

Conflict of interest

The authors declare no conflict of interest.

Author details

Enos Mirembe Masereka[1*], Clement Munguiko[2,3], Linda Grace Alanyo[1], Kenyonyozi Rubagumya[1], Brenda Nabawanuka[1], Julian Aryampa[1], Alex Tumusiime[4] and Emmanuel Kimera[1]

1 Faculty of Health Sciences, Department of Nursing and Midwifery, Mountains of the Moon University, Fort Portal, Uganda

2 Department of Nursing, School of Health Sciences, Soroti University, Soroti, Uganda

3 Faculty of Health Sciences, School of Medicine, Moi University, Kipkenyo, Cheptiret, Kenya

4 Department of Nursing and Midwifery, School of Medicine, Kabale University, Kabale, Uganda

*Address all correspondence to: mirembeenos@gmail.com

References

[1] World Health Organization. Preterm birth. 2018. Published February 19, 2018. Accessed January 1, 2022. Available from: https://www.who.int/news-room/fact-sheets/detail/preterm-birth

[2] De Costa A, Moller AB, Blencowe H, Johansson EW, Hussain-Alkhateeb L, Ohuma EO, et al. Study protocol for WHO and UNICEF estimates of global, regional, and national preterm birth rates for 2010 to 2019. PLoS One. 2021;**16**(10):e0258751. DOI: 10.1371/journal.pone.0258751

[3] Cao G, Liu J, Liu M. Global, regional, and national incidence and mortality of neonatal preterm birth, 1990-2019. JAMA Pediatrics. 2022;**176**(8):787-796. DOI: 10.1001/jamapediatrics.2022.1622

[4] Mabrouk A, Abubakar A, Too EK, Chongwo E, Adetifa IM. A scoping review of preterm births in sub-Saharan Africa: Burden, risk factors and outcomes. International Journal of Environmental Research and Public Health. 2022;**19**(17):10537. DOI: 10.3390/ijerph191710537

[5] Alamneh TS, Teshale AB, Worku MG, Tessema ZT, Yeshaw Y, Tesema GA, et al. Preterm birth and its associated factors among reproductive aged women in sub-Saharan Africa: Evidence from the recent demographic and health surveys of sub-Sharan African countries. BMC Pregnancy and Childbirth. 2021;**21**(1):1-11. DOI: 10.1186/s12884-021-04233-2

[6] Vissers KM, Feskens EJ, van Goudoever JB, Janse AJ. The timing of initiating complementary feeding in preterm infants and its effect on overweight: A systematic review. Annals of Nutrition and Metabolism. 2018;**72**(4):307-315. DOI: 10.1159/000488732

[7] Pados BF, Hill RR, Yamasaki JT, Litt JS, Lee CS. Prevalence of problematic feeding in young children born prematurely: A meta-analysis. BMC Pediatrics. 2021;**21**(1):1-15. DOI: 10.1186/s12887-021-02574-7

[8] Hack M, Estabrook MM, Robertson SS. Development of sucking rhythm in preterm infants. Early Human Development. 1985;**11**(2):133-140. DOI: 10.1016/0378-3782(85)90100-8

[9] Neiva FCB, Leone C, Leone C. Non-nutritive sucking scoring system for preterm newborns. Acta Paediatrica. 2008;**97**(10):1370-1375. DOI: 10.1111/j.1651-2227.2008.00943.x

[10] Miller JL, Kang SM. Preliminary ultrasound observation of lingual movement patterns during nutritive versus non-nutritive sucking in a premature infant. Dysphagia. 2007;**22**(2):150-160. DOI: 10.1007/s00455-006-9058-z

[11] Pickler RH, Chiaranai C, Reyna BA. Relationship of the first suck burst to feeding outcomes in preterm infants. The Journal of Perinatal & Neonatal Nursing. 2006;**20**(2):157. DOI: 10.1097/00005237-200604000-00010

[12] Iwayama K, Eishima M. Sucking behavior of normal full-term and low-risk preterm infants. No to Hattatsu=. Brain and Development. 1995;**27**(5):363-369. Available from: https://europepmc.org/article/med/7576781

[13] Daniels H, Devlieger H, Casaer P, Callens M, Eggermont E. Nutritive and non-nutritive sucking in preterm infants. Journal of Developmental Physiology. 1986;**8**(2):117-121. Available from: https://europepmc.org/article/med/3675720

[14] Amaizu N, Shulman R, Schanler R, Lau C. Maturation of oral feeding skills in preterm infants. Acta Paediatrica. 2008;**97**(1):61-67. DOI: 10.1111/j.1651-2227.2007.00548.x

[15] Mizuno K, Ueda A. The maturation and coordination of sucking, swallowing, and respiration in preterm infants. The Journal of Pediatrics. 2003;**142**(1):36-40. DOI: 10.1067/mpd.2003.mpd0312

[16] Law-Morstatt L, Judd DM, Snyder P, Baier RJ, Dhanireddy R. Pacing as a treatment technique for transitional sucking patterns. Journal of Perinatology. 2003;**23**(6):483-488. DOI: 10.1038/sj.jp.7210976

[17] Fucile S, Gisel E, Schanler RJ, Lau C. A controlled-flow vacuum-free bottle system enhances preterm infants' nutritive sucking skills. Dysphagia. 2009;**24**(2):145-151. DOI: 10.1007/s00455-008-9182-z

[18] Thoyre SM, Carlson J. Occurrence of oxygen desaturation events during preterm infant bottle feeding near discharge. Early Human Development. 2003;**72**(1):25-36. DOI: 10.1016/S0378-3782(03)00008-2

[19] Mathew OP. Respiratory control during nipple feeding preterm infants. Pediatric Pulmonology. 1988;**5**(4):220-224. DOI: 10.1002/ppul.1950050408

[20] Reynolds EW, Grider D, Caldwell R, Capilouto G, Vijaygopal P, Patwardhan A, et al. Swallow–breath interaction and phase of respiration with swallow during nonnutritive suck among low-risk preterm infants. American Journal of Perinatology. 2010;**27**(10):831-840. DOI: 10.3389/fped.2017.00214

[21] Thoyre SM, Brown RL. Factors contributing to preterm infant engagement during bottle-feeding. Nursing Research. 2004;**53**(5):304. DOI: 10.1097/00006199-200409000-00005

Chapter 11

Breastfeeding and Premature Newborn in the NICU

Alejandra Itzel Contreras Rivas, Gaston Eduardo Estudiillo Jiménez, Bernal Galicia Claudia, Gabriela Padilla Mendoza, Isaí Natan Yescas Osorio and Francisco Hernández Fragoso

Abstract

Today it is well known that the best gift that a mother can give her baby is breast milk. And what happens with all those children who for some reason are born premature, who cannot start breastfeeding either because of their severity, because they are separated from their breasts or simply because of their severity. For many years, the World Health Organization recommends exclusive human milk during the first 6 months of life, however, the premature newborn sent to the neonatal intensive care unit experiences a series of unfortunate events before starting enteral feeding many of them. They die during their stay. However, at the moment the importance has been given to the beginning of human milk from its mother or from a milk bank, and of the care around the family that the critically ill newborn must have. Unfortunately, Mexico and Latin America continue to have some areas with many lags in terms of nutrition and care of the newborn in the NICU. The success of breastfeeding with a baby in the NICU depends on the information and training provided to the mother about the expression, storage and transport of her milk. That the whole family be made aware that an essential part in the recovery of premature infants is to provide breast milk in a timely manner.

Keywords: breastfeeding, premature children, newborn, nicu, nutrition

1. Introduction

Worldwide, year after year, approximately 15 million premature children are born, a number that is increasing each year. And, adequate nutrition is currently considered a crucial factor for the survival of these babies as well as improving their neurological prognosis in the short and long term. His mother's milk, although it is premature milk, differs from the milk of mothers with full-term children. Far from being harmful to the patient, these differences have been shown to contain beneficial components and nutrients for the premature child. Many intensive care units have pasteurized milk, donated by mothers with sufficient milk production who for some reason did not give it to their babies (fasting children secondary to surgical pathologies, perinatal asphyxia, respiratory distress, deaths), these milk banks have become the only option in Latin American countries for the initiation of human milk in these premature children, demonstrating incredible benefits for all these children, so far from the benefits that their own mother's milk can give them given the weeks production management [1].

Human milk should be part of the daily medication of these critically ill premature infants or not. In the nutritional aspect, it is well known that it contains countless benefits than infant formulas, not to mention the danger that these substitutes can cause in the intestines of critically ill newborns. Not to mention the protection that human milk provides to reduce Skepsis, enterocolitis and retinopathy of prematurity. In current studies, children with extremely low birth weight, that is, under 1000 grams, human milk has shown to have multiple benefits in neurodevelopment, obtaining better results in the evaluation tests than those fed with substitute formulas. The American Academy of Pediatrics recommends starting your own mother's human milk as soon as possible or, in the case of pasteurized milk, fortifying it [2].

The bioactive components of your own mother's human milk enhance the immune system, improving gastrointestinal development. Containing abundant carbohydrate immunoglobulins, lactoferrins, enzymes and growth factors [3].

2. Epidemiology

In the past decade worldwide, the initiation of breast milk in neonatal intensive care units was 80% with a percentage of continuity at home from 35–54% [4]. however, year after year this percentage has been increasing. Thanks to the efforts of many governments with adequate public policies aimed at the protection of pregnant and lactating women. And so the standardization of perinatal health care was born in Europe, publishing the principles of family care for the newborn admitted to the neonatal intensive care unit. Emphasizing the early initiation of breastfeeding regardless of the severity of the baby. Giving rise to the 10 steps to help the mother to initiate breastfeeding in the NICU [5].

3. Human milk

The biochemical and bioactive components of human milk help the proper state of immunity, nutrition and growth in babies. The characteristics of these bioactive elements depend on genetic, demographic factors and of course lifestyles as well as exposure to pollutants, smokers. Having of course an impact on the health of the baby. For a woman to start breastfeeding after childbirth, a series of hormonal events occurs: when the placenta comes out and the uterus contracts, starting with milk production (many times it starts from the last weeks of pregnancy). The great advances in recent years regarding breast milk have also helped to improve infant formulas, currently many of the most important brands have added olisaccharides to the composition. But great benefits such as immunological as well as the plethora of bacteria that improve the baby's microbiota have not yet been possible to add to the substitutes. In the past it was thought that these bacteria were part of the skin of the breast or perhaps contaminated during extraction, storage or transport, which is not the case with multiple studies where the presence of an enteromammary route is evidenced [6, 7]. Being able to isolate the multiple probiotics contained in breast milk has opened a new frontier in research in order to demonstrate that these strains contained in human milk improve the immunological and intestinal development of babies, creating in the medical personnel in charge of the critically ill newborn, an easy-to-get, free weapon to improve the prognosis of these babies regardless of their underlying pathology or that their lives are in danger [7].

3.1 Breast milk with a premature child

Premature births, an event that is increasing worldwide, is associated with nutritionally and immunologically immature babies with a higher risk of complications, including necrotizing enterocolitis. And although the premature child needs caloric and protein contributions that exceed breast milk, the multiple benefits that it offers are not compared to the substitute, in addition to the fact that most of these babies have parenteral nutrition, which provides them with a sufficient amount of calories, protein, and lipids [8].

In addition, in recent studies, the analysis of the composition of breast milk with term babies and premature babies have shown that significantly the amount of protein, fat; as well as much higher levels of immunoglobulins, lactoferrin, growth factors and lysozyme [8, 9].

3.2 Lactating is a natural event

Providing the breast is the most natural way to provide all the clinical benefits of milk, however, on an emotional level, it creates a bond with your baby. In the intensive care unit, due to the severity of these babies, immediate attachment is often impossible, even They are children who spend months on invasive ventilation, which makes attachment to the mother's breast impossible. Currently, thanks to the importance that has been given to involving the family in the care of their critically ill child, there are therapies to improve the emotional aspect such as kangaroo mom or dad, the intention is that the emotional bond remains present and involves the family to favor the production of breast milk despite not having stimulated the baby, only breast pumps [10].

3.3 The popular phrase "human milk is pure gold"

The reason why the opportune initiation of breast milk despite the health status of the premature baby, is that the contribution of nutrients and immunoglobulins depends on the amount of milk that is provided, the greater the amount of milk, the greater the benefits, even more if it is from your own mother, which will have the gestational weeks with the fair benefits according to the gestational age. The great challenge in these units occurs when the mother is also in critical condition, since currently the main reason for premature birth is preeclampsia, leaving the mother in a state of vulnerability that of course makes it difficult to extract colostrum.

It has also been shown that the time of extraction, storage and transport of milk is vital for its conservation, it is advisable to extract it as close as possible to intensive therapy, and if this is not possible, follow the appropriate techniques of extraction to preserve your milk in the most hygienic way [11].

3.4 Differences between premature milk and term milk

As early as 1980, Shander et al. discovered that the protein content during the first two weeks of life was significantly higher than that of mature milk. At present, multiple meta-analyses have shown that milk from a breast with 28 weeks of gestation or less produces milk with a protein content of 2.3 g/100 ml, while the breast of

32–34 weeks produces between 1.8 to 1.9 grams. of protein per 100 ml. And not only is it the largest amount of protein, but also fat [12]. Of the free amino acids, 50% is made up of glutamine and glutamic acid in significantly higher quantities, so at the protein and free amino acid level, premature milk It is ideal to adapt to the growing needs of the premature child.

Regarding fats, these are also influenced by gestational age, mainly in the content of medium chain triglycerides and fatty acids. In a longitudinal study in 27 premature infants, it was found that the breast milk of premature infants had a much higher amount (between 0.8 and 0.5 grams/100 ml) of fats. As well as a greater contribution of saturated fats and medium chain lipids [13].

3.5 Oligosaccharides

Oligosaccharides are non-digestible carbohydrates that act as bioactive components in breast milk and provide a series of benefits such as improving microbiota colonization, reducing the pathogenesis of bacteria involved in enteral infections, and improving the immune system [14]. All oligosaccharides are produced in the mammary gland, demonstrating that in the early stages of lactation the concentration increases and gradually decreases over time. Among the many benefits of oligosaccharides, direct protection against enterocolitis (specifically flucosyltransferase 2) has been demonstrated. Another benefit that olisocarides have is that they do not lose effectiveness despite pasteurization, and their existence has been proven mainly between weeks 23 to 26 of gestation. Now, in comparison to premature babies fed with their own breast milk against those fed with pasteurized milk, it has been shown that those fed with their own breast milk have greater protection against enterocolitis, late sepsis, bronchopulmonary displasia and severe retinopathy, in a meta-analysis where 6 different studies were analyzed, 1472 babies and in observational studies where 14,950 babies were analyzed, a clear improvement in said pathologies was found in those fed with milk from their own breasts versus those fed with pasteurized milk [15].

In relation to the biocomponents of breast milk, the most significant element was the production of antioxidants found in colostrum and that decreases as lactation progresses. These levels are also much higher in the milk of breasts with premature babies than those of term. Finally, regarding the microbiota of breast milk with premature babies, it changes and is specific for each mother, providing the exact protection for the bacterial flora shared by mother and baby [16].

4. Gut microbiota of premature infants

The mode of birth, antibiotic administration, care environment and nutritional exposures, which particularly in intensive care are always present, and most notably breastfeeding, have all been shown to play important roles in the acquisition of the gut microbiome. Exposure to breast milk during infancy appears to be particularly important in shaping the microbiome. Among preterm infants, gestational age at birth and postnatal age have also been shown to be relevant to their microbiome characteristics. We also know that the microbiota of breastfed versus formula-fed infants has a more profound effect on genes in neonatal enterocytes that influence host protection and development [17].

Of the entire population of premature infants, those under 32 weeks are exceptionally more vulnerable, requiring full attention and human and material resources for a long time, with a higher risk of comorbidities that would complicate their evolution in the short, medium, and long term. 10% of these children will develop enterocolitis [18]. In a longitudinal study where the milk of their own mothers was analyzed, a considerable increase in the microbiota of babies was seen, mainly those with premature milk. Therefore, the Nutrition Committee of the European Society of Gastroenterology, Hepatology and Nutrition recommends early initiation of breast milk and preferably from your own mother [19].

5. Mothers of premature babies

Given the difficult circumstances these mothers live through, such as premature labor (most likely complicated by some circumstance), removing the mother from her baby, the poor suction that these babies present and the poor milk extraction technique, it seems consequently the failure of successful breastfeeding. Having a success rate in most countries of the world close to 25% (according to official UN records) [19]. Given the bad figures that exist worldwide, it is necessary not only to raise awareness among the medical personnel in charge of these children, but also to pay extra attention to these mothers. Feeling that there is an accompaniment during your breastfeeding from the staff who care for your baby, and sharing the experience with the whole family [20].

6. Nursing care and skills

The comprehensive care of a critically ill child is in charge of a multidisciplinary staff led by a neonatologist. However, also with the participation of the infectologist, nutritionist, neonatal surgeon and other specialists. But who is taking care of these babies 24 hours a day is the nursing staff. And they are the ones who provide advice and accompaniment to the mother for breastfeeding, and if they fail in their work, we will most likely not be able to maintain breastfeeding in the NICU. Fortunately, the knowledge of nurses has been improving over the years, with successful interventions at the beginning of the year 2000 barely 10–94% today [21]. And one of the most important and significant advances in these years was the timely start of the extraction of breast milk. The initial steps for the success of adequate breastfeeding in the neonatal intensive care unit is to begin with the education of the woman with a high-risk pregnancy, well aware of the possibility of having a premature birth, educating them with the necessary information about the use of the breast pump, the frequency, adequate nutrition and the nutrients that the mother needs to successfully carry out breastfeeding, regardless of the adverse situations that having her newborn in neonatal therapy implies [22].

7. Safe way of transportation of breast milk

7.1 Extraction

The physiological and emotional challenges associated with mother-infant separation, as well as inappropriate breast stimulation, can interfere with the establishment of lactation and increase the likelihood of complications. Consequently, for many mothers of preterm infants, the milk pathway begins with expressing rather than breastfeeding to initiate, build, and maintain lactation. And this milk expression can pose significant challenges for mothers of premature babies. If the initiation of lactation is delayed and the mother does not express milk consistently from the beginning, it is difficult to ensure adequate milk production in the long term. Therefore, having access to the right equipment and timely support is essential. It is important to recognize that the development of the mother's milk supply will require the mother to initiate, generate, and maintain lactation. And informing mothers that their milk supply will increase over time, thus setting the correct expectations, is the key to successful lactation. Necessary steps for expression: teach mothers to use their hands to massage the breasts, express milk during the first hour postpartum and keep it that way at least every 6 hours during the first 72 hours after birth, always start breastfeeding with a pump of milk (preferably bimanual), then express frequently, at least 6 times a day, express milk after skin-to-skin contact with your premature child, regardless of whether they have assisted ventilation [23].

7.2 Harvest

After expression, breast milk needs to be handled and stored, with attendant risks of nutrient loss and milk contamination. Therefore, it is essential to consider the best practices for handling human milk to ensure that the premature baby can access optimal nutrients. All certified intensive care units must standardize milk handling procedures in order to minimize losses (fewer containers) As well as loss of quality or integrity of milk components, milk contamination, risk of confusion between patients [23–25].

7.3 Labeling/tracking

It is very important to establish specific protocols to minimize errors in feeding with expressed milk. Giving a mother's expressed milk to a baby other than her own can have consequences for the baby in the NICU. The importance of providing milk from their own mother has already been discussed due to the difference in the weeks of gestation and in the days of life that the deceased children in the NICU have, therefore different nutritional needs. It is essential to control the feeding of the mothers and monitor expressed milk. This is to ensure that each patient has sufficient volume and receives the correct milk based on expression time and nutritional content, for each feed [24, 25].

7.4 Label expressed milk

Every institution must have a standard that must contain the milk label, giving priority to the baby's name, in this case their last names, the day and very importantly the time of extraction, as well as the quantity **Figure 1** [25].

7.5 Cold chain maintenance

The milk must be cooled immediately after expression and the cold chain must not be interrupted. Freezing the milk or simply chilling it is based on criteria such as

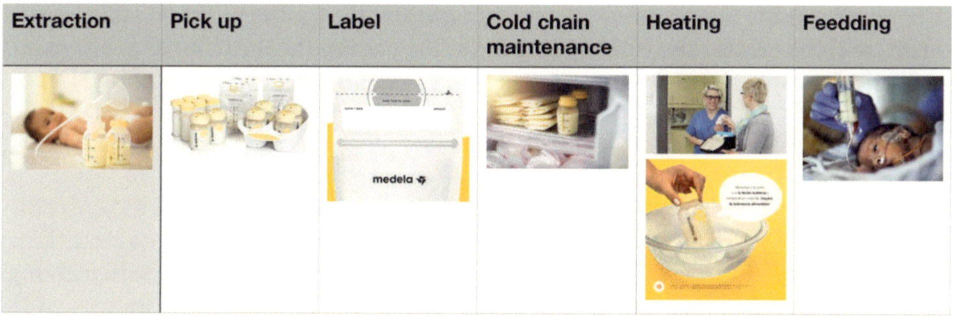

Figure 1.
Procedure to be followed for the collection and storage of breast milk as well as its transfer to the NICU until its ingestion.

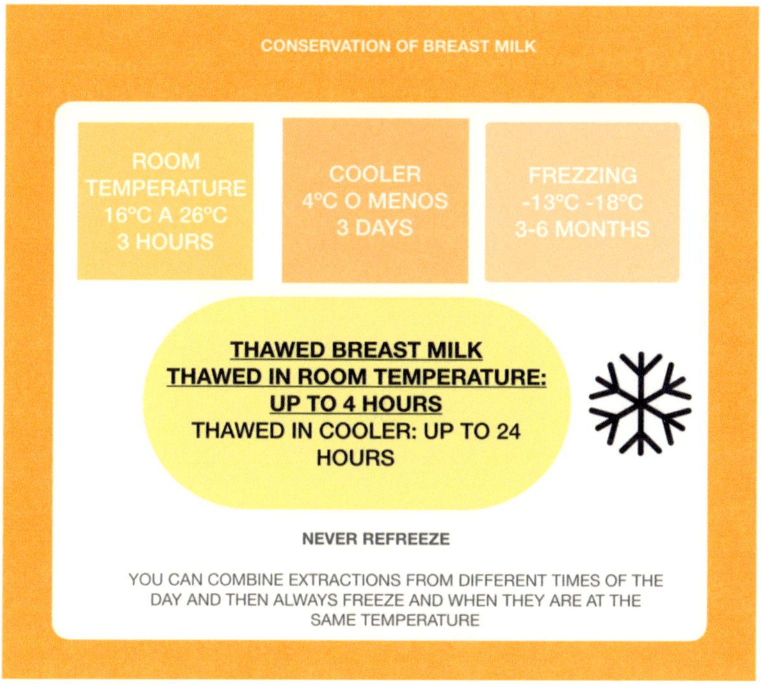

Figure 2.
Storage and conservation of breast milk.

the available distance from the home to the hospital, the amount of milk the mother already has in the NICU, and hospital policies. Freezing, although a necessary tool in the NICU, alters the integrity of the components of breast milk. Although most changes are now considered harmless, milk loses some of its value when fresh. For example, full-term infants ingest millions of live cells from breast milk every day. Unfortunately, these cells do not survive the freezing process [25].

To maximize the nutritional content between container transfers, the following should be considered: before handling the milk, it should always be shaken so that all the components are mixed homogeneously, consider the fat the most valuable component, and the greater the yellow coloration, the greater the nutritional components. and finally transport in the minimum number of containers (**Figure 2**) [26, 27].

7.6 Warming of breast milk in the NICU

I consider the science of heating milk and maintaining its properties to be the biggest challenge for nursing staff, milk must be gently heated to preserve its nutritional and immunological values. As well as the precaution that must be taken when giving it to the premature child. Due to the nature of the gastric and intestinal mucosa of the premature baby, the milk must have a certain temperature so as not to endanger his life and keep it as close as possible to fresh milk that has just been extracted.

8. Indications for use

This will depend 100 percent on the decision of the neonatologist and depending on his critical condition, as well as the weight of the baby to decide on the amount and frequency of administration.

9. Impact of breast milk on neurodevelopment

The biggest and most fearsome complication when we have a premature baby is that it has some type of delay, mainly motor [28].

The breastfed infant receives nutrients from breast milk which, once it crosses the intestinal barrier and ends up in the blood, with differences in phosphatidylcholine, sphingomyelin and triglycerides. This result is not necessarily related to the difference in triglyceride composition between breast milk and infant formula, but it may also be that neonatal nutrition has had additional effects on lipid metabolism. As we know the baby's brain and its entire peripheral nervous system is made up of fats, of course it does have a long-term impact on the fat intake provided by breast milk versus formula-fed [29]. The issue of breast milk in nutrition programming is really difficult to resolve. In fact, the interindividual variability of human milk and the heterogeneity of lactation times make it difficult to establish associations between a particular composition of breast milk and certain clinical parameters of the child who has received this milk. Breast milk lipids are the second most important macronutrient, it is rich in linoleic acid as well as alpha linoleic acid, important precursors of long-chain polysaturated acids essential for brain development [30]. At present, multiple associations between breast milk and neurodevelopment have been studied, mainly omega 3 and omega 6 [31]. We found a strong relationship between the growth of these premature infants during hospitalization and the presence of several lipid biomarkers in the In breast milk, faster growth was associated with milk containing more saturated medium-chain fatty acids and sphingomyelin, more phosphoethanolamine containing dihomo-ɣ-linolenic acid, and fewer oxylipins [32].

The oligosaccharide fraction of premature breast milk is probably the most interesting that raises challenging scientific questions [33]. The microbiome of children with severe growth delays is not refractory to nutritional supplementation with oligosaccharides. This opens up interesting perspectives for the care of premature newborns [34, 35].

After the battle that these preemies have in the NICU, when these preterm infants go home, they obtain a greater intestinal microbiota with greater bacterial diversity thanks to breast milk compared to formula-fed infants [36]. And for Of course we could not leave behind the economic benefit for the health system as well as for their families when they go home [37]. And, while it must be admitted that breast milk is not always perfect, the balance of benefits and risks tilts in the direction of benefits, especially for premature babies [38]. Epidemiologically speaking, morbidity and mortality in premature infants has decreased globally since more countries have joined breastfeeding programs, and of course better management of the nutrition of these babies improves their development. And, although it contains macronutrients with a fairly stable concentration, breast milk has a very diverse composition of micronutrients, which depends in particular on the physiology of the mother and her environment, so the question of whether it has an adaptive composition, according to the needs of the child, remains unanswered to this day [39].

10. Conclusion

Breast milk is a "natural" and "sustainable" food, without any impact on the environment, proving maternal attachment to be one more tool for these warriors to get ahead with the minimum of both physical and neurodevelopmental complications. And although the ideal will always be the direct suction of the mother, we are aware that for these babies the way of feeding is difficult; The important thing is that we are aware and that we are a team with the families, involve the family in the evolution of these babies by providing information that the best gift that can be given to a baby regardless of the week of gestation in breast milk.

Soon, all NICU units will be able to progress to a breastfeeding supplement or other device that will deliver expressed breast milk from a bottle or syringe through a small tube that is taped next to your nipple. With this method, all premature babies should begin feeding partly from the tube and partly from the breast while latching on to their mother's breast and actively feeding.

And what is the future of breastfeeding in neonatal intensive care units? The intention is not to have devices such as syringes or bottles to transport the milk, but rather devices that connect directly to the mother's nipple regardless of the baby's ventilatory support. And that the intensive care areas become a family environment involving the whole family in the care of their critically ill newborn.

Author details

Alejandra Itzel Contreras Rivas[1*], Gaston Eduardo Estudiillo Jiménez[2], Bernal Galicia Claudia[3], Gabriela Padilla Mendoza[4], Isaí Natan Yescas Osorio[5] and Francisco Hernández Fragoso[6]

1 Pediatrics - Neonatology, Biological and Health Sciences, Metropolitan Autonomous University Iztapalapa Campus, Neonatal Intensive Care Unit at Hospital General de Tlahuac, ISSSTE, Fetalvita Institute, Hospital San Ángel Inn University, Mexico

2 Gynecology and Obstetrics, Maternal Fetal Medicine, Fetal Surgery, CDMX Perinatal Health Program, Maternal Fetal Medicine Service, Dario Fernandez General Hospital ISSSTE, Perinatal/Genetic/Neonatal Diagnostic Center, Fetalvita Institute, CDMX, Mexico

3 Pediatric Nephrology Service Hospital General Doctor Dario Fernandez ISSSTE, Mexico

4 Pediatric Service Hospital General Doctor Dario Fernandez ISSSTE, Mexico

5 Gynecology and Obstetrics at the General Hospital, Dr. Jose Maria Rodriguez, Mexico

6 Gynecology and Obstetrics Hospital General Doctor Dario Fernandez ISSSTE, Hospital Administration, Mexico

*Address all correspondence to: alejandracontrerasr15@outlook.es

References

[1] Heller N, Rüdiger M, Hoffmeister V, Mense L. Mother's own Milk feeding in preterm Newborns admitted to the neonatal intensive care unit or special-care nursery: Obstacles, interventions, risk calculation. International Journal of Environmental Research and Public Health. 2021;**18**:4140

[2] Chowdhury R, Sinha B, Sankar MJ, Taneja S, Bhandari N, Rollins N, et al. Breastfeeding and maternal health outcomes: A systematic review and meta-analysis. Acta Paediatrica International Journal of Paediatrics. 2015;**104**:96-113

[3] Mitha A, Piedvache A, Glorieux I, Zeitlin J, Roué JM, Blondel B, et al. Unit policies and breast milk feeding at discharge of very preterm infants: The EPIPAGE-2 cohort study. Paediatric and Perinatal Epidemiology. 2019;**33**:59-69

[4] Wilson E, Edstedt Bonamy A-K, Bonet M, Toome L, Rodrigues C, Howell EA, et al. Room for improvement in breast milk feeding after very preterm birth in Europe: Results from the EPICE cohort. Maternal & Child Nutrition. 2018;**14**:e12485

[5] Mekonnen AG, Yehualashet SS, Bayleyegn AD. The effects of kangaroo mother care on the time to breastfeeding initiation among preterm and LBW infants: A meta-analysis of published studies. International Breastfeeding Journal. 2019;**14**:52-55

[6] Maastrup R, Walloee S, Kronborg H. Nipple shield use in preterm infants: Prevalence, motives for use and association with exclusive breastfeeding—Results from a national cohort study. PLoS One. 2019;**14**:e0222811

[7] Bonnet C, Blondel B, Piedvache A, Wilson E, Bonamy AKE, Gortner L, et al. Low breastfeeding continuation to 6 months for very preterm infants: A European multiregional cohort study. Maternal & Child Nutrition. 2019;**15**:e12657

[8] Casey L, Fucile S, Dow KE. Determinants of successful direct breastfeeding at hospital discharge in high-risk premature infants. Breastfeeding Medicine. 2018;**13**:346-351

[9] Bonet M, Forcella E, Blondel B, et al. Approaches to supporting lactation and breastfeeding for very preterm infants in the NICU: A qualitative study in three European regions. BMJ Open. 2015;**5**(6):e006973

[10] Lussier MM, Tosi L, Brownell EA. Predictors of Mother's own Milk feeding at discharge in preterm infants. Advances in Neonatal Care. 2019;**19**:468-473

[11] Gianni ML, Bezze EN, Sannino P, Baro M, Roggero P, Muscolo S, et al. Maternal views on facilitators of and barriers to breastfeeding preterm infants. BMC Pediatrics. 2018;**18**:283

[12] Hoban R, Bigger H, Schoeny M, Engstrom J, Meier P, Patel AL. Milk volume at 2 weeks predicts Mother's own Milk feeding at neonatal intensive care unit discharge for very low birthweight infants. Breastfeeding Medicine. 2018;**13**:135-141

[13] Herich LC, Cuttini M, Croci I, Franco F, Di Lallo D, Baronciani D, et al. Italian effective perinatal intensive Care in Europe (EPICE) network. Maternal education is associated with disparities in breastfeeding at time of discharge but not at initiation of enteral feeding in the

neonatal intensive care unit. The Journal of Pediatrics. 2017;**182**:59-65

[14] Meier PP, Johnson TJ, Patel AL, Rossman B. Evidence-based methods that promote human milk feeding of preterm infants: An expert review. Clinics in Perinatology. 2017;**44**(1):1-22

[15] Engstrom JL, Patel AL, Meier PP. Eliminating disparities in mother's milk feeding in the neonatal intensive care unit. The Journal of Pediatrics. 2017;**182**:8-9

[16] Aakko J, Kumar H, Rautava S, Wise A, Autran C, Bode L, et al. Humanmilkoligosaccharide categories define the microbiota composition in human colostrum. Beneficial Microbes. 2017;**8**:563-567

[17] Murphy K, Curley D, O'Callaghan TF, O'Shea C-A, Dempsey EM, O'Toole PW, et al. The composition of human milk and infant faecal microbiota over the first three months of life: A pilot study. Scientific Reports. 2017;7:1-10

[18] Lackey KA, Williams JE, Meehan CL, Zachek JA, Benda ED, Price WJ, et al. What's normal? Microbiomes in human milk and infant feces are related to each other but vary geographically: The INSPIRE study. Frontiers in Nutrition. 2019;**6**:45

[19] Kumar H, duToit E, Kulkarni A, Aakko J, Linderborg KM, Zhang Y, et al. Distinct patterns in human Milk microbiota and fatty acid profiles across specific geographic locations. Frontiers in Microbiology. 2016;7:1619

[20] Douglas CA, Ivey KL, Papanicolas LE, Best KP, Muhlhausler BS, Rogers GB. DNA extraction approaches substantially influence the assessment of the human breast milk microbiome. Scientific Reports. 2020;**10**:1-10

[21] Meyer KM, Pace RM, Mohammad M, Haymond M, Aagaard KM. 941: Composition of the breast milk microbiome is influenced by the method of 16S-amplicon sequencing used. American Journal of Obstetrics and Gynecology. 2019;**220**:S607-S608

[22] Houghteling P, Walker WA. Why is initial bacterial colonization of the intestine important to the infant's and child's health? Journal of Pediatric Gastroenterology and Nutrition. 2015;**60**:294-307

[23] Dominguez-Bello MG, Costello EK, Contreras M, Magris M, Hidalgo G, Fiere N, et al. Delivery mode shapes the acquisition and structure of the initial microbiota across multiple body habitats in newborns. Proceedings of the National Academy of Sciences of the United States of America. 2010;**107**(26):11971-11975

[24] Zeissig S, Blumberg RS. Life at the beginning: Perturbation of the microbiota by antibiotics in early life and its role in health and disease. Nature Immunology. 2014;**15**(4):307-310

[25] Brooks B, Firek BA, Miller CS, Sharon I, Thomas BC, Baker R, et al. Microbes in the neonatal intensive care unit resemble those found in the gut of premature infants. Microbiome. 2014;**2**(1):1

[26] Ardeshir A, Narayan NR, Méndez-Lagares G, Lu D, Rauch M, Huang Y, et al. Breast-fed and bottle-fed infant rhesus macaques develop distinct gut microbiotas and immune systems. Science Translational Medicine. 2014;**6**(252):252ra120

[27] Jost T, Lacroix C, Braegger CP, Chassard C. New insights in gut microbiota establishment in healthy breast fed neonates. PLoS One. 2012;7:e44595

[28] LaRosa P, Warner B, Zhou Y, Weinstock GM, Sodergren E, Hall-Moore CM, et al. Patterned progression of bacterial populations in the premature infant gut. Proceedings of the National Academy of Sciences of the United States of America. 2014;**111**(34):12522-12527

[29] Schwartz S, Friedberg I, Ivanov IV, Davidson LA, Goldsby JS, Dahl DB, et al. A metagenomic study of diet-dependent interaction between gut microbiota and host in infants reveals differences in immune response. Genome Biology. 2012;**13**(4):r32

[30] Patel RM, Kandefer S, Walsh MC, Bell EF, Carlo WA, Laptook AR, et al. Causes and timing of death in extremely premature infants from 2000 through 2011. The New England Journal of Medicine. 2015;**372**(4):331-340

[31] Zhou Y, Shan G, Sodergren E, Weinstock G, Walker WA, Gregory KE. Longitudinal analysis of preterm intestinal microbiome prior to necrotizing enterocolitis: A case-control study. PLoS One. 2015;**10**(3):e0118632

[32] Kostic AD, Gevers D, Siljander H, Vatanen T, Hyötyläinen T, Hämäläinen A-M, et al. The dynamics of the human infant gut min development and in progression towards type 1 diabetes. Cell Host & Microbe. 2015;**17**(2):260-273

[33] Chen EZ, Li H. A two-part mixed-effects model for analyzing longitudinal microbiome compositional data. Bioinformatics. 2016;**32**(17):2611-2617

[34] Working Group on Clinical Practice Guidelines. Clinical Practice Guide about Breastfeeding. Ministry of health social Services and Equality, Vasque Goverment. 2017. pp. 252-256. NIPO:680-16-068-2. Available: www.Euskadi.eus/publicaciones

[35] Christian P, Mullany LC, Hurley KM, Katz J, Black RE. Nutrition and maternal, neonatal, and child health. Seminars in Perinatology. 2015;**39**:361-372

[36] Oeschgera VV, Mazzaa CS, Araujoa MB, Sauré. Lineamientos en soporte nutricional en posoperatorio de cirugía cardiaca neonatal. Argent Pediatrics. 2014;**5**:443-450

[37] Koletzko B, Goulet O, Hunt J, Krohn K, Shamir R. Guidelines on paediatric parenteral nutrition of the European Society of Paediatric Gastroenterology, Hepatology and nutrition. Journal of Pediatric Gastroenterology and Nutrition. 2015;(41):8-16

[38] Jolin-Dahel K, Ferretti E, Montiveros C, Grenon R, Barrowman N, Jimenez-Rivera C. Parenteral nutrition-induced Cholestasis in neonates: Where does the problem lie? Gastroenterology Research and Practice. 2013;**13**:1-6

[39] Rice MS, Valentine CJ. Neonatal body composition: Measuring lean mass as a tool to guide nutrition management in the neonate. ASPEN. 2015;**XX**:1-8

Chapter 12

The Catch Up of Small for Gestational Age: Breast Milk Is It the Best?

Haythem Bachrouche

Abstract

Small for gestational age (SGA) is defined as a birth weight below the 10th percentile for gestational age. We can distinguish two categories of SGA: the first group is constitutionally programmed to be small despite a favorable maternal environment, the second group has a growth restriction due to a maternal condition leading to placental insufficiency. The burden of fetal growth-restricted (FGR) SGA is higher in resource-poor countries, and children born FGR SGA have a higher risk of mortality and morbidity during the neonatal period and beyond. To overcome this underweight and therefore the higher rate of early and late morbimortality, it seems logical that the weight gain in the first months of life (catch up phenomenon) have the optimal speed. Exclusive breastfeeding from birth until six months of age should be encouraged for all infants, including SGA infants, but the supplementation with standard formula or fortified formula until the 6th month of life is it not justified for an optimal catch up? Many authors believe that the "catch up" phenomenon would be the major etiological factors of obesity, cardiovascular disease, and metabolic syndrome in the future. It was demonstrated in many research that, SGA children who received fortified formula or standard formula whatever the reason, showed faster weight gain in the first months of life, which was related to increased body fat later in life. It was also revealed in several studies that, when exclusively breastfed, SGA achieved a catch-up growth slower, suggesting that the human milk can be the reference nutriment for healthy growth without nutritional impairment in children born SGA with effects persisting until adulthood.

Keywords: small for gestational age, breastfeeding, metabolic syndrome, overweight, standard formula, fortified formula

1. Introduction

Catch up growth (CUG) of small for gestational age (SGA) is a crucial determinant of short- and long-term health issues. Adequate nutrition and feedings practices during the early life are the key of an optimal growth rate.

Is exclusive breastfeeding from birth until six months of age (EBF) the best recommendation for preterm and term SGA? Would EBF be enough to prevent under-nutrition and to achieve optimal CUG of theses infants? Would EBF reduce morbidity and mortality during early life and later in this high-risk population? We will try to answer to these questions in this chapter according to the latest scientific evidences to guide health professionals to early preventive strategies.

2. Who is the small for gestational age?

Small for gestational age (SGA) is defined as a birth weight below the 10th percentile for gestational age.

During intrauterine life, the fetus may be constitutionally programmed to be small despite a favorable environment. It can also undergo adverse maternal conditions causing a placental insufficiency and leading to intrauterine growth restriction (IUGR) without achieving his genetic potential growth.

We distinguish the premature SGA (PT SGA) and full-term SGA (FT SGA) according to gestational age.

SGA infants represent about 10% of live births in developed countries [1]. Few years ago, this prevalence can be variable for the same population due to a lack of consensus on the definitions used for SGA, as well as on the reference standards for growth in the world.

To overcome this uniformity and due to a lack of evidence-based and internationally applicable tools, the International Consortium for Fetal and Newborn Growth in the 21st Century (INTERGROWTH-21e) published in 2014 standards for weight, height and head circumference at birth. The aim of this initiative is to monitor fetal growth and to standardize growth assessment, in order to provide compelling evidence for maternal and newborn health programs [2].

These fetal and neonatal references complement the WHO growth standards published in 2006 and represent the most appropriate framework for monitoring growth during the first 5 years of life.

Indeed, the WHO growth standards take an approach regardless of ethnicity or location and based on breastfed infants as the normative model of growth under optimal conditions, contrary to previous growth references like 1977 NCHS and 2000 CDC based on formula fed infants [3].

This evolution of growth assessment tools led to better harmonization of research and so a better quality of studies' conclusions.

3. The challenge of SGA nutrition in the early life

It is well known that a low birth weight is linked to the risk of perinatal and infantile morbidity and mortality [4].

There are many causes of SGA. A constitutionally small infant born to a small mother and/or father is the commonest cause of SGA. The commonest pathological cause of SGA is placental dysfunction leading to suboptimal nutrition and intrauterine growth retardation (IUGR).

This stressful environment during fetal development can cause epigenetic changes, abnormal vascularization and aberrant endocrine regulation. These conditions observed particularly in SGA with IUGR increase the risk of diseases later in life.

Prematurity is an additional factor, and the PT SGA has more complications in short and long-term life.

Prenatal monitoring can reduce the prevalence of SGA. The regular follow-up of pregnant women is a recommended universal action as a front-line strategy to prevent noncommunicable diseases in adulthood by decreasing the incidence of SGA.

But we know that not only the intrauterine period, but also the postnatal nutrition and growth interfere with future health issues. Indeed, human growth is the result of an interaction between genetic, hormonal, nutritional and environmental factors.

Due to evidence that one of the main factors for modulating the growth pattern in infancy is nutrition and, therefore, feeding policies are very important for the prognosis of these infants in the early life and later. So, the efforts can be directed to defining optimal feeding patterns for SGA.

Not long ago, we thought that the delay of weight at the start of life must be recovered as soon as possible to prevent cognitive issues by promoting rapid catch-up growth especially for head circumference.

We have encouraged in the past mothers and health professionals to supplement additional calories to SGA by administering a nutrient enriched formula to promote quick weight gain.

But from studies by Singhal and his team revealing that accelerated gain in weight with the supply of nutrient and calorie dense formulas to SGA was associated with increased total body fat in childhood [5], many other studies confirmed that this practice might be deleterious to infant born SGA and that who grew more rapidly were more likely to be obese later and have a specific increased risk of cardiovascular and metabolic diseases. In order to minimize the programmed disease risk (due to IUGR) and to reach optimal post-natal growth, the nutrition pattern in the first months of life is a real challenge.

4. Research limitations and proposals for standardization

As we described above the lack of uniformity and the need of standardization in SGA and CUG definitions made very difficult to complete metanalysis and to draw a valuable scientific conclusion.

Conjointly, for ethical reasons we cannot conduct randomized double-blind studies evaluating exclusively breastfed infants vs. exclusively formula fed infants.

For these reasons, researches in the literature about SGA nutrition are sparse and difficult to conduct and most current evidence is based on limited studies with low to medium study quality.

But after the INTERGROWTH-21 initiative coming to complete the WHO child and adolescent growth standards (2006–2007) we can propose the following, to improve globally the quality of our studies and to obtain more interpretable results:

- that the cut-off of the 10th percentile is the definition of SGA;
- that to standardize the identification of infants born SGA we recommend that the INTERGROWTH-21 birth-weight for-gestational-age standards be used;
- that the definition of CUG is a change of >0.67 in z score representing a clinically significant response;

- that the WHO Growth Standards be used to calculate z scores [2];
- that rapid CUG be defined as a postnatal centile crossing defined in terms of an upward change in weight z score during 1 month [6];

By applying these proposals, future metanalysis of small cohort's studies can be possible, and so we can obtain a better scientific quality recommendation.

5. Nutrition of FT SGA in the first months of life

To overcome the underweight at birth of FT SGA and to minimize a higher risk of early and late morbimortality, it seems logical that the weight gain in the first months of life (catch up phenomenon) have the optimal speed.

Many authors believe that the catch-up phenomenon would be the major etiological factors of obesity, cardiovascular disease, and metabolic syndrome in the future.

The challenge is how to nurture these FT SGA and achieve balance between risk of malnutrition (causing cognitive development impairment) and accelerated growth without increasing the risk of chronic non-communicable diseases in the future [4].

Exclusive breastfeeding (EBF) from birth until six months of age is strongly recommended by WHO for all infants (FT SGA, PT SGA, LBW and preterm infants) [1] but the supplementation with standard formula or fortified formula until the 6th month of life is it not justified for an optimal catch up?

Levels of overweight and obesity has increased remarkably worldwide and many studies found that infants who were grew rapidly were more likely to be obese in childhood, adolescence and early adulthood than other infants [7].

The study by Singhal et al. showed that the increased caloric supply in SGA infants, especially protein, led to a rapid early growth with fat mass accumulation. In the other hand, the breastmilk apart his nutritional components, contains adipokines (leptin and adiponectin) that lead to better appetite regulation, helping to achieve a healthier weight gain [8].

This fact was consolidated by other studies. After 3 months of age the growth diverges markedly between breastfed and formula fed infants with a difference in average of 600–650 g at 12 months. Differences in length tend to be less pronounced [3] which does not affect the prognosis of the size later. Furthermore, infant formula lacks growth mediators found in human milk and slower weight gain of breastfed infants was not associated with nutritional impairment in infancy or shorter size in adulthood.

In low and medium incomes countries, we note a virtual absence of studies of CUG, and to our knowledge the only research done by Bachrouche et al. was interesting [9]. They compared 2 groups (17 EBF FT SGA vs. 13 formula fed FT SGA) and there was a significant difference in the mean of weight at the age of 6 months suggesting that standard formula provided a faster weight gain and that EBF until 6 months ensured a slower CUG.

Also, Zegher et al. in his cohort study found that breastfed FT SGA had a higher insulin sensivity, normal serum fasting glucose, IGF 1 and adiponectin levels and a lower BMI and fat mass when compared to formula fed FT SGA suggesting a reduced risk of diabetes and obesity in adulthood [4].

Likewise, FT SGA exclusively breastfed until 6 months matched their genetic growth trajectory slower without nutritional impairment.

In the other hand, in a systematic review it was evidenced that, SGA showed higher insulin resistance and higher risk of diabetes [10], and additional to such risk and according to the result of latest studies, the early introduction during the first months of life of infant formulas or any other supplementation may induce a rapid catch-up growth of SGA that is considered as one of major etiological factors of obesity, cardiovascular diseases and metabolic syndrome in adulthood for these infants.

For all that, breastfeeding seems to be the best choice for FT SGA to reach an optimal catch-up growth with the best outcomes and this nutrition recommendation can prevent obesity and cardiovascular and metabolic diseases in this high-risk population.

6. Nutrition of PT SGA in the first months of life

The nutritional management of SGA associated to prematurity is more difficult in view of this double risk factor of morbidity and mortality. Postnatal nutrition of PT SGA must be safe, help to achieve optimal growth but also minimize the potential risk for later ill-health.

International pediatric societies recommend that postnatal growth should be close to that of the utero growing fetus. In neonatal period, we often need to hospitalize PT SGA in NICU for reasons of care and the staff has sometimes to limit nutrient intake.

Once again, Exclusive breastfeeding from birth until 6 months of age, is strongly recommended by WHO in PT-SGA, LBW and preterm infants, but is EBF enough to fulfill the nutritional requirements of this infants?

Energy and nutrient intakes for preterm based on weight and age of birth have been developed and published by several groups and notably by WHO (**Table 1**). Also, ESPEGHAN recommends to apply an enhanced nutrient strategy after discharge from hospital up to 52nd week of GA to all growth-restricted VLBW infants. Indeed, the breast milk or pasteurized donor milk as a first alternative milk source over standard and preterm infant formula are recommended for preterm and SGA [1].

This strategy improves feeding tolerance, reduces delay to enteral feeding and lead to a lower incidence of necrotizing enterocolitis (NEC). The breast milk (BM) or donor BM is usually fortified to achieve intake recommendations by preferably human milk (HM) originated fortifier better than cow milk-based protein or preterm formula.

Limited studies with low to medium quality had compared HM to HM fortified and HM to formula. Overall, only human milk compared to formula intervention had a positive effect on morbidity among preterm infants while no interventions had any effect on mortality. The Bovine/cow milk supplementation had unfavorable effects on morbidity and mortality. In a systematic review, 3 studies compared HM and formula in ELBW. 2 studies did not observe any effect on growth, and only the study of Manea et al. reported that breast milk was more effective than formula at improving the weight of these infants [11].

The higher caloric and protein intake for premature infants in general and especially for PT SGA has as arguments the immediate metabolic risks, the avoidance of malnutrition and the promotion of a better neurocognitive prognosis. Hence, nutrient fortification of HM is now standard clinical practice for VLBW babies in many settings.

However, it is important to note that these recommended intakes are for guidance and in 45 of 46 studies (summarized in 6 reviews) faster infant growth has

	Birth to 7 days	Stabilization to Term	Term
Energy Requirements			
Energy kJ/kg (kcal/kg)	292–334 (70–80)	438–563 (105–135)	417–501 (100–120)
Macronutrients			
Carbohydrates (g/kg)	5.0–20.0	7.5–15.5	7.5–15.5
Protein (g/kg)	1.0–3.0	3.0–3.6	2.2
Fat (g/kg)	0.5–3.6	4.5–6.8	4.4–7.3
Micronutrients per day			
Vitamin A (IU/kg)	700–1500	700–1500	600–1400
Thiamin (mg/kg)	0.04–0.05	0.04–0.05	0.05
Riboflavin (mg/kg)	0.36–0.46	0.36–0.46	0.05
Niacin (NEe /5000 IU)	8.6	8.6	8.6
Vitamin B6 (mg/g of protein intake)	0.015	0.015	0.015
Folate (μg)	50	50	25
Vitamin B12 (μg)	0.15	0.15	0.15

Table 1.
WHO recommended daily energy and nutrient intakes at birth for preterm infants (>1.0 kg). Adapted from Edmond, Karen and Bahl, (2006).

been associated with later obesity in both high- and low-income countries, in infants preterm or at term and born with normal or low birth weight.

In addition, the argument put forward that poor growth in preterm expose to neurocognitive impairment remains unproven according to a recent review [12].

That is why we can suggest that BM without any fortification can be the best choice for the PT SGA in neonatal period, based on its immunological advantages, its better digestive tolerance, the possibility of early introduction and the possibility of reducing hospital stays. After discharge and with a close monitoring of growth in PT SGA, EBF until 6 months can be advised with the aim to achieve a catch up with a slow and progressive weight gain without any rapid acceleration exposing to the obesity and others diseases in adulthood. Although in a recent systematic review, involving over 10,000 VLBW infants, we have found much of the evidence for the association between growth outcomes and HM intake to be inconclusive, largely due to the quality of the evidence [13].

In summary, the concept of EBF for PT SGA can be adopted worldwide, if efforts will be directed to conduct high quality studies that can prove that BM is safer for these infants in early life and also preventive later from adult diseases by a slower growth in the first months of life.

7. Breast milk values and actions to do for a successful breastfeeding of SGA

The benefits of breastmilk are innumerable. All efforts, before conception, during pregnancy and in postpartum should be focused on the success of breastfeeding, especially for SGA.

The unimpeachable high qualities of human milk have been well studied and still remain an area of research.

Breastmilk confers many immunological, bioactive, psychological benefits for mothers and infants. It improves neurologic maturation, protects against NEC, diarrhea and infections, and reduce morbimortality in all infants and notably in SGA. Recently, a relationship between breastfeeding and epigenetic regulation has been found. A study found a significantly lower DNA methylation in children exclusively formula fed compared to children exclusively breastfed [14].

DNA methylation is considered as one of the main epigenetic mechanisms responsible for gene regulation and a potential biomarker of a variety of pathologies, including cancers, metabolic disorders, and cardiovascular diseases. EBF seems to be an epigenetic regulator and a protective nutritional feeding from diseases through the DNA methylation.

In view of this major importance of BM for maternal and child health, and especially for SGA who are at high risk of morbidity and mortality during childhood and after, all care strategies must support the breastfeeding of these infants.

Many measures are recommended: continuous Staff training, clear information for parents, creating neonatal units with kangaroo rooms, creating BM and donor BM banks, providing places for breastfeeding and breast pumping in hospitals, public places and at work. Also preferring cup-feeding when direct BM is not possible and early progressive feeding instead of delayed feeding for PT SGA are recommended. Follow-up by breastfeeding consultants should be encouraged for a better chance to overcome hardships to succeed an EBF of SGA until 6 months of life.

8. Conclusions

Human milk (HM) is the gold standard for feeding all infants. SGA are a high-risk population of obesity, cardiovascular diseases and metabolic syndrome later in life. The strategy of nutrition in the first months of life is crucial modulator to prevent health issues. EBF is associated with slower growth of SGA, however formula fed interventions can lead to a rapid catch-up growth linked to a higher risk of diseases in infancy and adulthood. Our nutrition strategies in view of recent data must avoid increased caloric supply in the early life and EBF until 6 moths of life would be preferred even for PT SGA.

Finally, breastfeeding seems to be the best choice for all SGA to reach an optimal catch-up speed with the best outcomes.

Acknowledgements

All the team of Pediatrics and Neonatology department of Mohamed Tlatli Hospital, Nabeul, Tunisia.

Conflict of interest

The author declares no conflict of interest.

Author details

Haythem Bachrouche
Medicine School of Tunis, Tunis El Manar University, Nabeul, Tunisia

*Address all correspondence to: haythem.bachrouche@gmail.com

References

[1] Carducci B, Bhutta Z. Care of the Growth Restricted Newborn. Best Practice & Research Clinical Obstetrics & Gynaecology. 2018;**49**:103-116. DOI: 10.1016/j.bpobgyn

[2] Campisi SC, Carbone SE, Zlotkin S. Catch-up growth in full-term small for gestational age infants: A systematic review. Advances in Nutrition. 2019;**10**(1):104-111. DOI: 10.1093/advances/nmy091

[3] Laurie A, Nommsen-Rivers KG, Dewey. Growth of breastfed infants. Breastfeeding Medicine. 2009;**4**(1):S45-S49. DOI: 10.1089=bfm.2009.0048

[4] Santiago ACT, Martins LP, da Cunha M, de Lima Costa. Cardiometabolic evaluation of small for gestational age children: Protective effect of breast milk. Nutrición Hospitalaria. 2021;**38**(1):36-42. DOI: 10.20960/nh.03267

[5] Singhal A, Kennedy K, Lanigan J. Nutrition in infancy and long-term risk of obesity: Evidence from 2 randomized controlled trials. The American Journal of Clinical Nutrition. 2010;**92**:1133-1144. DOI: 10.3945/ajcn.2010.29302

[6] Phillip M, Turck D, Shamir R, Koletzko B, editors. Nutrition and growth. In: Yearbook 2022. Vol. 125. World Review of Nutrition and Dietetics. Basel: Karger AG; 2022. pp. 138-155. DOI: 10.1159/000521798

[7] Baird J, Fisher D, Lucas P, Kleijnen J. Being big or growing fast: Systematic review of size and growth in infancy and later obesity. BMJ. 2005;**331**(7522):929. DOI: 10.1136/bmj.38586.411273.EO

[8] Santiago AC, Cunha LP, Vieira NS, Moreira LM, Oliveira PR, Lyra PP, et al. Breastfeeding in children born small for gestational age and future nutritional and metabolic outcomes: A systematic review. Jornal de Pediatria. 2019;**95**:264-274. DOI: 10.1016/j.jped.2018.06.013

[9] Bachrouche H, Aissa MY, Chraiet K. Catch up growth in infants born small for gestational age: Breastfeeding vs standard formula feeding in Tunisia. In: EAPS8-0619 E-Poster Viewing. Paris: EAPS 2018; 2018

[10] Martín-Calvo N, Goni L, Tur JA. Low birth weight and small for gestational age are associated with complications of childhood and adolescence obesity: Systematic review and meta-analysis. Obesity Reviews. 2022;**23**(S1):e13380. DOI: 10.1111/obr.13380

[11] Rana R, McGrath M, Gupta P. Feeding interventions for infants with growth failure in the first six months of life: A systematic review. Nutrients. 2020;**12**:2044. DOI: 10.3390/nu12072044

[12] Singhal A. Long-term adverse effects of early growth acceleration or catch-up growth. Annals of Nutrition & Metabolism. 2017;**70**:236-240. DOI: 10.1159/000464302

[13] Suganuma M, Rumbold AR, Miller J. A systematic review and meta-analysis of human Milk feeding and short-term growth in preterm and very low birth weight infants. Nutrients. 2021;**13**:2089. DOI: 10.3390/nu13062089

[14] Koletzko B, El Sharkawy M. Epigenetics, nutrition, and growth. In: Yearbook 2022. Vol. 125. Basel, Karger: World Rev Nutr Diet; 2022. pp. 64-80. DOI: 10.1159/000521777

Chapter 13

Exclusive Breastfeeding in Infants with Ankyloglossia: Does the Tongue–Tie Interfere with Growth Patterns?

Christyann Lima Campos Batista and Alex Luiz Pozzobon Pereira

Abstract

The effect of ankyloglossia on breastfeeding remains unclear. Most studies focus on surgical procedures to correct aspects of breastfeeding, and few studies have focused on follow-up patients through. This chapter aims to analyze the influence of ankyloglossia on exclusive breastfeeding and the growth of infants up to the sixth month of life. A prospective cohort study was carried out with 225 mother–infant dyads who were followed up for the first six months of life. Full-term babies with and without ankyloglossia were followed up at a specialized breastfeeding center. Weight and length were measured and adjustments for age were calculated using the Body Mass Index and Z scores. Statistical analyzes were performed using descriptive statistics, and ANOVA for repeated measures. No significant differences were found in the growth measures of the following babies who remained exclusively breastfed ($p > 0.05$). Thus, compared with infants with the normal lingual frenulum, infants with ankyloglossia had no significant changes were observed in the growth measurements of babies with and without ankyloglossia. Infants should be followed and supported in initial difficulties to avoid unnecessary surgical procedures since the idea that tongue-tied babies could have a different milk flow rate is not supported.

Keywords: breastfeeding, ankyloglossia, infants, growth, failure to thrive

1. Introduction

The cumulative information about benefits in the current literature is massive [1]. Human milk is the optimal source of nutrition and protection for newborn infants [2]. Well-recognized as the gold standard for nutrition for infants, breastfeeding provides health benefits for infants, their mothers, and society [1, 3, 4].

Worldwide, major medical societies recommend breastfeeding exclusively for approximately the first six months of life and then continuing with the addition of complementary foods for as long as mutually desired by mother and child, potentially for two years [3]. This is the official recommendation by the World Health Organization [5, 6].

Several factors can hinder the establishment of breastfeeding and its exclusivity until the sixth month [7]. Among them, reports of low production or low perception of milk production by the mother, lack of support or knowledge about early difficulties, and pain when breastfeeding due to etiological changes such as nipple trauma, vasoconstriction, breast engorgement, ducts can be found in the literature. Obstructions, infections, and dermatitis [8, 9].

Thought recent years, a general increase in publications about ankyloglossia, popularly known as tongue–tie, emerged as one of the major factors that could interfere with exclusive breastfeeding [10].

Ankyloglossia is a congenital condition characterized by adhesion of the tongue to the floor of the mouth, resulting from the shortening or abnormality of the fixation of the Lingual Frenulum - a fold of mucous membrane - very close to the tip. of the tongue and/or on the upper surface of the gingiva or the alveolar crest [10–12]. The interest in this subject has increased due to considerable differences in diagnosis and treatment and management options around the world [13].

Recently, a systematic review of the literature, estimated a prevalence of 8% in babies under 1 year of age [14], with a higher prevalence being reported in male babies, in a ratio to a female sex of 1.5:1 to 2.6:1 [15]. Ankyloglossia can be clinically divided into two types: symptomatic when the frenulum directly impacts tongue movement and function; and asymptomatic, when the diagnosis is positive, but this does not result in major problems, especially in the neonatal period [16, 17].

Among the breastfeeding problems caused by ankyloglossia, authors have reported that a poor latch could result in low milk transfer, leading to failure to thrive in the exclusively breastfed infant [18, 19]. Although, most infants with tongue–tie can breastfeed without difficulty [20].

However, in the past years, the number of tongue–tie or ankyloglossia-related articles has increased dramatically, and among this research, few studies with robust methodological data support early surgical intervention [10]. The strength of evidence for the benefits of surgical treatment is limited; thus, other clinical therapies could be more beneficial if well implemented [21]. This treatment could be provided by a lactation specialist consultation and a speech therapist. Still, the optimal timing for surgery is controversial.

Evaluation by a speech pathologist is an essential component of the management of infants with breastfeeding problems and children that could have sound articulation problems [22].

Understanding that the general strategies for the infant should focus on supporting initiation and maintenance of breastfeeding and the remained controversies about the milk transfer rate and the possibility of failure to thrive of infants with ankyloglossia, this chapter is presented the result of a longitudinal study that assesses the growth of exclusive breastfeeding infants with and without ankyloglossia. The objective of this study was to analyze the influence of ankyloglossia on the growth evolution of infants up to the sixth month of life.

2. Methodology

A prospective cohort study was carried out at the University Hospital of the Federal University of Maranhao (Maternal–Infant Unit) - HUUFMA in the sectors of Rooming-in and Pediatric Follow-up Clinic at the Human Milk Bank (HMB), a center specializing in breastfeeding difficulties. HUUFMA is in the city of São Luís, the capital of a state in northeastern Brazil.

It is a high-complexity referral hospital for high-risk and habitual pregnancies. The estimated population of São Luís is 1.101,884 and an average income of 3.2 minimum wages. The data collection period was from January 2019 to December 2021.

To calculate the sample size, the level of alteration of the lingual frenulum reported in a previous prevalence study (8%) [14] was considered. In 2018, 15.959 live births were computed in the city, and the minimum number of participants calculated was 113 participants for a confidence level of 95% (population study with 80% power, 5% error). A total of 329 mother–infant dyads met the inclusion criteria at baseline. However, 225 remained followed up in the study, following the inclusion and exclusion criteria.

Mothers who expressed a desire to breastfeed, without medical contraindications for breastfeeding, and infants without health problems that could interfere with the growth or continuity of breastfeeding were included in the study. Babies with heart disease, pneumopathies, neuropathies, or those with genetic syndromes such as Pierre–Robin or Down syndrome, as well as twins, preterm newborns, and those with birth weight less than 2 kg were excluded.

Participants were recruited in two stages: initially in the rooming-in sector, through the "Tongue–tie Test Universal Screening (*Teste da Linguinha*)" performed by a qualified speech therapist. After a detailed assessment and completion of a positive diagnosis for ankyloglossia by a qualified speech therapist, those responsible were instructed to remain under follow-up in that sector and invited to participate in this research; for the group without ankyloglossia, they had to return to the outpatient clinic after 30 days of life to monitor growth and development until 6 months of age, and at that moment, those responsible were invited to participate in the study. The diagnosis was performed using the Bristol Tongue Assessment Tool [23].

Babies who for some reason met the criteria for surgical indication of ankyloglossia correction were removed from the study and referred for the procedure. All participants had the assistance of the multi-professional team to overcome the difficulties in breastfeeding and were properly instructed on the management of the nutritional aspect by a pediatrician and nutritionist.

Social and demographic data, as well as information regarding the type of diet declared by the mothers, were collected from the medical records. The birth-related variables were collected in the live birth declaration. Growth indicators were collected monthly as the dyads attended the follow-up appointment.

The measurements collected were weight in grams (with baby weighed in the morning, before feeding, without clothes and a diaper on a Balmak ELP25BB digital scale); length in centimeters (calm baby, lying on a rigid and fixed horizontal stadiometer model "Seca Mod. 416"). From these, the body mass index (BMI) (kg/m^2) was calculated. Adjustments regarding the Z score for age were calculated using the WHO Anthro software (v 3.2.2). All growth measurements were collected according to World Health Organization recommendations [24].

To analyze the evolution of the infants' growth, ANOVA for repeated measures was used in a general linear model, considering the Greenhouse–Geisser corrections to analyze the effects of time, the interaction time x ankyloglossia and ankyloglossia on the outcome variables, since the sphericity hypothesis in the Mauchly test was violated. In this analysis, only data from infants who remained on exclusive breastfeeding in all months were used.

The significance level adopted for all tests was 5% ($p < 0.05$). The analyzes were carried out using the IBM SPSS Statistics program (version 26).

This study was approved by the Ethics Committee for Research with Human Beings (local Institutional Review Board) under protocol no 3,052,208. The mothers and/or guardians of the newborns were informed about the objectives, risks, benefits, and procedures of the research and were invited to sign the Free and Informed Consent Form to participate in the study.

3. Results

A total of 225 dyads contained information on the outcome variable (weaning) in the study database and were entered into the final analysis. The median maternal age was 28 years (IQ 22–34).

It was observed that 27% of the sample presented early weaning and that, among infants with ankyloglossia, which represented 24% of the sample, the proportion of weaning rose to 51.9%. The general characteristics of the sample at the baseline are presented in **Table 1**.

The number of follow-up infants exclusively breastfed was presented in **Table 2**. The analysis showed no significant differences between the interaction of time x ankyloglossia

Variables	**N (%)**
Newborn sex	
Male	130 (57,8)
Female	95 (42,2)
Breastfed in the first hour	
Yes	138 (65,4)
No	73 (34,6)
Missing (14)	
Mother's age	
18 years old or less	18 (8,1)
Above 18 till 30 years	117 (52,7)
31 years old or more	87 (39,2)
Missing (3)	
Marital status	
Husband, live together	179 (79,6)
Single, widow	46 (20,4)
Mother's maximum educational level	
Elementary or less	31 (13,8)
High school	142 (63,1)
Graduate or more	52 (23,1)
Mother's occupation	
Jobless	104 (47,1)
Work	100 (45,2)
Just student	17 (7,7)

Variables	N (%)
Missing (4)	
Family income	
1 minimum wage (MW) or less	94 (42,2)
Above 1 till 3 MW	80 (35,9)
Above 3 till 5 MW	43 (19,3)
5 SM or more	6 (2,7)
Missing (2)	
Is the mother's first infant	
Yes	111 (49,3)
No	114 (50,7)
Delivery type	
Natural	103 (46)
C-section	121 (54)
Missing (1)	
Ankyloglossia	
Yes	54 (24)
No	171 (76)
Apgar Score	
1° minute, median - M, interquartile interval IQ	9 (8–9)
5° minute, M (IQ)	9 (9–9)
Birth weight, mean - m (standard deviation SD)	3212,9 (27)
Cephalic perimeter, M (IQ)	34,5 (33,5-35,3)
Thoracic perimeter, m (SD)	32,8 (0,3)
Length, M (IQ)	49 (47–50)

Table 1.
Social and demographic characteristics of mothers and infants in the baseline of the study, São Luís, Brazil, 2019–2021.

or isolated ankyloglossia on the reported measures ($p > 0.05$). For a better description of growth, only infants who were on exclusive breastfeeding were included in this analysis.

We observed that for the crude values in the intra-subjects (ANOVA) was a significant association that was not repeated for Z scores. This indicates that the infants followed in this study did grow positively and the adjustment for age was considered normal. In the other words, the infants did grow in the normal velocity and rhythm, ankyloglossia does not affect these measures.

When we observed the values for ankyloglossia isolated, none of the variables has an association with the grown measures, that is, the presence of tongue-tie does not affect the growth when we compare the groups ($p > 0,05$).

Figure 1(A–F) visually shows the growth curves between the groups analyzed, reporting no differences between the curves. All growth measurements were considered within the normal range according to the WHO growth curves.

Month	First		Second		Third		Fourth		Fifth		Sixth		ANOVA for repeated measures (p-value)		
Report Ankyloglossia	**Yes (36)**	**No (198)**	**Yes (21)**	**No (169)**	**Yes (27)**	**No (155)**	**Yes (20)**	**No (152)**	**Yes (18)**	**No (137)**	**Yes (18)**	**No (136)**	**Intra-subjects**	**Between subjects**	**Ankyloglossia isolated x time**
Weight (g; mean, SD)	4349,1 (116,7)	4341,7 (45,6)	5407,0 (151,8)	5477,2 (54,5)	6274,8 (177,5)	6297,7 (69,3)	7184,2 (217,8)	7010,1 (78,9)	7673,1 (201,8)	7542,2 (87,9)	7984,1 (181,4)	8000,8 (95,7)	<0,001	0,817	0,597
Length (cm; mean, SD)	53,41 (2,11)	53,30 (2,37)	57,16 (2,18)	56,90 (2,49)	60,32 (2,88)	60,20 (2,49)	62,80 (2,64)	62,70 (2,40)	65,07 (2,09)	64,72 (2,39)	66,27 (2,29)	65,95 (3,09)	<0,001	0,396	0,771
BMI (Mean, SD)	15,17 (1,68)	15,21 (1,56)	16,51 (1,61)	16,88 (1,67)	17,15 (1,63)	17,32 (1,71)	18,16 (1,65)	17,79 (1,86)	18,10 (1,68)	17,93 (1,83)	18,15 (1,76)	18,39 (2,35)	<0,001	0,778	0,624
Z scores for age															
Weight (Mean, SD)	−0,05 (1,20)	−0,00 (1,08)	−0,04 (0,98)	0,14 (0,94)	0,01 (1,31)	0,22 (1,06)	0,39 (1,17)	0,27 (1,09)	0,42 (0,92)	0,31 (1,10)	0,29 (1,00)	0,33 (1,13)	0,054	0,832	0,539
Length (Mean, SD)	−0,43 (1,09)	−0,42 (1,19)	−0,37 (1,08)	−0,41 (1,18)	−0,28 (1,37)	−0,15 (1,14)	−0,22 (1,27)	−0,17 (1,08)	−0,04 (1,03)	−0,12 (1,06)	−0,26 (1,02)	−0,35 (1,30)	0,112	0,406	0,718
BMI (Mean, SD)	0,23 (1,24)	0,32 (1,10)	0,23 (1,06)	0,53 (1,07)	0,22 (1,14)	0,43 (1,07)	0,71 (1,06)	0,51 (1,15)	0,60 (0,97)	0,50 (1,12)	0,59 (1,08)	0,73 (1,37)	0,559	0,819	0,628

BMI: body mass index; SD: standard deviation
Linear generalized model, ANOVA for repeated measures. The Mauchly test indicates that the sphericity hypothesis was always violated, therefore, the degrees of freedom were corrected using the estimation of sphericity of Greenhouse–Geisser ($p > 0,05$).

Table 2.
Analysis of variance of variables related to the growth of infants evaluated according to the month of follow-up and ankyloglossia, São Luís, Brazil, 2019–2021.

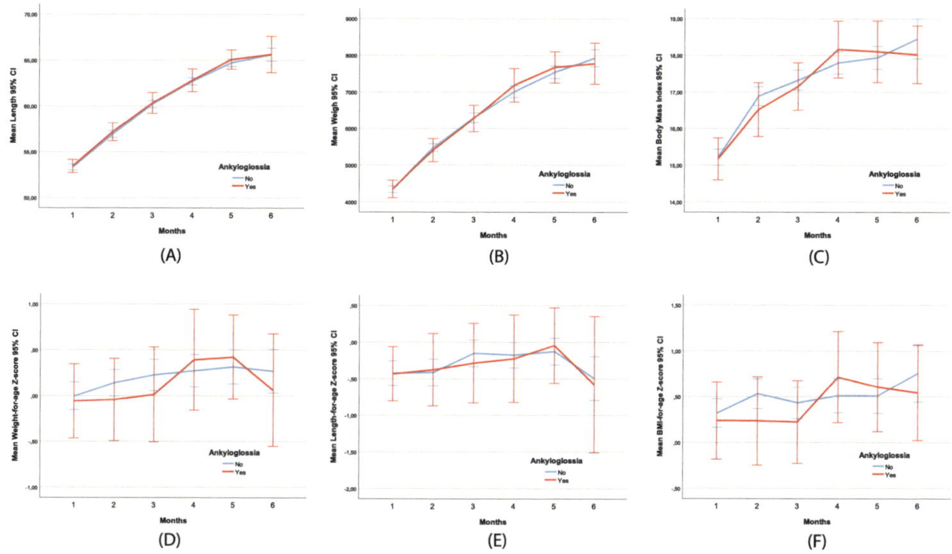

Figure 1.
(A–F) Graphics showing the monthly evolution of infant growth indicators, according to ankyloglossia. Curves: Mean (95% CI) of weight in kg for age (A); length in cm for age (B); body mass index for age (C); weight-for-age Z score (D); length for age (E) and body mass index for age (F).

4. Discussion

The main findings of this study, which analyzed the influence of ankyloglossia on aspects of growth, suggest that tongue–tie did not interfere with the growth of healthy full-term infants diagnosed when compared to infants without the normal tongue when they were exclusively breastfed until the sixth month of life. Life. This finding corroborates the hypothesis that ankyloglossia does not interfere with the milk flow transmitted during sucking and that babies with and without ankyloglossia can breastfeed exclusively and have the same growth rate and speed.

To this date, this is the first long-term follow-up study in early life to report the influence of ankyloglossia on growth indicators. Other studies [25–27], below, were similar in pointing out how ankyloglossia can act on the sucking and swallowing mechanisms, thus being able to affect the ingestion of human milk from the mother's breast.

In a retrospective study carried out in Austria, low weight gain was observed, for example, among effects on breastfeeding of infants aged 0–12 months such as breast pain, irritability, cracked nipples, reduced milk production, and poor attachment. However, this effect was not measured, being only reported by parents in the presentation of symptoms for frenotomy/frenectomy [26]. A systematic review of the literature by Manipon [25] states that weight loss is a common problem, but the isolated relationship of ankyloglossia with this outcome, or the age of presentation of these indicators, was not evidenced. A study by Livingstone et al. [27] reported cases of dehydration after massive weight loss caused by breastfeeding problems, citing ankyloglossia among adjacent disorders, but without mentioning its direct effect on the outcome.

The concern with the adequate growth of the baby is constant for families that seek medical help for breastfeeding problems in the first months of life and adequate multidisciplinary follow-up can be requested [28, 29].

The growth velocity seems to be more linked to the feeding method, and the effects of weaning can be corrected by the use of formulas, generally more caloric in advance in babies with this alteration [30]. Thus, this study analyzed only infants who remained on exclusive breastfeeding until the 6th month. A longer duration of exclusive breastfeeding can impact overall growth [31].

It is observed that breastfeeding problems should be the criteria to be taken into account when deciding on the frenotomy/frenectomy correction procedure, and in the current scientific literature, concerns about growth indicators are not mentioned. It is theorized that problematic breastfeeding resulting from ankyloglossia can generate low weight gain and consequent hypodevelopment.

Among the benefits reported after surgical intervention are the reduction of pain when breastfeeding and the improvement in the quality of breastfeeding [29, 32, 33]. Attention must be given to a precise clinical indication, as complications, although rare, can be found in the literature. A study carried out in New Zealand found an incidence of 13.9 problems per 100,000 procedures, such as feeding difficulties, respiratory events, pain, bleeding, and weight loss [34].

Therefore, it is evident that a reduction in frenotomy/frenectomy rates may result from the establishment of a multi-professional consensus with continued education and improvement of diagnostic methods for tongue–tie [35]. For this, the determination of comorbidities associated with ankyloglossia, such as alterations in growth indicators, can prove efficient to avoid unnecessary procedures.

This research was conducted in a center specializing in breastfeeding, which may lead to selection bias or bias in the reported rates, as mothers were continually instructed to continue with exclusive breastfeeding and were helped when they reported problems. However, this situation can be seen as a strong point since, even for the group with the alteration, the total breastfeeding time was longer than the national average, demonstrating that adequate monitoring and guidance can be decisive for reducing the chance of weaning, thus highlighting clinical and non-surgical measures as a protective effect of breastfeeding.

5. Conclusions

In EBF infants, no differences were observed in the measures of growth assessed up to the sixth month of age, demonstrating that, for all groups, the studied indicators were equivalent.

Adequate follow-up by a specialized team can help in the early diagnosis and treatment of ankyloglossia, which may result in a decrease in weaning rates and improve children's health indicators. Thus, in this way, early surgery could be unnecessary if the mother–infant dyad has the correct support and guidance on breastfeeding.

Acknowledgements

I would like to thank the University Hospital of the Federal University of Maranhao for providing the structure and materials for the research. Also, thanks for the Post-Graduation in Dentistry from where part of this chapter was developed. To Alex Luiz Pozzobon Pereira (DDS, Ph.D.) who supervised this research.

Funding information: the author developed this study in a public health facility. All the resources were provided by the author.

Conflict of interest

The author declares no conflict of interest.

Acronyms and abbreviations

HUUFMA	University Hospital of the Federal University of Maranhao
HMB	Human Milk Bank
EBF	Exclusive Breastfeeding
BF	Breastfeeding
BMI	Body Mass Index

Author details

Christyann Lima Campos Batista[1*] and Alex Luiz Pozzobon Pereira[2]

1 University Hospital, Federal University of Maranhão, São Luís, Brazil

2 Department of Dentistry, Federal University of Maranhão, São Luís, Brazil

*Address all correspondence to: christyann.batista@huufma.br

References

[1] Victora CG, Bahl R, Barros AJD, França GVA, Horton S, Krasevec J, et al. Breastfeeding in the 21st century: Epidemiology, mechanisms, and lifelong effect. Lancet. 2016;**387**(10017):475-490

[2] Singh KS, Singh BP, Rokana N, Singh N, Kaur J, Singh A, et al. Bio-therapeutics from human milk: Prospects and perspectives. Journal of Applied Microbiology. 2021;**131**(6):2669-2687

[3] Meek JY, Noble L. Section on breastfeeding. Policy statement: Breastfeeding and the use of human milk. Pediatrics. 2022;**150**(1):e2022057988

[4] Salone LR, Vann WF, Dee DL. Breastfeeding: An overview of oral and general health benefits. Journal of American Dental Association. 2013;**144**(2):143-151

[5] World Health Organization. Baby-Friendly Hospital Initiative: Revised, Updated and Expanded for Integrated Care. Geneva: World Health Organization; 2009 [citado 26 de novembro de 2022]. (WHO Guidelines Approved by the Guidelines Review Committee). Disponível em: http://www.ncbi.nlm.nih.gov/books/NBK153471/

[6] Kramer MS, Kakuma R. Optimal duration of exclusive breastfeeding. Cochrane Database of Systematic Reviews. 2012;**2012**(8):CD003517

[7] Anderson L, Kynoch K, Kildea S, Lee N. Effectiveness of breast massage for the treatment of women with breastfeeding problems: A systematic review. JBI Database System Review Implement Report. 2019;**17**(8):1668-1694

[8] Bergmann RL, Bergmann KE, von Weizsäcker K, Berns M, Henrich W, Dudenhausen JW. Breastfeeding is natural but not always easy: intervention for common medical problems of breastfeeding mothers – a review of the scientific evidence. Journal of Perinatal Medicine. 2014;**42**(1):26. Available from: https://www.degruyter.com/document/doi/10.1515/jpm-2013-0095/html

[9] Karacam Z, Saglik M. Breastfeeding problems and interventions performed on problems: Systematic review based on studies made in Turkey. Turk Pediatri Ars. 2018;**53**(3):134-148

[10] Bin-Nun A, Kasirer YM, Mimouni FB. A dramatic increase in Tongue tie-related articles: A 67 years systematic review. Breastfeed Medicine. 2017;**12**(7):410-414

[11] O'Shea JE, Foster JP, O'Donnell CP, Breathnach D, Jacobs SE, Todd DA, et al. Frenotomy for tongue-tie in newborn infants. Cochrane Database System Review. 2017;**3**:CD011065

[12] Mills N, Keough N, Geddes DT, Pransky SM, Mirjalili SA. Defining the anatomy of the neonatal lingual frenulum. Clinical Anatomy. 2019;**32**(6):824-835

[13] Jin RR, Sutcliffe A, Vento M, Miles C, Travadi J, Kishore K, et al. What does the world think of ankyloglossia? Acta Paediatric. 2018;**107**(10):1733-1738

[14] Hill RR, Lee CS, Pados BF. The prevalence of ankyloglossia in children aged <1 year: A systematic review and meta-analysis. Pediatric Research. 2021;**90**(2):259-266

[15] Hall DMB. Tongue tie. Archives of Disease in Childhood. 2005;**90**(12):1211-1215

[16] Brzęcka D, Garbacz M, Micał M, Zych B, Lewandowski B. Diagnosis, classification and management of ankyloglossia including its influence on breastfeeding. Developmental Period Medicine. 2019;**23**(1):79-87

[17] Buck LS, Frey H, Davis M, Robbins M, Spankovich C, Narisetty V, et al. Characteristics and considerations for children with ankyloglossia undergoing frenulectomy for dysphagia and aspiration. American Journal of Otolaryngology. 2020;**41**(3):102393

[18] Forlenza GP, Paradise Black NM, McNamara EG, Sullivan SE. Ankyloglossia, exclusive breastfeeding, and failure to thrive. Pediatrics. 2010;**125**(6):e1500-e1504

[19] Ballard JL, Auer CE, Khoury JC. Ankyloglossia: Assessment, incidence, and effect of frenuloplasty on the breastfeeding dyad. Pediatrics. 2002;**110**(5):e63

[20] Messner AH, Lalakea ML, Aby J, Macmahon J, Bair E. Ankyloglossia: Incidence and associated feeding difficulties. Archieves of Otolaryngological Head and Neck Surgery. 2000;**126**(1):36-39

[21] Walsh J, Tunkel D. Diagnosis and treatment of ankyloglossia in newborns and infants: A review. JAMA Otolaryngology Head and Neck Surgery. 2017;**143**(10):1032-1039

[22] Lalakea ML, Messner AH. Ankyloglossia: Does it matter? Pediatric Clinical North America. 2003;**50**(2):381-397

[23] Ingram J, Johnson D, Copeland M, Churchill C, Taylor H, Emond A. The development of a tongue assessment tool to assist with tongue-tie identification. Archieves Disease Child and Fetal Neonatal Edition. 2015;**100**(4):F344-F349

[24] World Health Organization. WHO Child Growth Standards: Training Course on Child Growth Assessment. 2nd ed. Geneva: World Health Organization; 2008. Available from: https://apps.who.int/iris/handle/10665/350477

[25] Manipon C. Ankyloglossia and the breastfeeding infant: Assessment and intervention. Advances in Neonatal Care. 2016;**16**(2):108-113

[26] Ramoser G, Guóth-Gumberger M, Baumgartner-Sigl S, Zoeggeler T, Scholl-Bürgi S, Karall D. Frenotomy for tongue-tie (frenulum linguac breve) showed improved symptoms in the short- and long-term follow-up. Acta Paediatric. 2019;**108**(10):1861-1866

[27] Livingstone VH, Willis CE, Abdel-Wareth LO, Thiessen P, Lockitch G. Neonatal hypernatremic dehydration associated with breast-feeding malnutrition: a retrospective survey. CMAJ. 2000;**162**(5):647-652

[28] Ray S, Hairston TK, Giorgi M, Links AR, Boss EF, Walsh J. Speaking in tongues: What parents really think about Tongue-tie surgery for their infants. Clinical Pediatric. 2020;**59**(3):236-244

[29] Muldoon K, Gallagher L, McGuinness D, Smith V. Effect of frenotomy on breastfeeding variables in infants with ankyloglossia (tongue-tie): A prospective before and after cohort study. BMC Pregnancy Childbirth. 2017;**17**(1):373

[30] Azad MB, Vehling L, Chan D, Klopp A, Nickel NC, McGavock JM, et al. Infant feeding and weight gain: Separating breast Milk from breastfeeding and formula from food. Pediatrics. 2018;**142**(4):e20181092

[31] Patro-Gołąb B, Zalewski BM, Polaczek A, Szajewska H. Duration of breastfeeding and early growth: A systematic review of current evidence. Breastfeed Medicine. 2019;**14**(4):218-229

[32] Slagter KW, Raghoebar GM, Hamming I, Meijer J, Vissink A. Effect of frenotomy on breastfeeding and reflux: Results from the BRIEF prospective longitudinal cohort study. Clinical Oral Investigation. 2021;**25**(6):3431-3439

[33] Ghaheri BA, Cole M, Fausel SC, Chuop M, Mace JC. Breastfeeding improvement following tongue-tie and lip-tie release: A prospective cohort study. Laryngoscope. 2017;**127**(5):1217-1223

[34] Hale M, Mills N, Edmonds L, Dawes P, Dickson N, Barker D, et al. Complications following frenotomy for ankyloglossia: A 24-month prospective New Zealand paediatric surveillance unit study. Journal of Paediatric Child Health. 2020;**56**(4):557-562

[35] Dixon B, Gray J, Elliot N, Shand B, Lynn A. A multifaceted programme to reduce the rate of tongue-tie release surgery in newborn infants: Observational study. International Journal of Pediatric Otorhinolaryngology. 2018;**113**:156-163

Section 4

Breastfeeding Interventions

Chapter 14

Cost-Effectiveness and Equity Trade-Off for Breastfeeding Interventions

Sinead M. Hurley, Kathy Whyte and Jan Sorensen

Abstract

Many factors influence mothers' decisions to begin and continue breastfeeding (BF). These include individual, societal and policy factors. In this chapter, we address these factors including the social differences in BF practice among Irish women and discuss important policy implications (efficiency and equity). It is well-documented that BF practice is different for mothers with different social backgrounds. Traditionally, evaluations of BF support interventions have focused on either the effectiveness or the equity issues, but rarely analysed both in a joint framework. The aim of this chapter is to discuss the cost-effectiveness and equity trade-off for BF interventions. We identify different BF support interventions and focus on social differences and their influence for maintaining BF practices. We illustrate how the "Distributional cost-effectiveness (DCEA) framework" can be applied to these interventions and how some interventions may be more effective in changing behaviour and outcomes for mothers with different social-economic status (SES), which may change the inequality in effectiveness and reduce the health equity.

Keywords: breastfeeding, socioeconomic, cost-effectiveness, interventions, inequality, equity

1. Introduction

Ireland has the lowest breastfeeding (BF) rate among Western countries at about 61% compared to rates of 94% in Sweden, 95% in Australia, 81% in the UK, and 79% in the USA [1–5]. The Irish proportion of babies being exclusively BF on discharge from hospital is even lower at 44% [3]. **Figure 1** shows a slowly growing proportion of babies are breastfed on discharge from hospital from 2011 to 2020, although around two out of five babies are still being fed with artificial feed. Ireland has introduced many BF strategies and actions such as; the European Perinatal Health reports, reports documenting BF actions from collaborations with the WHO Baby Friendly Hospital Initiative and the BF in the Healthy Ireland Health Service Executive Action Plan 2016–2021 [6]. However, Irish BF rates still continue to lag behind Western counterparts.

It is widely recognised that BF provides health benefits to both the baby and the BF mother [7]. It is reasonable to assume that there will be some form of

IntechOpen

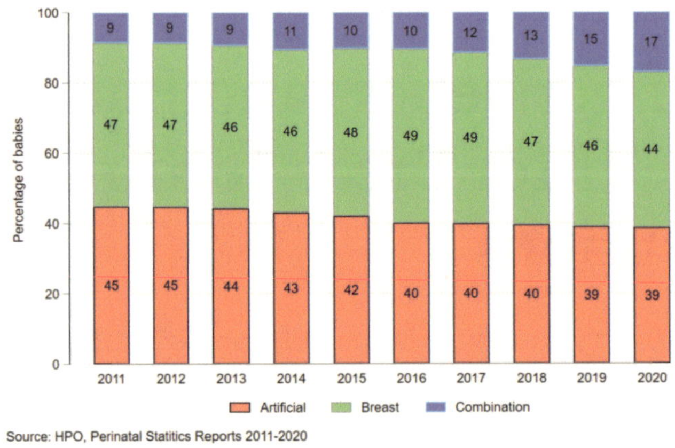

Figure 1.
Types of infant feeding at discharge from hospital, Ireland 2011–2020.

exposure-response relationship, although it may be difficult to quantify based on observational data. Indeed, systematic reviews have identified that studies use different methodologies to analyse this relationship, and the empirical results show great variation, dependent on the intensity (exclusive or partial) and duration of the BF practice [8]. Systematic reviews have reported evidence that suggests that babies who are exclusively breastfed over 6 months have lower risks of developing infections and other complications in comparison with babies who have been exclusively fed with artificial feeding [9]. Studies have identified that BF reduces the risk of a range of infectious diseases and BF has a preventive effect against developing obesity [10].

The types of infectious diseases being present from mothers who don't BF versus those who do include otitis media, gastroenteritis, childhood pneumonia, as well as childhood obesity, type 1 and type 2 diabetes and cancers [8, 11]. The duration of BF is essential in terms of the child health outcomes. BF for greater than 6 months has protecting influences from childhood overweight/obesity [10]. Child intellectual activity such as reading and remembering has been shown to improve with higher rates and longer BF duration [12]. A recent study in 2022 demonstrated that longer BF duration was associated with improved cognitive score of children from age 5 up to age 14 [13]. Breastmilk contains antibodies and protective factors that transfers cytokines and growth factors to the infant which can stimulate the infant's immune system and reduce the risk of infection. Lactoferrin has anti-inflammatory, antioxidant, antiviral and antimicrobial effects and lactoferrin supplementation has been shown recently to reduce the cytokine IL6 and associated systemic inflammation [14]. BF over a long period reduces the risk of breast cancer in comparison with mothers who have not been BF their babies [15].

Beyond the health benefits of BF, a higher BF rate can offer substantial financial savings in the long term by reducing infant infections such as gastrointestinal and respiratory infections as well as otitis media, necrotising enterocolitis and breast cancer, which are all significantly reduced in women who are BF the infant [16]. In addition, in a review article from 2022 we identified BF as a mediator for youth adiposity in Ireland and the UK [17]. In the UK for example the cost to the economy from infant infections alone was £89 million and approx. £959 million for breast cancer treatments [18, 19]. Not many papers have studied the cost-effectiveness of promoting BF in Ireland, but one reported that BF for low-birth weight babies was associated with lower costs and greater health benefits [20].

2. Factors relating to Irish women's decision to BF

Irish women's decision to BF are influenced by individual, societal and political factors as illustrated in **Figure 2**.

Individual factors relating to BF decisions include women's perceptions of healthcare professionals (HCP), level of education and awareness among others. Building trust with HCPs is important for women to feel more supported in their BF choice and more in control during their pregnancy. Individual factors are influenced by women's SES. SES reflects an individual's position in society and is determined by an individual's social and economic status such as income, education level, occupation and area of residence. BF rates vary between urban and rural settings. This variation is partly explained by the level of maternal education and household income [21]. In Ireland, women living in socioeconomically disadvantaged areas are less likely to BF compared to those living in a more socioeconomically advantaged area, and they are also less likely to continue BF [22]. The proportion of babies that are artificially fed are lowest for women in higher professional work, indicative of educational attainment (**Figure 3**).

Societal factors include advice offered to women from HCPs during pre and post pregnancy care. Immigrant women living in Ireland felt that HCPs "did not sufficiently stress the importance of BF in Irish hospital setting" [23]. They made a number of suggestions for governments and HCPs to support women to exclusively breastfeed in Ireland including BF counselling, more advice from HCPs, and that governments should develop better BF facilities in public places such as public parks or shopping malls. The health service executive (HSE) published the National Standards for Antenatal Education which identifies elements that should be included in all antenatal education programmes [24]. One of the themes of this was having an educated workforce to provide BF skills to women. More of these supports are needed for BF women in Ireland. In a study in three countries: Australia, Ireland and Sweden, exploring women's perceptions of what best encouraged them to BF, the main factors were support and social networks which included face-to-face or online informal support, societal support from HCPs, and the supportive BF culture of the particular country [25].

Societal factors include the culture of a country which has an important role as to whether BF practices take place and for how long. Ireland's BF culture reported women "feeling embarrassed" about BF in public [26]. In a comparison study with Sweden and Australia, Ireland ranked highest for having a "BF environment not suitable" [27]. The cultural views on BF practices differ in other EU states. Swedish culture for example is reported to be supportive towards public BF practices, where Swedish women found engaging in BF practices in public to be "easy and enjoyable" [28]. In order to create

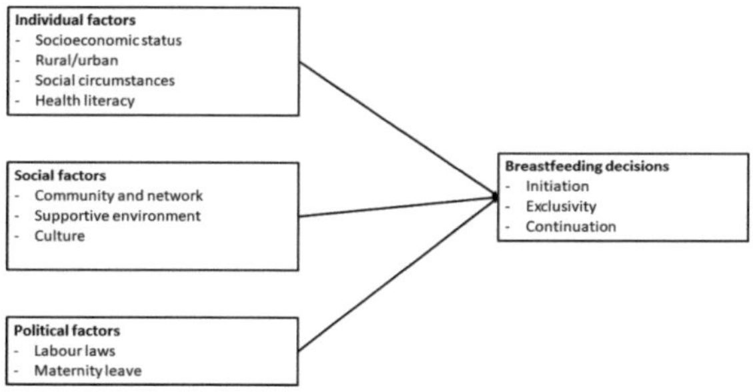

Figure 2.
Factors influencing BF decisions.

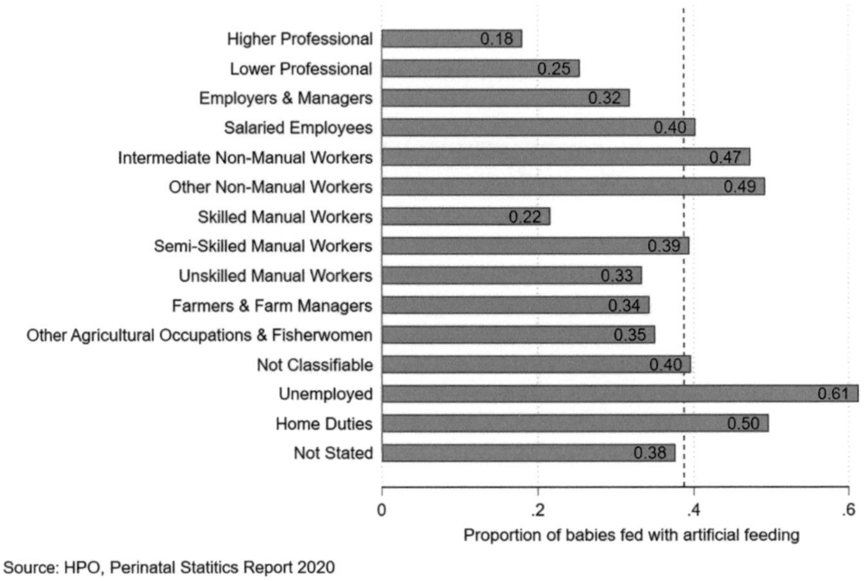

Figure 3.
Proportion of babies fed with artificial feeding by mothers' socioeconomic status, Ireland, 2020.

a BF-supportive culture it is essential to instil positive attitudes towards BF women early on and encourage continued self-efficacy, beliefs in their ability to breastfeed. Supportive environments that promote increased BF include, more social, family and partner supports. Women should feel empowered, supported and look favourability on BF practices in public.

Policy factors influencing BF decisions include: National policies i.e. maternal and parental leave policies, Irish marketing practices including the marketing of infant formula, BF promotion policies and policies related to the level of resources and supports provided to women returning to the work environment after leave [29]. Other policies are hospital/HCP guidelines i.e. the baby friendly hospital initiative (BFHI), educational policies i.e. healthcare staff educational requirements and individual policies such as those providing one-to-one support to women.

Paid maternity and parental leave policies have a role in BF decisions. Evidence has demonstrated that the longer the period of paid maternity or parental leave, the higher the rates of BF and the higher the odds of initiating BF in the first instance [30, 31]. BF has been associated with multiple positive benefits for both mother and child and it is recommended by the World Health Organisation (WHO) and HSE to exclusively breastfeed for a minimum of 6 months [32]. The duration of maternity leave and sharing parental leave, has also been associated with longer BF rates [33]. Ireland has the fourth shortest period of paid parental and maternity leave compared to other European countries [34]. In Ireland women can take 26 weeks (182 days) paid maternity leave with up to an additional 16 weeks of unpaid leave [35]. Maternity leave is paid by the Irish government or by employers, but employers in Ireland are not under obligation to pay maternity leave [35]. The duration of leave means that many Irish women feel compiled to begin work sooner than they wish leading to discontinuation of BF practices [36]. A study in three Organisation for Economic Co-operation and Development (OECD) countries ranked Sweden as the country providing the longest paid maternity and parental leave from all three countries and having the highest proportion of women returning to full time work after leave [37]. In contrast to Ireland, Swedish parental leave is paid up to 68 weeks (480 days) and each parent is entitled to 120 days each which they can either choose to divide between them or take solely by one parent [38]. The OECD report indicated that 77.8% of women return to full-time employment after parental leave in Sweden versus 61.5% in the US and just 44.4% in Ireland [37].

The marketing and advertising of infant formula can discourage women from BF which may contribute to the low BF rates in Ireland. Ireland is one of the biggest producers of infant formula in the world which results in higher advertising and marketing of infant formula contributing to lower BF practices [39]. The Code of Marketing of Breast-milk Substitutes (BMS) from the WHO states that marketing of breast milk substitutes should not be allowed up to 36 months, and EU food law states that companies are not allowed to make health claims about infant formula or compare breast milk and infant formula or imply it is superior to BF [40]. The Food Safety Authority of Ireland (FSAI) audits the labelling of infant formula in Ireland. However, breaches of milk formula marketing rules do occur. Milk formula manufacturers also sponsor certain helplines and other agencies and offer free gifts for health care workers (HCWs). The result of this is negligible on patients attending care during pregnancy. Governments and other policy-makers are urged to do more. A proposed amendment to the Online Safety bill was recently made to restrict marketing of infant formula and follow on formula [41]. This would legally restrict the marketing of follow-on infant formula as a proposed alternative to BF practice.

3. Interventions to support BF

Interventions to support BF include Individual, Societal, and Policy-based interventions.

For Societal (environment, education, counselling and support) interventions, different approaches have been studied. Some previous reviews indicated that methods such as one-to-one education, counselling and support provided to women over a long time period is an effective method of promoting BF [42, 43]. This may be even more effective for women of lower SES. Internet support may be a useful adjunct to face-to-face care. The settings where the interventions were conducted varied, as did the training which was provided to those performing the interventions. For peer support, there are considerable differences which include the study populations, the definition of peers, and the definition of counsellors, peer counsellor training protocols, peer visit schedules, and outcome ascertainment methods between trials. In the majority of studies, the interventions were compared to 'routine care', the definition of which seems to vary considerably between countries.

The acute maternity care settings are central for implementation of structured programmes to support BF. The content of such programmes could replace an existing programme, such as the BFHI, in full or in part, or be specifically developed to reflect local needs. A review of 21 studies (mostly observational) and five systematic reviews observed the introduction of a structured BF programme which offered some improvement in the duration of BF but these structured programmes were not always statistically significant [44]. A Cochrane review of 52 randomised control trials (RCTs) indicated that providing support to women during BF is effective in increasing the rates of exclusive BF [42, 45]. Having the appropriate supports in place would be effective in health care for increasing BF initiation, however support mechanisms should be offered at all heath care settings. Support may be offered by professional health care staff, through peer to peer support groups either in person or online. The media also plays a role in relaying evidence based supportive advice to women on BF. Support that is offered face-to-face is more likely to be the most effective.

Providing professional support to women has been shown to promote BF for a longer period of time [46]. Support should be tailored to the setting and the needs of the population group. In the same Cochrane review, a subgroup analysis of two studies (162 women) evaluating the effect of repeated informal BF education programmes personalised to each woman's needs showed a statistically significant increase in the number of women starting to breastfeed as a result of the intervention. The reviews that addressed interventions among adolescent mothers showed mixed results, but it is clear that peer support and educational interventions improve BF rates, especially when these are targeted at individuals.

Exclusive BF during hospital stay also significantly increases BF duration outside the hospital irrespective of SES [47–49]. In addition, regardless of SES, BF mothers generally need practical knowledge and experienced support in order to attain BF success, however disadvantaged mothers may require extra support in order to overcome BF problems [50–52]. Education for women should be aimed at increasing their knowledge of BF practice and to acknowledge the possible lack of exposure to BF they may be engaging in along with trying to allay fears that their baby will not be satisfied by breastmilk alone. All new mothers need support from professionals and others to reassure them that exclusively BF will provide sufficient nutrition for their infants. Education about the benefits of BF should also be extended to their partners and the community [53]. Developing healthcare professionals' capabilities to educate disadvantaged groups, their social networks and the public about BF is crucial [54].

Educational resources and BF supports for women should include adequate lactation consultant visits. In New Zealand for example at 3,650 annual births, there were 3 full-time lactation consultants in the Women's Health Service and 0.8 full-time in the Neonatal Intensive Care Unit at the hospital setting in 2017, which if applied to Irish figures of 62,039 births would equate to approximately 50 full time lactation consultants to meet demands in the Women's Health Service [55]. In Ireland there are significantly less numbers of lactation consultants and there is a significant need for additional lactation consultants in hospitals, with some having no specialist lactation posts in lactation [55]. In order to increase the availability and affordability of lactation consultant services for BF women, more public funding should be made available. In addition, private demand could be increased by health insurance plans providing coverage for lactation consultant services. There are a number of volunteer support groups across Ireland that support women and offer guidance and advice on BF practices. Some of these support groups include: La Leche League of Ireland, Friends of Breastfeeding, and Cuidiú support groups, among others. Many of these groups were set up by women wanting a better understanding of BF and more supports and better accessibility to these supports for Irish women. While there are many groups setup, some areas of Ireland are still limited in terms of accessibility and location. More advice from HCPs, more resources and encouragement to attend these groups early in an infant's stage of growth are needed.

Policy interventions can further support BF practices. A barrier is a lack of resources and supports to BF women returning to work. The Work Life Balance and Miscellaneous Provisions Bill (2022) was recently proposed in Ireland to provide parents with rights to better support a work life balance including, extending BF breaks by allowing women to take paid time from work each day for BF [56]. This will assist women and support BF practices but much more needs to be done [25]. BF duration and pressure to return to work due to poor pay is forcing women to stop BF early or to not begin at all [36].

For policy-based interventions under hospital and HCP guidelines, the BFHI guidelines indicate that interventions including structured programmes to promote BF are required as well as promoting early skin-to-skin contact (SSC), the practice of rooming-in, where the baby's crib is kept beside the mother for mother-infant contact, and avoiding supplementary infant feeding are important [57].

4. Other factors to consider in relation to BF interventions

It is also important to consider other influencing factors such as the timing of the intervention with respect to the pregnancy, who delivers the intervention, the target group, and the use of e-health technology as an add on to in-person supports. With technology and telephone support forming an ever increasing integral part of health-care delivery, the development of web-based, text messaging, electronic prompts and interactive computer interventions promote and support BF [58]. Technology for assisting women in public to find facilities and services for BF are very useful. Further investment in technology is also needed to support women to find facilities that are available in their area. A study conducted demonstrated the advantages of the "FeedFinder App" whereby women shared views on various facilities and level of privacy [59]. Women should feel empowered to breastfeed in public and technology also can have a positive role. Business owners may also become more motivated to have positively reviewed facilities as it may enhance their customer numbers and instil more awareness on the benefits of BF facilities in public.

5. Demonstrating health economic value of BF interventions

Whether BF interventions are offering better opportunities, better knowledge or developing a supportive environment, the end result of these programmes is determined by the women's willingness to engage and continue BF. Evaluations of these interventions must therefore consider to which extent they are able to influence women's BF inclinations. This may be observed in the proportion of women who begin BF and continue to exclusively breastfeed their babies which should be for at least 6 months as recommended in various guidelines and recommendations e.g. by the WHO. Women's BF practices are difficult to monitor and systematically observe. Most data collection about BF will rely on accurate self-reporting and holds a risk of misclassification. This would imply that there are various errors in reports of the duration of exclusive and partial BF periods.

In an Irish context, there is a National Perinatal Reporting System (NPRS), which captures all births and this system obtains data on the infants' feeding at the time of discharge from the birth hospital or midwifery service [3]. Three categories of feeding are used: Artificial feed, Breast, or Combined artificial and breastfeed (see **Figure 1**). The accurate reporting of this variable requires that the researchers have access to information about the real BF practice. Such information may be obtained through direct observation or conversation with the woman, through qualitative studies or through analysing and reporting records in the medical charts. It is clear that the time of discharge from hospital will be between one-three days after the birth [3]. After discharge from hospital, BF practice may depend on the women's level of knowledge and support provided.

"Growing Up in Ireland" (GUI) is a national longitudinal study of children in Ireland. This represents a different way of collecting data about BF. The first data collection point is when the child is 9 month old. Questions about BF are included in the personal interviews of predominantly the mothers. An analysis of BF practices sampled 11,134 infants out of 41,185 born during December 2007 and 2008, and 65% of the sampled families agreed to take part [60]. The BF initiation rate was 56% and reduced to 48% when the baby was brought home from hospital. In all, 44% of the babies were reported to be ever exclusively breastfed and 8% were reported to be breastfed 9 months after the birth [60]. The study reported substantially lower BF initiation rates for mothers born in Ireland (48.8%) in comparison with mothers born elsewhere (82.3%). The study reported higher BF rates for women aged over 30 years (~60%) and women of higher SES (>75%) [60].

Although the full picture of BF practice in Ireland is not conveyed through these data sources, it is clear, that the WHO recommendations of exclusively BF during the first 6 month of the infant's life, is not followed for all babies. It would appear that there continues to be scope for further public programmes, to support BF practices in Ireland. With limited resources allocated to healthcare and with competing demands for these resources, it is relevant to analyse and document the value from investments to better support BF practice.

To inform decisions about what might be appropriate investments, the target groups, configuration, content and organisation of BF support programmes should be clearly specified to enable a careful analysis of their potential costs, effects, cost-effectiveness and potential impact on social equality.

6. Models for BF support

It is worth carefully considering different models for how health interventions can be implemented especially across different social groups. One model could be providing BF support to all women who have given birth. It is then crucial to consider whether the acceptance of the BF service will be similar for all social groups. This is unlikely to be the case especially if the mothers have to make an active effort themselves to get contacts with the BF support. There may be mothers who are well experienced with approaching HCPs and following their advice, and there may be mothers who find it much more difficult. This difference may relate to the mothers' social and cultural background including demographic and social factors and health literacy.

It is likely that mothers with lower health literacy may be less likely to get in contact with the BF support, and if that is the case, there may be an unequal effect of the programme across different social groups. A universally available intervention is thus likely to be more favorable for mothers with higher health literacy and less favourable for mothers with lower health literacy. This will be expressed as variation in the uptake of BF support and by implication, the proportion of mothers who successfully initiate BF after the birth. When having established contacts between the BF support and mothers, there may also be variation among social groups in their acceptance, and willingness and opportunities to follow the advice and recommendations to breastfeed. Mothers from some social groups may find it easier and more appropriate than mothers from other social groups. This will in particular be expressed in social variation in the duration of BF (e.g. the proportion who is exclusively BF 6 months after the birth).

The health benefit of BF for both the baby and the mother may also be different for different social groups. Very little empirical research has explored this. It is generally challenging to demonstrate the positive health benefits of BF, in different social groups although several meta-analyses have identified health benefits. The causal inference is generally challenging. The challenges relate partly to whether the effect found in studies from different populations and jurisdictions can be assumed to apply in other contexts. Furthermore, there may be different valuations of the health benefits from different social groups. If there is social variation in the health benefits from BF by social groups, then that is also something that should be considered when evaluating BF interventions.

7. Models for outcomes

An American group of clinicians developed a model framework to estimate the impact of changes in BF practice on population health and costs [61, 62]. They analysed the health impact of higher BF rates on a range of maternal diseases including number of cases, deaths and costs related to pre-menopausal ovarian cancer, breast cancer, hypertension, diabetes, and myocardial infarction. For the baby they considered cases, deaths and costs related to acute lymphoblastic leukaemia, crohn's disease, ulcerative colitis, sudden infant death syndrome, otitis media, gastrointestinal illness, obesity, lower respiratory tract infection and necrotizing enterocolitis. They modelled the outcomes for 21 different BF scenarios specified by monthly rates of exclusive or any BF until 12 months after the birth. They employed BF rates for different US states and reported results separately for the non-Hispanic white, non-Hispanic blacks and Hispanic sub-populations.

Behind their analysis was a mathematical model, which probably represents the most detailed approach to simulating the health outcomes from BF. The results should be interpreted with due consideration of the underlying assumptions and their validity in relation to the analysed population. Similar, although less comprehensive models of BF outcomes have been reported for Mexico and the UK [63–65].

8. Costing BF support programmes

8.1 Gross-costing approach

Costs of BF support programmes can be determined using either a gross-costing or a micro-costing approach. The gross-costing approach determines the cost of the programme by identifying the aggregated amount of resources required to implement and run the programme. The cost analysis of the programme will need to consider which resources are required and their associated cost. The costs may relate to the salary, consumables, transport and overheads. The gross-cost of a programme could be determined based on assumptions of the number of staff and related resources as illustrated with fictitious numbers in **Table 1**.

These total costs can then be apportioned to participants or activities conducted as part of the programme in order to assess the average cost per:

- Peer-support groups established.
- Mothers offered BF support.
- Individual and group contacts.

Resource	Cost per month (€]
Salary (10.0 full time lactation consultant)	60,000
Secretarial support (2 FT)	8000
Consumables	2000
Transport	5000
Consultation and office space	10,000
Overhead 40% of above	30,000
Total cost	115,000

Table 1.
Illustrative gross-costing of a BF support programme.

	Peer-support (groups of 8)	6-month BF support of mothers initiating LC services	Single, individual contacts	Group contacts
Initiation	2 h	1 h	0.5 h	2 h
Contacts	1 h	5 contacts @1 h	5 contacts @1 h	
Number of participants	8	1 over 6 months	1	6 per group
Facilities	Private homes/ public space	Hospital and private home	Hospital	Meeting space
Transport cost	€20	€40	€0	€0
Total cost per woman	€100	€300	€250	€50

Table 2.
Illustrative micro-costing of a BF support programme.

8.2 Micro-costing approach

The alternative micro-costing approach is based on explicit assumptions of resource use for different activities in the programme. Four different activities are outlined in **Table 2** with number of activities included in each.

Each activity is specified by nominal (ideal) numbers of contacts in a month or year, or number of contacts for mothers who enter the programme (e.g. 3–5 contacts during the first 12 months after the birth). The contacts may be counted as individual sessions or as group sessions.

9. Cost-effectiveness of BF support programmes

When there is information about the cost of different configurations of BF support programmes and the associated outcomes can be modelled based on descriptions of the target group, uptake and adherence to the programme, the cost-effectiveness and "value for money" can be assessed.

In cost-effectiveness analyses, different programmes are compared against a base case, which often is the current situation. The required cost of the programmes is related to the health outcomes and the potential downstream healthcare costs in so-called incremental cost-effectiveness ratios (ICER). The incremental cost is the additional cost of the BF programme and the cost of future healthcare (which might be savings, if the BF programme is successful in reducing the disease incidence for the babies and their mothers). These incremental costs should be related to a valid measure of effect, which could be gains in the proportion of exclusively 6-month breastfed babies, time without disease for the baby or mother, life expectancy, health-related quality of life, or quality-adjusted life years (QALYs).

By comparing the ICERs for different configurations of the BF programmes, it is possible to identify those programmes which are more cost-effective (lower cost per unit of effect) and should be preferred over the less cost-effective programmes (higher cost per unit of effect) [20]. If decision makers want to assess to what extent a BF programme represents "good value for money" in comparison with investments in other healthcare interventions, there is a need for an effect measure that can be used to compare health outcomes across different populations and interventions. The QALY measure is a composite indicator that combines health-related quality of life with life expectancy. This outcome measure can also be used in the modelling of health outcomes from BF programmes. If the incremental cost per QALY is less than €35,000 the programme is traditionally considered to represent "good value for money" and would be recommended to be implemented [66]. The QALY outcome measure was used in a UK analysis and was enumerated separately for the baby and the mother, and combined into an ICER at €52,000 per QALY, which is not considered to represent "good value for money" [64].

A number of additional cost-effectiveness analyses have been reported. A Mexican model-based cost effectiveness study compared two optimal BF scenarios with 95% of all babies being breastfed for the first 6-months exclusively and 95% of all babies being breastfed between 12 and 36 months of their life in comparison with the suboptimal practice reported in 2012 [63]. A microsimulation model was developed to follow a synthetic cohort of 100,000 15-year-old women in terms of their fertility, BF practice, and incidence of breast cancer, treatment costs, mortality rates, employment and income status over their remaining life time. The two scenarios were simulated and the difference in outcomes from the base case were interpreted as the potential impact of more frequent and longer BF practice. The base case model was calibrated with best local data from available sources. The impact of BF on breast cancer risk was expressed in terms of relative risk rates obtained from previous meta-analyses. An increase of 6-month exclusive BF rate from 14 to 95% was modelled to avoid 573 breast cancer cases and 126 premature deaths per 100,000 women during their lifetime. This resulted in a gain in 2629 DALYs and a total cost saving at US$14 Mio. If the BF during 12 and 36 months increased from 33 to 95%, the analysis showed a lower, but still positive effect on health outcomes and costs.

A different UK-based model assessed the costs-effectiveness of BF for preterm infants [65]. They used a cohort of 51,700 preterm infants (2013, in England and Wales) and compared health outcomes and healthcare costs in a scenario where all premature infants were fed with human milk during their first 6-month lifetime in comparison with a scenario where all premature infants were fed formula milk. From literature reviews, they identified odds ratios and costs of the infants experiencing any of the following outcomes: sepsis, necrotising enterocolitis, sudden infant death syndrome, acute otitis media, childhood leukaemia, childhood obesity and the associated impact of developing type-2 diabetes and coronary heart disease, neurodevelopment impairment and disability. They found that the BF scenario provided better health outcomes and lower healthcare costs with a potential saving per infant at £583 and a mean QALY gain at 0.088.

A more recent UK-based model was developed to inform the national guidance on postnatal care in England [64]. A decision-analytic cost-effectiveness model was developed to evaluate a range of interventions added to standard care. These interventions aimed at increasing BF included different models of education, advice and support provided by professionals or peers before or immediately after, or within the first 8 weeks after the birth. The primary outcome was "any BF, 16-26 weeks after birth". The derived outcomes for the infant related to gastrointestinal infection, respiratory tract infection, acute otitis media, and mortality due to infections disease and due to sudden infant death syndrome. The derived outcome for the mother was breast cancer. The assumed impact from BF were obtained from comprehensive literature reviews conducted on behalf of the Lancet BF Support Group [67]. In the base-case analysis, the BF support model reduced the number of disease episodes in both infants and mothers. The QALY gain per 1000 babies and women were modelled at 0.16 for infants and 1.09 for mothers. However, the modelled intervention cost at £84 per baby exceeded the modelled cost-savings £10, resulting in an ICER of £52,000 per QALY which is normally not considered to be cost-effective. By changing the assumptions related to e.g. intervention cost and effects, the model indicated situations where the ICER might suggest cost-effectiveness and dominance.

In their discussion of the results, the authors point out that the quality of data regarding the associations between BF and avoidance of certain diseases are relatively low, due to studies with risk of bias related to the randomisation process, selective reporting and missing outcomes. They also comment on the variations related to the models of interventions. BF interventions may vary in model of delivery (face-to-face, telephone, individually vs. groups, or combinations), the number of contacts, the duration of the intervention, the place of delivery (home, hospital, community setting or combinations), the person delivering the intervention (peer supporter, lactation consultant, midwife, health visitor or combinations). Furthermore, there might be variations in the target group, and their recruitment and motivation to breastfeed. Finally, they remark that their definition of "any BF" as an outcome and the definition of standard care generally are poorly described.

10. Distributional cost-effectiveness

In traditional cost-effectiveness analysis, the focus is on the efficiency of the whole programme delivered to a specified target group. This assumes that each individual who receives the services have similar rates of uptake, adherence and effect. This is a strong assumption for BF programmes. In practice, the base case BF rate, the uptake, the adherence and effect may vary for different social groups. Younger mothers might have lower BF rates than older mothers, and they might be less likely to take part in BF programmes, and may be less likely to adhere to the recommendations. Therefore, both babies and the younger mothers may experience poorer health outcomes from BF than older mothers. A cost-effective BF programme may have potential for increasing the inequality in the health outcomes, and thus reduce the health equity in the population. Economists describe this situation as the trade-off between efficiency and equity.

This efficiency-equity trade-off is particularly relevant to consider for BF programmes as the reviewed material clearly have demonstrated, there are variations in

BF practice by sub-populations defined by age, geography, rural/urban, nationality, culturally, educational and labour market position. These factors: which can be denoted as SES, increase the complexities of the economic analysis. This is particularly related to the validity of data that not only need to be related to the whole population but also should consider differences between social groups. However, recent developments in methods for health economic evaluations have developed frameworks that enables these trade-off analyses [68]. With the application of model-based analysis, it is possible to conduct systematic analyses of the efficiency-equity trade-off and provide additional insight, which may support the development of appropriate programmes for BF interventions. The model-based analysis may also be used to highlight the need for data analyses.

The definition of relevant social groups represents a major challenge. The previous section has identified studies that have used different characteristics to define social groups. This is a specific research area and is beyond the focus of this chapter. Education or labour market position is often used as an indicator for social groups. It may also work well for BF interventions and has the advantage that national data are available on birth and BF practice for different educational groups.

The principles of analysing the efficiency-equity trade-off for a BF-intervention is first to assess the difference in cost-effectiveness of the intervention for the different SES groups and then analyse the distribution of health outcomes among these groups. The idea is to represent interventions in a so-called health equity impact plane, where the X-axis represents incremental change in equity and the Y-axis represents incremental change in efficiency (**Figure 4**). There are thus four situations identified by the four quadrants. The NE quadrant (denoted A) represents programmes that both increase efficiency and improve equity. The SW quadrant (B) represents programmes that are both inefficient and harms equity. Programmes in the NW and SE quadrant (C and D) are either efficient or improve equity at the expense of the other [69].

There is clear evidence that mothers with different social backgrounds have different propensity to start BF and continue when they have started. If such variations are to be considered when designing and implementing BF intervention programmes, there is a risk of increasing the inequality in efficiency and inequity in health. This could for example arise if a peer-to-peer programme was introduced as a general

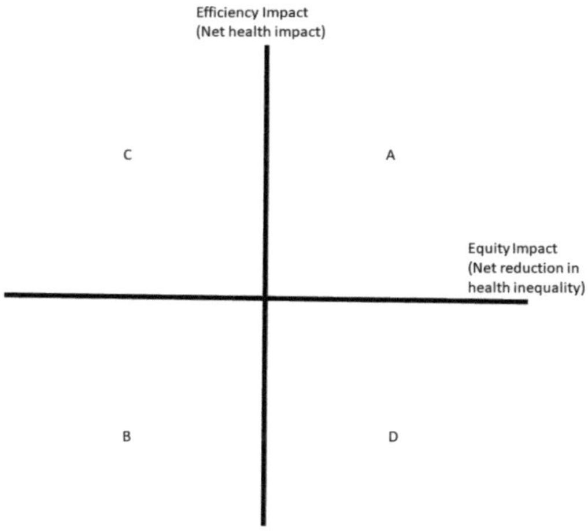

Figure 4.
Equity-efficiency impact.

offer. Women with certain backgrounds would enjoy and adhere to such programmes while others will identify barriers for taking part and have difficulties in overcoming these barriers. The result might be that they refuse to take part and thus experience no or little support to begin and maintain BF practices.

It is well documented that higher educational attainments are associated with increased BF [70]. Higher educational attainment leads to better job mobility and wealth, which may facilitate BF through increased financial support. Mothers with higher income can afford private lactation consultations, breast pumps and paid support of childcare and other household duties that may facilitate BF. Therefore, active BF practice is more common in groups of mothers with higher education.

As studies have shown, BF is associated with positive outcomes for both the baby and mother. When the practice of BF is different in different groups of mothers, the outcomes from BF will also be different. The implication is that the difference in BF practice adds to an inequitable health distribution. If a BF intervention (e.g. community lactation consultants) is made available as a general offer to all mothers, there may be variation in how groups of mothers perceive the desirability of the offer. Mothers who are motivated and well-acquainted with using the services offered by the ante-natal hospital service, may be more likely to seek the advice from the lactation consultants. The implication could be that none of the BF support models may fit all, resulting in variation in behavioural change, costs and outcomes. If such variation exists, then it becomes relevant to assess which BF support models are a better fit to certain groups, and assess their implications in terms of efficiency and equity.

11. Analysing the distributional cost-effectiveness of BF

Figure 5 below illustrates different elements of the analysis of distributional cost-effectiveness. For simplicity, there are three social groups, which could be mothers outside the labour market and mothers with different positions in the labour market.

To analyse the potential benefit in terms of efficiency and equity of a new programme, there needs to be a base case situation. The illustration would be the proportion of mothers in each social group who are exclusively or partially BF their babies at particular times after the birth. Both the proportion who initiate BF and the duration may be different for different social groups and thus the average time with BF will vary.

For each group, the BF practice will result in health outcomes for the babies and mothers. It is likely, there is a relationship between the duration of BF and the occurrence of adverse events such as infections for the baby and positive effects such as reduced risk of obesity for the baby and reduced risk of breast and ovarian cancer for the mother. These relationships can be used to model the health outcomes for the babies and mothers. Unless there is a clear indication that the health effects may differ for different social groups, it is reasonable to assume that the health effects occur independently of social characteristics.

It is clear, that the assumptions about the relationship between BF practice and health effects are crucial for any analysis and pose a major challenge for any analysis. However, as has been shown above, there are a number of examples where researchers have developed such models to predict health outcomes from BF.

Based on the modelling of health effects for different social groups, the distribution of health outcomes can be assumed to be representing the base case situation.

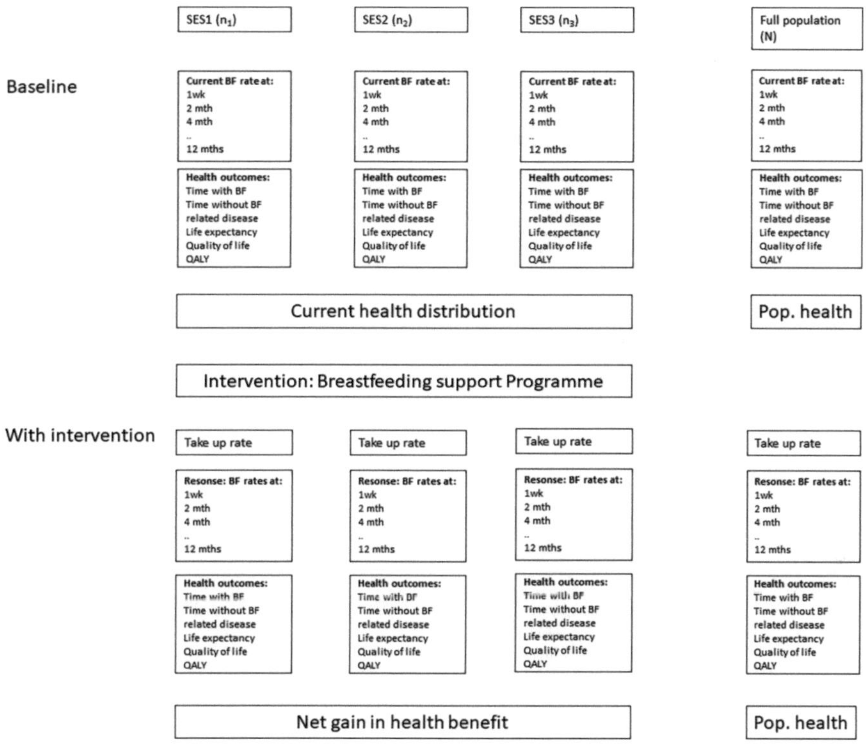

Figure 5.
Illustration of the modelling of potential health impact from BF support programmes.

The social variation in health outcomes could be described in terms of absolute or relative gaps between the group with the best outcomes and other groups. This could express the mean difference in the composite QALY measure between the groups – e.g. the most disadvantaged group experience on average 5 fewer QALYs than the best group. This could also be expressed in relative terms, e.g. the most disadvantaged group experience 10% less QALYs than the best group. There also are a number of equality indices based e.g. on Lorenz-curves, where the index can be interpreted as a measure of deviation from a fully equal distribution.

The next part in the analysis is to specify the design and effect of the BF programme. In some analyses, it could be expected that several different designs could be envisaged and specified in terms of their target group, the organisation and provision of the intervention. Each design or model of care would be associated with different use of resources and costs and will have different consequences in terms of the proportion of mothers who initiate and continue BF their babies.

The consequences of these alternative models of care can then be analysed using the same modelling framework as was used in the baseline situation. This implies that the change in health benefits is determined by the change in BF practice as specified as part of the model of care. The health benefits with the intervention and without the intervention is compared across the social groups. The distribution of health gains (e.g. in terms of QALYs) for each social group can be calculated and the total cost-effectiveness can be compared for the whole population in terms of the ICER. The distribution of outcomes across social groups may be expressed as the health gain in each social group or by using one of the proposed equity indices. The net gain in health benefit (QALYs) may be expressed as the net gain, where the cost of the intervention programme is expressed in forgone health gains as the opportunity cost of the intervention programme.

When several models of BF support programmes are compared in terms of their efficiency-equity trade-off, they may be represented in the equity-efficiency impact plane as shown in **Figure 4**. Models in quadrant A have positive impact on both equity and efficiency. Models in quadrant B have negative impacts on both equity and efficiency, while models in quadrant C and D have positive impact on either efficiency or equity but not both. Interventions in quadrant A are clearly preferable. When several models are in quadrant A, decision makers can make an assessment on which model best satisfy policy objectives.

12. Conclusion

Individual, societal and policy factors influence mothers' decisions to begin and continue BF and interventions targeted towards these factors are essential, in particular the cost-effectiveness and equity trade-off components associated with them. BF may be encouraged through social interventions where the perception, understanding and culture around BF is influenced, e.g. by offering information and advice on proper BF technique and maintenance of BF for a period of time after the birth. In addition, specifically targeted programmes may be devised to support and encourage women to breastfeed. These can be offered as part of maternity services that are offered by public, private and voluntary organisations at different phases during the ante and post-natal care. There may be programmes that are targeted to individual women during the immediate post-natal phase or to groups of women in a peer-support programme. Interventions may include high-level policies such as labour market regulations which makes continuous BF easier for mothers e.g. by extending periods of maternity leave and offering good facilities for BF. BF legislation and BF practices should be revisited in Ireland and further BF supporting policy implementations should be considered with e.g. a law stating that mothers have a right to breastfeed or a law requiring employers to prove BF facilities at work [71].

Some interventions may be more effective in changing the BF behaviour for mothers with different SES. Universally provided interventions are likely to be more effective for some SES groups because their willingness to initiate and continue BF will be impacted differently. Investments in BF support therefore have the risk of providing an unequal health benefit and may increase the inequity in health. To address both the efficiency and equity issues, it is relevant to evaluate future and current BF interventions using the "Distributional cost-effectiveness framework". The framework will enable evaluation of the impact on efficiency and equity of more targeted BF interventions. This will provide decision-makers with stronger arguments for offering differentiated BF interventions to different SES groups.

Conflict of interest

The authors declare no conflict of interest.

Appendices and nomenclature

BF	Breastfeeding
BMS	Breast-milk Substitutes
HCP	Healthcare professionals
DCEA	Distributional cost-effectiveness analysis
BFHI	The Baby Friendly Hospital Initiative
SES	Socioeconomic status
SSC	Skin-to-Skin Contact
FSAI	Food Safety Authority of Ireland
HSE	Health Service Executive
HIQA	Health Information Quality Authority
RCTs	Randomised control trials
GUI	Growing Up in Ireland
QALYs	Quality-adjusted life years
ICER	Incremental cost-effectiveness ratios
WHO	World Health Organisation
OECD	Organisation for Economic Co-operation and Development
HCWs	Health Care Workers
NPRS	National Perinatal Reporting System

Author details

Sinead M. Hurley*, Kathy Whyte and Jan Sorensen
School of Population Health, RCSI University of Medicine and Health Sciences, Dublin, Ireland

*Address all correspondence to: sineadhurley@rcsi.ie

References

[1] Socialstyrelsen, the National Board of Health and Welfare. Statistics on Breastfeeding 2019. 2021. Retrieved from: https://www.socialstyrelsen.se/globalassets/sharepoint-dokument/artikelkatalog/statistik/2021-12-7694.pdf. [Accessed: March 20, 2023]

[2] Statistics ABo. Breastfeeding. 2022. Available from: https://www.abs.gov.au/statistics/health/health-conditions-and-risks/breastfeeding/latest-release [Accessed: November 30, 2022]

[3] Healthcare Pricing Office (HPO), Health Service Executive (HSE). Perinatal Statistics Report 2020. Report No.: 978-1-78602-209-7. 2020. Available from: http://www.hpo.ie/latest_hipe_nprs_reports/NPRS_2020/Perinatal_Statistics_Report_2020.pdf

[4] Prevention CfDCa. Breastfeeding Rates: National Immunization Survey (NIS) 2012-2019. Available from: https://www.cdc.gov/breastfeeding/data/nis_data/results.html#print.

[5] England N. Maternity and Breastfeeding. 2022. Available from: https://www.england.nhs.uk/statistics/statistical-work-areas/maternity-and-breastfeeding/.

[6] Health Service Executive. Breastfeeding in a Healthy Ireland: Health Service Breastfeeding Action Plan. 2016-2021. Available from: https://www.hse.ie/eng/about/who/healthwellbeing/our-priority-programmes/child-health-and-wellbeing/breastfeeding-healthy-childhood-programme/policies-and-guidelines-breastfeeding/breastfeeding-in-a-healthy-ireland-report.pdf

[7] Kinoshita M, Doolan A, Crushell E. A Position Paper on Breastfeeding. Ireland: Faculty of Paediatrics, Faculty of Public Health Medicine, Institute of Obstericians and Gynaecologists, Royal College of Physicians of Ireland; 2021

[8] Duijts L, Ramadhani MK, Moll HA. Breastfeeding protects against infectious diseases during infancy in industrialized countries. A systematic review. Maternal & Child Nutrition. 2009;**5**(3):199-210

[9] Theurich MA, Davanzo R, Busck-Rasmussen M, Diaz-Gomez NM, Brennan C, Kylberg E, et al. Breastfeeding rates and programs in Europe: A survey of 11 National Breastfeeding Committees and representatives. Journal of Pediatric Gastroenterology and Nutrition. 2019;**68**(3):400-407

[10] Pattison KL, Kraschnewski JL, Lehman E, Savage JS, Downs DS, Leonard KS, et al. Breastfeeding initiation and duration and child health outcomes in the first baby study. Preventive Medicine. 2019;**118**:1-6

[11] Stuebe A. The risks of not breastfeeding for mothers and infants. Reviews in Obstetrics and Gynecology. 2009;**2**(4):222-231

[12] McCrory C, Layte R. The effect of breastfeeding on children's educational test scores at nine years of age: Results of an Irish cohort study. Social Science & Medicine. 2011;**72**(9):1515-1521

[13] Pereyra-Elías R, Quigley MA, Carson C. To what extent does confounding explain the association between breastfeeding duration and cognitive development up to age 14? Findings from the UK millennium cohort study. PLoS One. 2022;**17**(5):e0267326

[14] Berthon BS, Williams LM, Williams EJ, Wood LG. Effect of Lactoferrin supplementation on inflammation, immune function, and prevention of respiratory tract infections in humans: A systematic review and meta-analysis. Advances in Nutrition (Bethesda, Md). 2022;**13**(5):1799-1819

[15] Chowdhury R, Sinha B, Sankar MJ, Taneja S, Bhandari N, Rollins N, et al. Breastfeeding and maternal health outcomes: A systematic review and meta-analysis. Acta Paediatrica. 2015;**104**(Suppl. 467):96-113

[16] Frank NM, Lynch KF, Uusitalo U, Yang J, Lönnrot M, Virtanen SM, et al. The relationship between breastfeeding and reported respiratory and gastrointestinal infection rates in young children. BMC Pediatrics. 2019;**19**(1):339

[17] Cronin FM, Hurley SM, Buckley T, Mancebo Guinea Arquez D, Lakshmanan N, O'Gorman A, et al. Mediators of socioeconomic differences in overweight and obesity among youth in Ireland and the UK (2011-2021): A systematic review. BMC Public Health. 2022;**22**(1):1585

[18] Kwan ML, Bernard PS, Kroenke CH, Factor RE, Habel LA, Weltzien EK, et al. Breastfeeding, PAM50 tumor subtype, and breast cancer prognosis and survival. JNCI: Journal of the National Cancer Institute. 2015;**107**(7):djv087

[19] Pokhrel S, Quigley MA, Fox-Rushby J, McCormick F, Williams A, Trueman P, et al. Potential economic impacts from improving breastfeeding rates in the UK. Archives of Disease in Childhood. 2015;**100**(4):334-340

[20] Camacho EM, Hussain H. Cost-effectiveness evidence for strategies to promote or support breastfeeding: A systematic search and narrative literature review. BMC Pregnancy and Childbirth. 2020;**20**(1):757

[21] Wallenborn JT, Valera CB, Kounnavong S, Sayasone S, Odermatt P, Fink G. Urban-rural gaps in breastfeeding practices: Evidence from Lao People's Democratic Republic. International journal of public health. 2021;**66**:1604062

[22] Greene S, Mc Crory C, Mc Nally S. Growing up in Ireland: Review of the Literature Pertaining to the Second Wave of Data Collection with the Infant Cohort at Three Years. Dublin: Department of Children and Youth Affairs; 2014

[23] Chen H, Li C, Zhou Q, Cassidy TM, Younger KM, Shen S, et al. How to promote exclusive breastfeeding in Ireland: A qualitative study on views of Chinese immigrant mothers. International Breastfeeding Journal. 2021;**16**(1):10

[24] Health Service Executive. National Standards for Antenatal Education in Ireland. 2020. Available from: https://www.hse.ie/eng/about/who/healthwellbeing/our-priority-programmes/child-health-and-wellbeing/antenatal-ed.pdf

[25] Hauck YL, Blixt I, Hildingsson I, Gallagher L, Rubertsson C, Thomson B, et al. Australian, Irish and Swedish women's perceptions of what assisted them to breastfeed for six months: Exploratory design using critical incident technique. BMC Public Health. 2016;**16**(1):1067

[26] Stewart-Knox B, Gardiner K, Wright M. What is the problem with breast-feeding? A qualitative analysis of infant feeding perceptions. Journal of Human Nutrition and Dietetics. 2003;**16**(4):265-273

[27] Hauck YL, Kuliukas L, Gallagher L, Brady V, Dykes C, Rubertsson C. Helpful and challenging aspects of breastfeeding in public for women living in Australia, Ireland and Sweden: A cross-sectional study. International Breastfeeding Journal. 2020;**15**(1):38

[28] Claesson IM, Larsson L, Steen L, Alehagen S. "you just need to leave the room when you breastfeed" breastfeeding experiences among obese women in Sweden - a qualitative study. BMC Pregnancy and Childbirth. 2018;**18**(1):39

[29] Desmond D, Meaney S. A qualitative study investigating the barriers to returning to work for breastfeeding mothers in Ireland. International Breastfeeding Journal. 2016;**11**(1):16

[30] Ogbuanu C, Glover S, Probst J, Liu J, Hussey J. The effect of maternity leave length and time of return to work on breastfeeding. Pediatrics. 2011;**127**(6):e1414-e1427

[31] Hawkins SS, Griffiths LJ, Dezateux C, Law C. The impact of maternal employment on breast-feeding duration in the UK millennium cohort study. Public Health Nutrition. 2007;**10**(9):891-896

[32] Health Services Executive. Extended Breastfeeding. 2022. Available from: https://www2.hse.ie/babies-children/breastfeeding/stopping-extending/extended-breastfeeding/

[33] Grandahl M, Stern J, Funkquist EL. Longer shared parental leave is associated with longer duration of breastfeeding: A cross-sectional study among Swedish mothers and their partners. BMC Pediatrics. 2020;**20**(1):159

[34] European Commission, Directorate-General for Employment, Social Affairs and Inclusion, Stewart K, Janta B. Paternity and parental leave policies across the European Union: assessment of current provision. Publications Office. 2018. Available from: https://data.europa.eu/doi/10.2767/51284

[35] Maternity Protection (Amendment) Act 2004 (Revised 2020); 1994

[36] Russell H, Watson D, Banks J. Pregnancy at Work: A National Survey, Dublin: HSE Crisis Pregnancy Programme and the Equality Authority. 2011. Available from: https://www.esri.ie/publications/pregnancy-at-work-a-national-survey

[37] Brown CA, Poag S, Kasprzycki C. Exploring large employers' and small employers' knowledge, attitudes, and practices on breastfeeding support in the workplace. Journal of Human Lactation. 2001;**17**(1):39-46

[38] Koslowski A, Blum, S., Dobrotić, I., Kaufman, G, Moss, P. 18th International Review of Leave Policies and Related Research. 2022

[39] IrishExaminer. Ireland's complicated relationship with infant formula 2021. Available from: https://www.irishexaminer.com/news/spotlight/arid-40339367.html

[40] Fund WHOaUNCs. The Impact of Marketing of Breast-Milk Substitutes on Infant Feeding Decisions and Practices. Fund WHOaUNCs; 2022

[41] Online Safety and Media Regulation Bill. Houses of the Oireachtas. 2022. (6). Act. 41. Available from: https://www.oireachtas.ie/en/bills/bill/2022/6/

[42] Renfrew MJ, McCormick FM, Wade A, Quinn B, Dowswell T. Support for healthy breastfeeding mothers with healthy term babies. Cochrane Database of Systematic Reviews. 2012;**5**(5):Cd001141

[43] Smith JPCA, Iellamo A, Javanparast S, Atchan M, et al. Review of Effective Strategies to Promote Breastfeeding. An Evidence Check Rapid Review Brokered by the Sax Institute for the Department of Health, 2018; 2018

[44] Beake S, Pellowe C, Dykes F, Schmied V, Bick D. A systematic review of structured compared with non-structured breastfeeding programmes to support the initiation and duration of exclusive and any breastfeeding in acute and primary health care settings. Maternal & Child Nutrition. 2012;**8**(2):141-161

[45] Health Research Board MS et al. Interventions That Promote Increased Breastfeeding Rates and Breastfeeding Duration among Women. 2016. Available from: https://www.hrb.ie/fileadmin/publications_files/Interventions_that_promote_increased_breastfeeding_rates_2016.pdf

[46] Sikorski J, Renfrew MJ, Pindoria S, Wade A. Support for breastfeeding mothers: A systematic review. Paediatric and Perinatal Epidemiology. 2003;**17**(4):407-417

[47] Manganaro R, Marseglia L, Mamì C, Paolata A, Gargano R, Mondello M, et al. Effects of hospital policies and practices on initiation and duration of breastfeeding. Child: Care, Health and Development. 2009;**35**(1):106-111

[48] Merten S, Dratva J, Ackermann-Liebrich U. Do baby-friendly hospitals influence breastfeeding duration on a national level? Pediatrics. 2005;**116**(5):e702-e708

[49] Murray EK, Ricketts S, Dellaport J. Hospital practices that increase breastfeeding duration: Results from a population-based study. Birth. 2007;**34**(3):202-211

[50] Simard I, O'Brien HT, Beaudoin A, Turcotte D, Damant D, Ferland S, et al. Factors influencing the initiation and duration of breastfeeding among low-income women followed by the Canada prenatal nutrition program in 4 regions of Quebec. Journal of Human Lactation. 2005;**21**(3):327-337

[51] Haslam C, Lawrence W, Haefeli K. Intention to breastfeed and other important health-related behaviour and beliefs during pregnancy. Family Practice. 2003;**20**(5):528-530

[52] Dubois L, Girard M. Social determinants of initiation, duration and exclusivity of breastfeeding at the population level: The results of the longitudinal study of child development in Quebec (ELDEQ 1998-2002) Canadian Journal of Public Health. 2003;**94**(4):300-305

[53] Li R, Fein SB, Chen J, Grummer-Strawn LM. Why mothers stop breastfeeding: mothers' self-reported reasons for stopping during the first year. Pediatrics. 2008;**122**(Suppl. 2):S69-S76

[54] Dyson L, McCormick F, Renfrew MJ. Interventions for promoting the initiation of breastfeeding. Cochrane Database of Systematic Reviews. 2005;**2**:Cd001688

[55] Executive HS. The Mapping Project 2017. 2017. Available from: https://www.hse.ie/file-library/mapping-report.pdf

[56] Department of Children, Equality, Disability, Integration and Youth. General Scheme of a Work Life Balance and Miscellaneous Provisions Bill. Department of Children, Equality, Disability, Integration and Youth; 2022

[57] Johantgen M, Fountain L, Zangaro G, Newhouse R, Stanik-Hutt J, White K.

Comparison of labor and delivery care provided by certified nurse-midwives and physicians: A systematic review, 1990 to 2008. Women's Health Issues. 2012;**22**(1):e73-e81

[58] Lau Y, Htun TP, Tam WS, Klainin-Yobas P. Efficacy of e-technologies in improving breastfeeding outcomes among perinatal women: A meta-analysis. Maternal & Child Nutrition. 2016;**12**(3):381-401

[59] Simpson E, Garbett A, Comber R, Balaam M. Factors important for women who breastfeed in public: A content analysis of review data from FeedFinder. BMJ Open. 2016;**6**(10):e011762

[60] Ladewig EL, Hayes C, Browne J, Layte R, Reulbach U. The influence of ethnicity on breastfeeding rates in Ireland: A cross-sectional study. Journal of Epidemiology and Community Health. 2014;**68**(4):356-362

[61] Stuebe AM, Jegier BJ, Schwarz EB, Green BD, Reinhold AG, Colaizy TT, et al. An online calculator to estimate the impact of changes in breastfeeding rates on population health and costs. Breastfeeding Medicine. 2017;**12**(10):645-658

[62] Bartick MC, Nickel NC, Hanley LE. Evidence for the baby-friendly hospital initiative to support breastfeeding. Journal of the American Medical Association. 2017;**317**(7):770-771

[63] Unar-Munguia M, Meza R, Colchero MA, Torres-Mejia G, de Cosio TG. Economic and disease burden of breast cancer associated with suboptimal breastfeeding practices in Mexico. Cancer Causes & Control. 2017;**28**(12):1381-1391

[64] Mavranezouli I, Varley-Campbell J, Stockton S, Francis J, Macdonald C, Sharma S, et al. The cost-effectiveness of antenatal and postnatal education and support interventions for women aimed at promoting breastfeeding in the UK. BMC Public Health. 2022;**22**(1):153

[65] Mahon J, Claxton L, Wood H. Modelling the cost-effectiveness of human milk and breastfeeding in preterm infants in the United Kingdom. Health Economics Review. 2016;**6**(1):54

[66] Health Information and Quality Authority. Guidelines for the Economic Evaluation of Health Technologies in Ireland. Dublin: HIQA; 2020

[67] Victora CG, Bahl R, Barros AJ, Franca GV, Horton S, Krasevec J, et al. Breastfeeding in the 21st century: Epidemiology, mechanisms, and lifelong effect. Lancet. 2016;**387**(10017):475-490

[68] Cookson R, Mirelman AJ, Griffin S, Asaria M, Dawkins B, Norheim OF, et al. Using cost-effectiveness analysis to address health equity concerns. Value in Health. 2017;**20**(2):206-212

[69] Cookson R, Griffin S, Norheim OF, Culyer AJ, Chalkidou K. Distributional cost-effectiveness analysis comes of age. Value in Health. 2021;**24**(1):118-120

[70] Standish KR, Parker MG. Social determinants of breastfeeding in the United States. Clinical Therapeutics. 2022;**44**(2):186-192

[71] Book. Electronic Irish Statute. Maternity Protection (Amendment) Act; 28. 2004

Chapter 15

Breastfeeding Support

Yeshimebet Ali Dawed, Shambel Aychew Tsegaw and Erkihun Tadesse Amsalu

Abstract

Supporting mothers to continue breastfeeding is a public health priority. Scientific studies identify challenges to optimal breastfeeding practice. Exclusive breastfeeding is one of the core indicators of infant and young child feeding, among strategies for reducing infant morbidity and mortality. It determines future growth and development of the infants both in physical and mental health. As the principle of implementation science designing evidence-based intervention strategies and support addressing individual and community level factors associated with exclusive breastfeeding practice through policies and programs was essential to improve infant feeding practice and quality of life. Therefore, emphasis should be given to encouraging women to be educated, employed, and empowered to have ANC and PNC follow-ups, and to improve their decision-making power on themselves and their infant health care for saving lives of the infants and reduction of economic losses of a country. Breastfeeding support mainly focuses on empowering women, providing emotional, instrumental, information, flexible working time, appraisal of their performance, support at individual, community, and policy level interventions with the concept of implementation science need to be implemented. This chapter intended to provide evidence-based infant feeding intervention strategies for mothers, students, health professionals, and policymakers for better implementation.

Keywords: breastfeeding support, breastfeeding interventions, exclusive breastfeeding, under six infants, infant and young child feeding practices, optimal breastfeeding, implementation sciences in breastfeeding, implementation science

1. Introduction

This chapter is intended to address basics of breastfeeding support for designing sustainable, efficient, and effective breastfeeding interventions with the concept of implementation science for the well-being of the future generation. Improving knowledge and skills in proper infant feeding practice is not an overnight activity and needs intensive intervention and support from pregnancy till two years of postnatal period. The components of breastfeeding support in this chapter include; the importance of breastfeeding, the existing breastfeeding practice, and its factors, breastfeeding support intervention strategy from pregnancy to the first two years of life, breastfeeding support in a special situation, emotional, information, social, physical, economic supports, advocacy and involving multisectoral stakeholders are some of the contents included in this chapter.

Breastfeeding is the best start in life and is used as a foundation for child health, development, and survival. The World Health Organization (WHO) has recommended optimal breastfeeding that; should be initiated within an hour after birth, exclusive breastfeeding till 6 months of life, and continued breastfeeding till 24 months and more with appropriate complementary feeding practice [1].

Breastfeeding is an unrivaled method of providing ideal food for infants' healthy growth and development; it is also an essential part of nutrition and the reproductive process, with significant implications for the mother's health as well. It mainly prevents breast cancer and the risk of acquiring cardiovascular disease [2].

Breastfeeding is a natural gift for mothers, but it is also a learning behavior. Almost all mothers can breastfeed if they have accurate information and support from their families, communities, and health care system. They should also have access to skills from trained health workers and peer counselors who can help to build mothers' confidence, improve feeding techniques, and prevent or resolve any breastfeeding problems [3].

Breastfeeding support is an intervention to improve early initiation of breastfeeding immediately after birth, enhancing exclusive breastfeeding practice and continuing breastfeeding with timely initiation of appropriate complementary feeding but its implementation was challenging and needs special focus for evidence-based interventions [4].

For the first six months of life, breast milk provides all of the nutrients required for survival, growth, and development, as well as immunologic, antimicrobial, and anti-inflammatory factors [5, 6].

1.1 Why breastfeeding support

Optimal breastfeeding practice is the best solution for prevention of infant and child mortality. However, exclusive breastfeeding practice substantially decreased over time. According to the "Convention on the Rights of the Child," every infant and child has the right to adequate nutrition but undernutrition is highly prevalent and responsible for 45% of all child deaths. In 2020, the global estimate of exclusive breastfeeding practice was 44%, and malnutrition on under five years children was 149 million stunted (too short for their age), 45 million were wasted (too thin for their height), and 38.9 million were overweight or obese [7].

Optimal breastfeeding saves the lives of more than 823,000 under five children, prevent mother from acquiring breast cancer, and 20,000 annual deaths from breast cancer. It also improves school attendance and Intelligent Quiescent (IQ), and it is associated with lowering the occurrence of non-communicable diseases and higher income in adult life. Breastfeeding results in economic gains for both individual families and the nation as a whole contributing as one of the poverty reduction methods [7, 8]. Hence breastfeeding support promote child survival, growth, and development and reduce the incidence of non-communicable disease in their adult life. Thus, it needs intensive action at individual, community, health care system, and policy levels.

1.2 Factors for exclusive breastfeeding practice

The global nutrition targets for 2025 recommend improving the rate of exclusive breastfeeding practice at least by 50% [9] but the rate of exclusive breastfeeding was low many infants and children do not receive optimal breastfeeding. Over the 2015–2020 period, only about 44% of infants aged 0–6 months worldwide were exclusively breastfed [7]. The contributing factors for this low rate of exclusive breastfeeding include individual, interpersonal, social, cultural, commercial, media, community, health service-related factors and poor knowledge of breastfeeding [9].

A systematic review of mothers' knowledge, attitude, and practice in East Africa identified that exclusive breastfeeding practice in the first 6 months was 55.9%, only 49.2% knew the duration of exclusive breastfeeding, 66.1% of them disagree with giving breastfeeding immediately after birth and only 47.9% of them disagreed that discarding colostrum is important [10].

In Ethiopia, the rate of exclusive breastfeeding practice was 58% for this the individual level determinants were infant age and gender, the presence of co-morbidities, antenatal care, and wealth index, whereas contextual region, community level of postnatal visit, and community level of maternal employment were community level factors [11]. A similarly systematic review of exclusive breastfeeding practice identified that full-time employed mothers in the first 6 months were 57% less likely to practice exclusive breastfeeding [12].

A systematic review of implementation science in maternity care identified factors enabling the implementation of evidence-based intervention includes; knowledge, service providers' motivations, training, effective multilevel coordination, effective communication, leadership and limited knowledge, practice and experience of researchers, and implementers to use theory, model or framework to guide implementation [13].

In addition, Equitable access to breastfeeding programs guided by evidence-based policies and programs delivered via infrastructures that promotes, protects, and supports breastfeeding should be considered a human right and social justice. Any social, economic, legal, political, or biomedical barrier that prevents women from exercising their right to breastfeed should be seen as a social injustice, a threat to their health, and ultimately a violation of their human rights. To address all factors designing evidence-based interventions to support breastfeeding with the concepts of implementation and behavioral science needs to be integrated and implemented with the existing policies and programs [14].

2. The concepts of implementation science on breastfeeding

Implementation science is an emerging science in nutrition focusing on the implementation of evidence-based intervention strategies to alleviate malnutrition and nutrition-related health problems. It is the young science to fill the gaps between what we know and what we practice [15].

Implementation science in nutrition (ISN) is defined as "*an interdisciplinary body of theory, knowledge, frameworks, tools, and approaches whose purpose is to strengthen implementation quality and impact. It includes a wide range of methods and approaches to identify and address implementation bottlenecks; means to identify, evaluate, and scale up implementation innovations; and strategies to enhance the utilization of existing knowledge, tools, and frameworks based on the evolving science of implementation*" [16].

Designing a breastfeeding intervention strategy supported by the concepts of implementation science is constructive step to achieve an effective outcome. Since

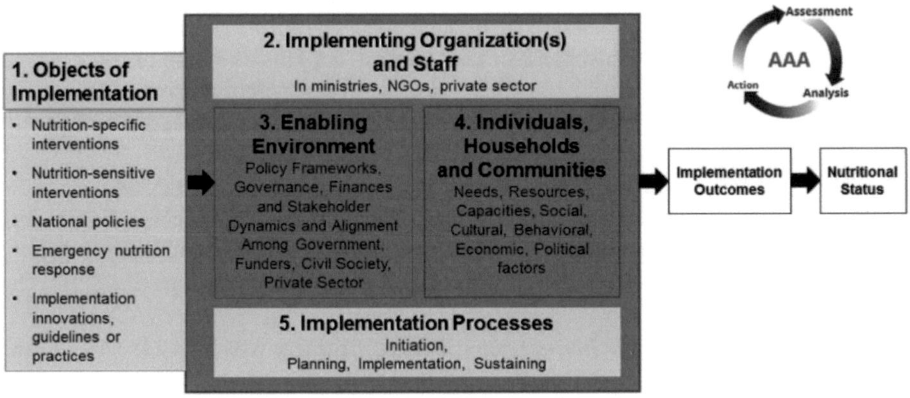
1. Objects of Implementation
Nutrition-specific interventions
Nutrition-sensitive interventions
National policies
Emergency nutrition response
Implementation innovations, guidelines or practices
2. Implementing Organization(s) and Staff
In ministries, NGOs, private sector
3. Enabling Environment
Policy Frameworks, Governance, Finances and Stakeholder Dynamics and Alignment Among Government, Funders, Civil Society, Private Sector
4. Individuals, Households and Communities
Needs, Resources, Capacities, Social, Cultural, Behavioral, Economic, Political factors
5. Implementation Processes
Initiation, Planning, Implementation, Sustaining
Implementation Outcomes
Nutritional Status
AAA
Assessment
Analysis
Action

Figure 1.
The five domains of implementation science in nutrition: Adapted from reference [16].

theories, models, and concepts can educate researchers and practitioners about contextually relevant factors and processes suitable for the successful implementation of breastfeeding interventions [17].

In this regard, the breastfeeding support intervention written here is using the concepts of implementation sciences in nutrition, previous research findings, and standard international guidelines on breastfeeding recommendations. The five domains of implementation science were used as a framework for designing the intervention (**Figure 1**).

3. Breastfeeding support

It is much recommended that evidence-based breastfeeding support using the five domains of implementation science integrated with the World Health Organization's (WHO) ten steps for successful breastfeeding recommendations at each level and stage of life. Breastfeeding support aims to promote nutrition-sensitive interventions on optimal breastfeeding practice for sustainable improvement in childhood nutrition status and development for further productivity later in life.

The implementing organization for breastfeeding supports are almost all ministries of a given country, nongovernmental organizations, public and private sectors need to take full responsibility to organize, implement monitoring, and evaluation of each intervention strategy. The implementation process started with the initiation of the intervention starting from need assessment, identification of the existing problem on optimal breastfeeding practice, and implementer and beneficiaries. Then planning the intervention should consider multisectoral collaborations and all possible factors at all stages. There are countless enabling factors starting from individual to policy level which need to design sustainable evidence-based implementation. Finally, the effectiveness of implementation should be monitored and evaluated using its indicators to measure optimal breastfeeding practice as an outcome and nutritional status as an impact indicator. These all processes should be guided by the triple A's cycle; Assessment, Analysis, and Action in order to measure the effectiveness and revise implementation strategies [16].

3.1 The 10 steps, for successful breastfeeding support

These steps should be addressed and implemented in all health care institutions with the aim to protect, promote and support breastfeeding for the well-being of future generations. The first two steps are critical management procedures and the remaining 8 steps are key clinical practices [17, 18].

3.2 Designing breastfeeding policy and routinely communicating to all healthcare staff

Policies to enhance exclusive breastfeeding in the first six months are the cornerstone interventions for the promotion of child survival and development. These include 6 months of paid maternity leave allowing women to continue breastfeeding for longer periods of time, designing strong legislation to control marketing on breast-milk substitutions, and prohibition of bottle feeding [7, 9]. All regulatory legislation must be shared with the respective health institutions and healthcare workers for its effective implementation and follow-up.

Findings from research show that longer maternity leave is associated with a longer duration of exclusive breastfeeding practice [18]. Countries with effective control on the marketing of breast milk substitutes and bottle feeding had a high rate of exclusive breastfeeding practice [9, 18]. Countries need to design strong policies and implementation plan with comprehensive programs, guidelines, and strategies that dramatically increase the rate of exclusive breastfeeding and the overall optimal breastfeeding practice.

The driving force for optimal breastfeeding practice at the policy level was multi-sectoral participation with political commitment, effective coordination of programs and strategies, designing contextualized intervention strategies, effective communication, advocacy and media coverage, adequate resource mainly finance, manpower, and time for implementation [18].

1. Ensure that health care providers at each level should have sufficient knowledge, competence and skills to support breastfeeding. Invest in exclusive breastfeeding protection, promotion, and support through training and capacity-building for health care providers [9].

2. Discuss the importance and management of breastfeeding with pregnant women and their families.

   Breastfeeding counseling should be provided during antenatal follow-up for pregnant women and their families at the institution and community level using community health workers/ health extension workers like Ethiopia to enhance optimal breastfeeding practice for better nutrition [7, 9].

3. Facilitate immediate and uninterrupted skin-to-skin contact and support mothers to initiate breastfeeding as soon as possible after birth.

4. Support mothers to initiate and maintain breastfeeding and manage common difficulties.

5. Give infants no food or drink other than breast milk in the first six months of life, unless medically indicated.

6. Practice rooming in – enable mothers and infants to remain together 24 hours a day in the first two years of life.

7. Support mothers to recognize and respond to their infant's cues for feeding.

8. Counsel mothers on the use and risks of feeding bottles, teats, and pacifiers.

9. Coordinate discharge so that parents and their infants have timely access to on-going support and care at home and community level [7, 18].

3.3 Breastfeeding support during pregnancy

Breastfeeding counseling during pregnancy has been linked to an increase in the likelihood of meeting breastfeeding intentions and practices during the postnatal period. Women who experienced supportive antenatal care practices were more likely to fulfill their prenatal breastfeeding intentions mainly initiation of breastfeeding within one hour and giving only breast milk in the first six months [19].

Counseling on breastfeeding during pregnancy improves maternal self-efficacy and knowledge and also helps in motivating the mother on early initiation and exclusive breastfeeding and timely initiation of complementary feeding. Such a knowledge change played a significant role in women's breastfeeding decisions and significantly improve optimal breastfeeding practices [20, 21].

The principles of implementation science need to be applied to learn how to scale up and sustain effective breastfeeding interventions while taking into account the needs and desires of women mainly focusing on the minority. Improvements in breastfeeding outcomes for women are likely to come from policy and community-level interventions provided through women's infant and child (WIC), healthcare facilities, and community agencies starting from pregnancy [22].

Comprehensive prenatal professional breastfeeding education for the mother and family plays a significant role in helping mothers' proficiency in breastfeeding attachment, proper positioning, and preventing nipple damage [23].

In general breastfeeding counseling and education during pregnancy have a significant role in improving knowledge, skill, and self-efficacy on optimal breastfeeding practice in the postnatal period as emotional, social, and cognitive domains play a substantial role in women's breastfeeding decisions and solve most breastfeeding problems later on. Such education should be provided using social behavior change models like the Health Belief Model, social cognitive theory, and theory of planned behavior by skilled professionals with compassionate and respectful care [20, 23, 24].

3.4 Breastfeeding support during labor and delivery

The place of delivery was the integral component for the promotion and actual implementation of optimal breastfeeding practices. Effective breastfeeding support during labor and delivery hospitalization is crucial for mothers to be able to achieve their breastfeeding goals [19].

For improving early initiation of breastfeeding encouraging women to give birth at public health institutes have a significant contribution. A study done on Cambodian women identified that the odds of timely initiation of breastfeeding were 57% times lower among women who gave birth at home compared to those who gave birth in public health facilities [25].

The global survey on early initiation of breastfeeding (EIBF) and its factors reported that only 57.6% of newborn starts breastfeeding immediately after birth. Complications during pregnancy, Cesarean delivery, and absence of postnatal/neonatal care guidelines at hospitals were factors affecting EIBF. Risk identification during pregnancy, minimizing elective cesarean delivery, and adhering to postnatal care guideline is the best intervention to support breastfeeding during labor and delivery [26].

Care immediately after birth in the health institution needs to make the hospital mother and baby friendly, encourage to start breastfeeding as soon as possible within an hour, encourage skin-to-skin contact for providing heat to the newborn, and to start effective breastfeeding [9, 18].

3.5 Breastfeeding support during post-natal period

Breastfeeding counseling is an effective public health intervention for optimal breastfeeding practice. Face-to-face repeated counseling starting from the prenatal period was mandatory. Breastfeeding counseling delivered at least four times in postnatal period was more effective than counseling delivered antenatally only and/or fewer than four times [27].

Breastfeeding support and education provided to mothers by health professionals and peers were associated with an increase in the duration of any and exclusive breastfeeding practices [28].

Breastfeeding counseling in postnatal period should include encouraging the mother to give breastmilk only day and night as often as the child wants or on average 8–12times in every 24 hours, providing practical breastfeeding support, checking position, attachment and suckling, helping the mother with breastfeeding problems and allowing mothers and infants to remain together 24 hours a day [7]. Empowering women through training and education to make them decision-makers on their life and get adequate and nutritious food for themand their child health.

Encouraging to empower community support, including mother support groups and community-based health promotion and education activities [7, 9]. Advise the mother to continue frequent, on-demand breastfeeding until 2 years of age or beyond [7].

3.6 Breastfeeding in exceptionally difficult circumstance

Children and families facing difficulty in breastfeeding require extra care and practical assistance. In such cases, mothers and infants should stay together and receive the assistance they require to use the best feeding technique. In almost all challenging circumstances, breastfeeding is still the preferred method of infant feeding option [7].

3.6.1 Breastfeeding support in HIV-infected women

One of the most important ways to increase infant survival is through breastfeeding, especially early and exclusive breastfeeding. WHO now advises that all HIV-positive individuals, including pregnant and nursing women, begin taking antiretroviral therapy (ART) as soon as they know they are infected with HIV [7].

Recommendations have been improved to take infants born to mothers who are HIV-positive into account. These infants can now breastfeed exclusively for at least six months and up to 12 months with a significantly lower risk of HIV transmission [7, 9].

3.6.2 Breastfeeding support in low-birth-weight or premature infants

Most low birth weight and preterm infants were admitted to Neonatal Intensive Care Unit (NICU) for further life and breastfeeding support. Despite the fact that breastfeeding is a top priority for low birth weight and preterm infants admitted to NICU, the hospitalized neonates' exclusive breastfeeding rates at 6 months were quite low and fell short of World Health Organization (WHO) recommendations. Families and mothers of hospitalized newborns should receive integrated counseling and support for breastfeeding on both a practical and psychological level [29].

Having baby friendly hospital to enhance breastfeeding adoption among mothers of low birth weight or preterm infants by interventions to improve early postpartum lactation and breastfeeding techniques like early initiation of milk expression significantly improves breastfeeding practice and the survival of infants. Support at the community and policy levels also have a significant role to improve breastfeeding, and the well-being of infants and their mothers [30, 31].

3.6.3 Breastfeeding support during illness

Optimal breastfeeding in general and exclusive breastfeeding for infants up to six months of age is recommended in preventing diarrhea and Acute Respiratory Infections (ARI)-specific morbidity and mortality. Infant with any illness should frequently breastfeed [32]. Exclusive breastfeeding with special protection is recommended during any illness of mother or infants including COVID-19 and HIV infection. Continued breastfeeding may offer passive immunity against any infection including COVID 19 and protect the infant, and vaccination against COVID-19 is safe and effective for pregnant and nursing women [33]. Breast milk sample from COVID-19 infected mothers finds negative result and most of the infant from infected mother has a negative result from COVID-19 infection. In this case, breastfeeding with general prevention precautions is recommended [34].

A systematic review on breastfeeding during infectious disease identified that breastfeeding in all infectious diseases is safe even in the case of HIV infection with adequate antiretroviral therapy (ART). Finally, it is recommended that initiating and continuing breastfeeding should continue to protect both mothers' and babies' health [35].

In general, breastfeeding practice can be affected by individual and community-level factors [11] and also policy-level factors [7]. Supporting breastfeeding in a sustainable way needs to implement with multisectoral participation in future research, policies, and practices in increasing breastfeeding rates in women and children [36]. Mothers who practiced exclusive breastfeeding should have higher information support from health facilities and the community [37].

Health care interventions that can be used to encourage and support breastfeeding includes two major areas; individual-level and system/ policy-level interventions. Individual-level interventions given to women and their supporters as well as system-level policies or maternity care practices aimed at fostering an environment supportive of breastfeeding are examples of interventions that can take place during pregnancy (prenatal), during labor and delivery (peripartum), or even after giving birth (postpartum) [28].

Individual-level interventions may consist of structured education, and professional or peer support. Breastfeeding support is typically provided in addition to general education and can take the form of direct support during breastfeeding observations as well as psychological and social support (encouraging the mother, assuring her, and discussing her questions and problems) [28]. Emotional, practical skill transfer and information support also have great contributions [37].

System-level interventions include policies or maternity care practices like the implementation of baby-friendly hospital initiatives or all or some of the 10 Steps to Successful Breastfeeding are examples of system-level interventions.

A written breastfeeding policy for the facility, provider or staff training in breastfeeding support, policies for implementing breastfeeding support groups, providing adequate maternity leave of at least for 6 months, encouragement of rooming-in, restrictions on using breastfeeding substitute, maintenance of skin-to-skin contact between the mother and child after birth, and encouragement of early breastfeeding initiation are some examples of these interventions [28].

4. Conclusion

Breastfeeding promotion and support are core indicators of infant and young child feeding practices for reducing infant morbidity and mortality. It can determine both the physical and mental growth and development of infants. Breastfeeding is highly recommended during illness and in any difficult situations to save the lives of the infant and promote maternal health. Breastfeeding support needs to be implemented at individual, community, and policy levels to improve the overall optimal breastfeeding practice for the well-being of the coming generation. It should be provided starting from pregnancy, during labor and delivery, and after birth.

Individual level intervention provided through counseling and education of the mother by professional or peer education and support. Structured education can include psychological, social, and direct support.

Community-level intervention includes improving knowledge of the importance and duration of breastfeeding, and promoting community-level antenatal and postnatal care service utilization. These all are demanded improving the lives of the infants and reduction of economic loss of the country.

Policy or system-level breastfeeding interventions should be focused on designing policies and strategies to improve breastfeeding practices such as maternity care practices, and implementation of all or some of the 10 steps to successful breastfeeding. Policies for six months of maternity leave, empowering women through education and employment, restriction in breast milk substitutes and bottle feeding, community breastfeeding support and promotion, worksite and child care policies and family leave policies.

Acknowledgements

The deepest gratitude goes to our family for their patience, support and unconditional love provided to us on writing this paper.

Funding

The authors received no specific funding for this work.

Conflict of interest

The authors declare no conflict of interest.

Acronyms and abbreviations

AAU	Addis Ababa University
ARI	Acute Respiratory Infections
ART	Antiretroviral Therapy
COVID-19	Coronavirus Disease 2019
EBF	Exclusive Breastfeeding
EIBF	Early Initiation of Breastfeeding
EPHA	Ethiopian Public Health Association
HIV	Human Immunodeficiency Virus
IQ	Intelligent Quiescent
NICU	Neonatal Intensive Care Unit
WHO	World Health, Organization
WIC	Women Infant Child

Author details

Yeshimebet Ali Dawed[1*], Shambel Aychew Tsegaw[2] and Erkihun Tadesse Amsalu[3]

1 Department of Nutrition and Dietetics, School of Public Health, College of Medicine and Health Sciences, Wollo University, Dessie, Ethiopia

2 MPH in Epidemiology and Biostatistics, Dessie Health Science College, Dessie, Ethiopia

3 MPH in Epidemiology and Biostatistics, Department of Epidemiology and Biostatistics, School of Public Health, College of Medicine and Health Sciences, Wollo University, Dessie, Ethiopia

*Address all correspondence to: ymaali32@gmail.com

References

[1] WHO. Guideline: Counselling of Women to Improve Breastfeeding Practices. Geneva: World Health Organization; 2018 Licence: CC BY-NC-SA 3.0 IGO

[2] Tschiderer L, Seekircher L, Kunutsor SK, Peters SAE, O'Keeffe LM, Willeit P. Breastfeeding is associated with a reduced maternal cardiovascular risk: Systematic review and Meta-analysis involving data from 8 studies and 11 92 700 parous women. Journal of the American Heart Association. 2022;**11**(2):e022746. DOI: 10.1161/JAHA.121.022746

[3] Fentahun M, Berhane Y, Tsui AO, et al. The Text Book of Reproductive and Child Health with Focus on Ethiopia and Other Developing Countries. First ed. Ethiopia: EPHA, AAU and JOHNSHOPKINS University; 2014. pp. 137-167

[4] WHO. Protecting, Promoting and Supporting Breastfeeding in Facilities Providing Maternity and Newborn Services: The Revised Baby-friendly Hospital Initiative 2018 Implementation Guidance. Frequently Asked Questions. Geneva: World Health Organization and the United Nations Children's Fund (UNICEF); 2020 Licence: CC BY-NC-SA 3.0 IGO

[5] WHO. Protecting, Promoting and Supporting Breastfeeding in Facilities Providing Maternity and Newborn Services. Geneva: World Health Organization; 2017

[6] Thomas JV. Barriers to Exclusive Breastfeeding among Mothers during the First Four Weeks Postpartum; 2016

[7] World Health Organization. Key Facts on Infant and Young Child Feeding. Geneva: World Health Organization; 2021. pp. 1-6. Available from: https://www.who.int/news-room/fact-sheets/detail/infant-and-young-child-feeding

[8] Victora CG, Bahl R, Barros AJ, França GV, Horton S, Krasevec J, et al. Breastfeeding in the 21st century: Epidemiology, mechanisms, and lifelong effect. Lancet. 2016;**387**(10017):475-490. DOI: 10.1016/S0140-6736(15)01024-7

[9] World Health Organization. Global nutrition targets. Breastfeeding Policy Brief. Geneva: World Health Organization; 2025. pp. 1-8. Available from: https://apps.who.int/iris/handle/10665/149022

[10] Dukuzumuremyi JPC, Acheampong K, Abesig J, Luo J. K knowledge attitude and practice of exclusive breast feeding among mothers in East Africa: A systematic review. International Breast-feeding Journal. 2022;**15**(70):1-17. DOI: 10.1186/s13006-020-00313-9

[11] Tsegaw SA, Dawed YD, Amsalu ET. Individual level and community level factors affecting exclusive breast feeding among infants under-six months in Ethiopia using multilevel analysis. Italian Journal of Pediatrics. 2021;**47**:106. DOI: 10.1186/s13052-021-01062-z

[12] Wake GE, Mittiku YG. Prevalence of exclusive breast feeding and its association with maternal employment in Ethiopia: A systematic review and meta-analysis. International Breastfeeding Journal. 2021;**16**(86):1-14. DOI: 10.1186/s13006-021-00432-x

[13] Dadich A, Piper A, Coates D. Implementation science in maternity

care: A scope review. Implementation Science. 2021;**16**(16):1-20. DOI: 10.1186/s13012-021-01083-6

[14] Vilar-Compte M, Perez-Escamilla R, Ruano AL. Interventions and policy approaches to promote equity in breast feeding. International Journal for Equity in Health. 2022;**21**:63. DOI: 10.1186/s12939-022-01670-z

[15] Brown M, Rosenthal M, Yeh DD. Implementation science and nutrition: From researchto practice. Nutrition in Clinical Practice. 2021;**36**(3):586-597. DOI: 10.1002/ncp.10677

[16] Tumilowicz A, Ruel MT, Pelto G, Pelletier D, Monterrosa EC, Karin Lapping K, et al. Implementation science in nutrition: Concepts and frameworks for an emerging field of science and practice. ASN, Current Developments in Nutrition. 2018:1-11

[17] Amoo BT, Popoola T, Lucas R. Promoting the practice of exclusive breast feeding: A philosophic scope review. BMC Pregnancy and Childbirth. 2022;**22**(1):380. DOI: 10.1186/s12884-022-04689-w

[18] WHO. Implementation Guide on Protecting, Promoting and Supporting Breastfeeding in Facilities Providing Maternity and Newborn Services: Implementing the Revised Baby-friendly Hospital Initiative. Geneva: World Health Organization (WHO); 2018

[19] Beauregard JL, Nelson JM, Li R, Perrine CG, Hamner HC. Maternity care practices and breastfeeding intentions at one month among low-income women. Pediatrics. 2022;**149**(4):e2021052561. DOI: 10.1542/peds.2021-052561

[20] Anaba UC, Johansson EW, Abegunde D, et al. The role of maternal ideations on breastfeeding practices in northwestern Nigeria: A cross-section study. International Breastfeeding Journal. 2022;**17**:63. DOI: 10.1186/s13006-022-00500-w

[21] Ahmad MO, Sughra U, Kalsoom U, Imran M, Hadi U. Effect of antenatal counselling on exclusive breastfeeding. Journal of Ayub Medical College, Abbottabad. 2012;**24**(2):116-119

[22] Segura-Pérez S, Hromi-Fiedler A, Adnew M, Nyhan K, Pérez-Escamilla R. Impact of breastfeeding interventions among United States minority women on breastfeeding outcomes: A systematic review. International Journal for Equity in Health. 2021;**20**(1):72. DOI: 10.1186/s12939-021-01388-4

[23] Gao H, Wang J, An J, et al. Effects of prenatal professional breastfeeding education for the family. Scientific Reports. 2022;**12**:5577. DOI: 10.1038/s41598-022-09586-y

[24] Shafaei FS, Mirghafourv M, Havizari S. The effect of prenatal counseling on breastfeeding self-efficacy and frequency of breastfeeding problems in mothers with previous unsuccessful breastfeeding: A randomized controlled clinical trial. BMC Women's Health. 2020;**20**(1):94. DOI: 10.1186/s12905-020-00947-1

[25] Harriott RM, Haile ZT, Chertok IRA, Haider MR. Association between place of birth and timely breastfeeding initiation among Cambodian women: A population-based study. International Breastfeeding Journal. 2022;**17**(1):54. DOI: 10.1186/s13006-022-00496-3

[26] Takahashi K et al. Prevalence of early initiation of breastfeeding and determinants of delayed initiation of breastfeeding: Secondary analysis of the WHO Global S. Scientific Reports. 2017;7:44868. DOI: 10.1038/srep44868

[27] McFadden A, Siebelt L, Marshall JL, Gavine A, Girard LC, Symon A, et al. Counselling interventions to enable women to initiate and continue breastfeeding: A systematic review and meta-analysis. International Breastfeeding Journal. 2019 Oct;**21**(14):42. DOI: 10.1186/s13006-019-0235-8

[28] Patnode CD, Henninger ML, Senger CA, Perdue LA, Whitlock EP. Primary Care Interventions to Support Breastfeeding: Updated Systematic Review for the U.S. Preventive Services Task Force. Rockville, MD: Agency for Healthcare Research and Quality; 2016

[29] Sokou R, Parastatidou S, Ioakeimidis G, Tavoulari EF, Makrogianni A, Isaakidou E, et al. Breastfeeding in neonates admitted to an NICU: 18-month follow-up. Nutrients. 2022;**14**(18):3841. DOI: 10.3390/nu14183841

[30] Dong D, Ru X, Huang X, Sang T, Li S, Wang Y, et al. A prospective cohort study on lactation status and breastfeeding challenges in mothers giving birth to preterm infants. International Breastfeeding Journal. 2022;**17**(1):6. DOI: 10.1186/s13006-021-00447-4

[31] Ward LP, Tonnis R, Otuneye AT, Clemens N, Akinbi H, Morrow AL. Impact of institutional breastfeeding support in very low-birth weight infants. Breastfeeding Medicine. 2021;**16**(3):238-244. DOI: 10.1089/bfm.2020.0137

[32] Abdulla F, Hossain MM, Karimuzzaman M, Ali M, Rahman A. Likelihood of infectious diseases due to lack of exclusive breastfeeding among infants in Bangladesh. PLoS One. 2022;**17**(2):e0263890. DOI: 10.1371/journal.pone.0263890

[33] Sakalidis VS, Perrella SL, Prosser SA, Geddes DT. Breastfeeding in a COVID-19 world. Current Opinion in Clinical Nutrition and Metabolic Care. 2022;**25**(3):188-194. DOI: 10.1097/MCO.0000000000000821

[34] Liu X, Chen H, An M, et al. Recommendations for breastfeeding during coronavirus disease 2019 (COVID-19) pandemic. International Breastfeeding Journal. 2022;**17**:28. DOI: 10.1186/s13006-022-00465-w

[35] Yeo S, Yang L, Ong K, Yong TT. Breastfeeding with infectious diseases. SAGE Journals Proceedings of Singapore Healthcare. 2022;**2022**:31. DOI: 10.1177/20101058221123395

[36] Houghtaling B, Byker Shanks C, Jenkins M. Likelihood of breastfeeding Within the USDA's Food and Nutrition Service Special Supplemental Nutrition Program for Women, Infants, and Children Population. Journal of Human Lactate. 2017;**33**(1):83-97. DOI: 10.1177/0890334416679619

[37] Agrina A, Afandi D, Suyanto S, Erika E, Dewi YI, Helina S, et al. Analysis of supporting factors associated with exclusive breastfeeding practice in the urban setting during the COVID-19 pandemic. Children (Basel). 2022;**9**(7):1074. DOI: 10.3390/children9071074

Chapter 16

Breastfeeding, the Importance of Education during Neonatal Hospitalization

Patricia Triviño Vargas

Abstract

In this chapter, scientific evidence is compiled in relation to the level of education that mothers need during their breastfeeding period and the importance of it. Studies are presented from a base on the promotion and protection of breastfeeding as well as from the publication of UNICEF, defends with conviction the rights of children in the promotion of parental care from around the world constituting the basis of human development to nursing care models for direct care. The nutrition, center of this work, which plays a key role in this development through the dietary needs of the organism since its inception and the way in which we, as health professionals, produce behavioral changes in lactating mothers. UNICEF in 2017 suggests a point of view of the wealth of nations to emphasize the promotion of health and invest in the development of breastfeeding. Therefore, breastfeeding is one of the most effective and cost-effective investments that nations can make for the health of their youngest members and the future health of their economies and societies. The tools that health professionals have for promotion and prevention of optimal nutrition from the newborn stage are those who through studies and research based on scientific evidence, such as Ramona Mercer's theory, they conclude that the mother achieves knowledge through multiple interventions highlighting the importance of health education. Consequently, health education and programs to promote breastfeeding constitute vital support to develop parental skills for parents.

Keywords: breast feeding, health education, infant nutrition, nursing model, neonatal hospitalization

1. Introduction

According to the Convention on the Rights of the Child, all infants and children have the right to good nutrition. The estimated number of child deaths due to malnutrition is 2.7 million, which represents 45% of all infant deaths. Infant and young child feeding is critical to improving child survival and promoting healthy growth and development. Accordingly, approximately 40% of infants from 0 to 6 months are exclusively breastfed. Optimal breastfeeding is of great importance as it saves the lives of more than 820,000 children under 5 years of age every year [1].

The World Health Organization (WHO) and UNICEF are concerned about the low prevalence of breastfeeding worldwide, despite the promotional campaigns they carry out. It is undoubtedly a challenge for health teams to focus their efforts on promoting this precious food from one human to another to create mutual benefit.

Breastfeeding is an unbeatable issue that provides perfect nutrition for infants, promoting healthy growth and development, reducing, and limiting the risk of contracting serious infectious diseases, therefore, reducing infant mortality and morbidity. As a result of that, it also favors women's health by reducing the risk of breast and ovarian cancer, and increasing pregnancy periods since it is a natural contraceptive method. In this sense, breastfeeding provides social and economic benefits to the family nucleus and why not say it, to a particular nation. For all that has been stated in the previous paragraphs, it is possible to provide most mothers with a feeling of satisfaction when it is carried out successfully and, according to recent research, they have found that these benefits increase with the exclusive nutrition of breastfeeding during the first few months, 6 months of life and later with solid and liquid food supplements [2].

The interventions of an educational program can result in positive behaviors toward exclusive and complementary breastfeeding. It has significantly influenced adherence to it and has collaborated in postponing feeding with infant formulas.

This review involves based on the latest and historical research that breastfeeding implies that it is not just a one-woman job, it requires encouragement and support from trained counselors, supportive family members, health care providers, employers, legislators, and others.

2. The importance of the promotion of breastfeeding

The publication of the Global Breastfeeding Collective in 2017 gives an account of the reasons why you should invest in the promotion of natural breastfeeding from a mother to her infant. It proposes that meeting this investment goal could save the lives of 520,000 children under the age of five and potentially create $300 billion in economic gains over 10 years because of reduced illnesses and costs of medical care, and the increase in the productivity of the population due to the cognitive development that is generated in this fundamental nutrition for the neuronal cell strengthening of the child population [3].

In this sense, within the statements issued by non-profit and governmental institutions, it is highlighted that breastfeeding from one human being to another is one of the most powerful and profitable investments that countries can manage in favor of health of people in their economies and societies. By not investing in breastfeeding, one is failing to provide ethical well-being to mothers and their babies and consequently generating lost lives and opportunities [4].

Consequently, through decades, the World Health Organization (WHO) actively promotes breastfeeding as the best source of nutrients for infants and young children, since it is an ideal way to provide them with the necessary nutrients for growth and development healthy. Exclusive breastfeeding is recommended for the first 6 months of life [5].

Breastfeeding upto the 6th month of life favors adequate growth and development, impacting avoidable causes of infant morbidity and mortality, regardless of socioeconomic level or maternal work. Infants who are not fully breastfed during the first 3–4 months of life are more likely to develop infections of the stomach and intestines, respiratory tract, and lungs, or develop ear infections. In addition, non-breastfed infants are more likely to be overweight or have diabetes later in life, and non-breastfeeding mothers are at increased risk of breast and ovarian cancer. For all this, a better knowledge of the benefits of breastfeeding is associated with earlier and greater initiation of lactation. Other practical benefits of breastfeeding include saving money in the purchase of breast milk substitutes and, for society, in the treatment of diseases [6].

2.1 Health education

On the other hand, health education and educational programs for fathers and mothers constitute one of those supports that the family needs to develop parental skills or abilities that allow them to face the vital task of being a father and mother.

Therefore, health education is developed in specific areas: prenatal intentions, breastfeeding experiences and support for the mother, this education affects the initiation or early suspension of breastfeeding.

The World Health Organization, already in 1989, specified that the recommendation and educational intervention on breastfeeding in support of mothers and their babies, carried out by health professionals, is related to the decision-making process, overcoming difficulties, and implementing adequate feeding practices. The key to the success of these processes is the interaction that occurs between the mother and the health professional.

Therefore, the educational recommendation and intervention is an example of a preventive connotation that emphasizes the interaction between mother/infant and a health worker, rather than the top-down approach often more characteristic of intervention-based types in education. Therefore, all counseling can be considered supportive, but not all supportive interventions include counseling [7].

WHO describes supportive counseling for mothers and infants by health workers to assist in decision-making, overcoming difficulties, and implementing optimal feeding practices [8].

Breastfeeding takes place during the postpartum period, which is a transition state from the stage of that close relationship between the mother and her daughter and the period of greater autonomy for both. The postpartum period is essential for the development of children, for the recovery of the mother, for learning parental functions, and for establishing the affective bond between newborns and their parents.

It is striking that various studies show the importance of certain predictive factors, determinants, barriers, influences, and contributing factors that act together and affect breastfeeding practices. These factors that influence maternal decisions are described at 3 levels, such as: individual, group, and social.

In turn, as a team that provides care, we must have a better understanding of how effective and functional it is to maintain exclusive breastfeeding at the time of neonatal discharge, focusing on health promotion and prevention for women, their families, and society. With this, we will have healthy and fit children for the society of the future. With the appropriate strategies to achieve an impact on the motivation and understanding of providing natural milk to infants, we solve and take charge of the questions of mothers who the potential donors of human milk for another human being.

The context is described, but not the problem, because you want to investigate this phenomenon, what is the need to investigate the subject?

2.2 Breastfeeding and its importance of historical evolution

Breastfeeding is an unparalleled way of providing excellent food for beneficial growth and development of infants, it is also an additional part of the reproductive process, with transcendental repercussions on the health of mothers. The analysis of scientific data has discovered that, at the population level, exclusive breastfeeding for 6 months is the imponderable form of feeding for the child population. They should subsequently start receiving additional foods, but not stop breastfeeding until 2 years or older [9].

Likewise, it determines a decrease in morbidity and mortality in the infant and the mother herself. Research in recent years shows that children who are breastfed have an increase in their cognitive capacity and present less frequently with different diseases such as bronchial asthma, atopic and gastrointestinal diseases, obesity, type I and II diabetes mellitus, and autoimmune diseases. Mothers benefit in the short and long term through natural contraception, greater recovery of weight prior to pregnancy, lower incidence of osteoporosis, and lower incidence of breast and ovarian cancer [10].

From a historical context, breastfeeding has been observed with many changes in relation to infant feeding. In ancient times, the only feeding alternative for newborns and infants was breast milk; if for some reason the biological mother could not breastfeed or decided not to, wet nurses or "nurses of pups" were used to fulfill that function.

While some cultures assumed breastfeeding in a natural and exclusive way, in Europe, between the 16th and 17th centuries, the use of wet nursing was encouraged among women from more affluent social classes, since it was not well seen that they breastfed, because this work gave them it took away beauty and negatively affected her figure. The wet nurses usually corresponded to low-income women, who lived with the family of the newborn, they were given lodging, food, and a salary for their services [11].

In the 19th century, there was an important change in relation to infant feeding, since mothers began to feed their children in a general way and, only in case of need, they sought out the wet nurse, who used to be highly valued. The feeding guidelines gained increasing concern since it was related to infant mortality. There was a movement in support of breastfeeding and human milk was defined as the healthiest food.

At the Academy of Medicine in Paris (1870) [12], there was a discussion about wet nurses and the promotion of breastfeeding by the mother herself to reduce infant mortality. The mother was held responsible for the direct upbringing of the children and mothers who did so were praised. It was accepted that milk could be affected both in quality and quantity, depending on the maternal diet, the characteristics of the home in which the mother lived, genital disorders, temperament, age, and the exclusivity of the child which was fed.

In the year 1890, the "Infant Clinics" and "The Drop of Milk" were created, these were two French initiatives based on an idea by Pierre Budin. They consisted of providing parents with information on food and hygiene issues in general so that they could care for their newborn and infant children. Then they spread throughout Europe. Sterilized mammalian milk subsidized partly by municipalities and partly by private charity was supplied daily, free, or semi-free [13].

At the end of the 19th century, when scientific development was in full swing, artificial milk formulas appeared, which claimed to satisfy all the nutritional needs of infants. In its beginnings, they were highly valued since they were chemically manufactured using all the available technology, which supported the quality of the preparations. The commercialization of these types of products and the medicalization of childcare established a propitious environment so that formula feeding was not only acceptable but also something desirable and normal.

During the 20th century, other factors were added that promoted the use of artificial milk, to the detriment of breastfeeding: urbanization, the incorporation of women to work, changes in family patterns, with smaller families and isolated generations. Previous; the appearance of the Human Immunodeficiency Virus (HIV), among others. The wet nurse disappears completely, especially in developed countries, and breastfeeding is very low. All these sociodemographic and cultural changes led to the lowest rates of breastfeeding in the United States at the beginning of the 1970s, reaching 25% at hospital discharge and close to 5% at 6 months of life.

Since the 1990s, breastfeeding has been increasing and currently, most mothers already choose this practice to feed their baby. However, its duration is short since after 3 months they switch to artificial feeding in a general way.

At the beginning of the 21st century, it is certain that breastfeeding will be compatible with modern and industrialized society, but social awareness is necessary, and the proven scientific advantages of breastfeeding are known, both for the newborn and for the mother. The media have a very important role in the transmission of aspects related to breastfeeding, in the education and awareness of people, and the dissemination of the laws and recommendations established by international organizations such as the WHO and UNICEF [14].

For several decades, work has been done to promote exclusive breastfeeding for up to 6 months of the child's life and up to 2 years of age, complemented with non-dairy food. The evidence gives an active position, aimed at the promotion and protection of breastfeeding [15].

2.3 Strategies for the promotion of breastfeeding in the field of public health

From the point of view of international evidence to promote breastfeeding, multiple studies have been conducted to assess the effectiveness of various interventions to promote the initiation and maintenance of breastfeeding. Those with the best methodological quality have been in systematic reviews, with or without meta-analyses, which take a critical look at primary studies and evaluate the weighted effect of interventions to promote breastfeeding [6].

According to the Balogun study, an updated review that includes 28 randomized controlled studies with 107,362 women, they analyzed interventions to promote breastfeeding in primiparous women in high-income developed countries: Australia, 1 study; UK, 4 studies and the USA, 14 studies and one middle-income country: Nicaragua, 1 study. Three studies studied the effect of an intervention to increase the number of women who started breastfeeding early, within one hour after birth. 76,373 women from Malawi, Nigeria, and Ghana participated in them. The Malawi study was large, with 55,931 participants.

It can be inferred from these studies that health education by health professionals, especially doctors and nurses, and peer counseling and support by trained volunteers, optimized the number of women who attempted to breastfeed their babies. Five investigations with 564 women reported in their results that women who received breastfeeding education and support from health professionals were more likely to start breastfeeding compared to women who received standard or conventional care. Four of these investigations were conducted in low-income or ethnic minority women in the United States, where baseline breastfeeding rates are generally low. Eight trials involving 5712 women showed better rates of breastfeeding initiation with volunteer-trained interventions and support groups compared with women receiving standard conventional care.

Breastfeeding health education and intervention delivered by trained volunteers could also improve rates of early initiation of breastfeeding within one hour after delivery in low-income countries [16].

Continuing with this study, it was concluded that health professionals with training in breastfeeding, including midwives, nurses, doctors, and trained volunteers can conduct educational sessions and provide peer counseling and support to increase the number of women who start breastfeeding their babies. More studies are needed in low- and middle-income countries to find out which strategies will encourage women to start breastfeeding right after birth.

On the other hand, in our country, the use of promotion strategies is a resource that has had positive consequences in the improvement of lactation rates. Since 1990, Chile has implemented different regular programs that promote breastfeeding, such as the WHO/UNICEF "Friendly Hospital for Children and Mothers," prenatal education workshops for pregnant women and their companions on breastfeeding issues. Breastfeeding, in addition to the Child Protection Program, called "Chile Crece Contigo" of Law 20,379, and finally training of health teams and creation of a breast milk bank, among other state and private benefits [16].

In 2011, the parental postnatal leave was increased from 12 to 24 weeks of maternity leave through parliamentary law 20.54514. National surveys that measure the prevalence of breastfeeding in Chile conducted between 1993 and 2002 revealed an increase in the prevalence of exclusive breastfeeding at the 6th month of life from 25% in 1993 to 43% in 2002. Significantly very auspicious and encouraging from a public health standpoint [17].

It was also observed that the prevalence of exclusive breastfeeding at the 6th month in women who worked outside the home was half that of those who stayed at home [18].

The last national survey on breastfeeding carried out by the Ministry of Health (MINSAL) in 2013, carried out in children aged 6–24 months who were cared for in the public health system, showed a national average of exclusive breastfeeding at the 6th month of 56%. These results show an increase in the duration of exclusive and complementary breastfeeding when comparing data from 1993 to 2013 [19].

There are other strategies that are probably effective, among them, the promotion of early attachment in maternity wards promoted by the Chile Crece Contigo Comprehensive Protection System and counseling or visits focused on breastfeeding carried out by professionals within the family health model. Investing in printed material and promotional packages for the population seems to be an ineffective strategy to promote breastfeeding. These resources should be redirected toward other strategies with a greater cost-effectiveness ratio, such as peer support, a modality that has not been implemented at the national level.

A systematically searched European study found that a mother's own maternal education is a protective factor in the decision-making of the type of breastfeeding that mothers will offer their children and that it will improve the maintenance of breastfeeding. The experience is better valued when this education is carried out by midwives through audiovisual methods in the first prenatal control visit, ideally to be carried out in the preconception visit, paying special attention to women with a lower level of education. The inclusion and participation of pregnant women in spaces where satisfactory breastfeeding is practiced help to start and maintain breastfeeding, as well as the distribution of simple guides to resolve doubts and complications during the first days. This is a type A recommendation after analyzing the studies carried out [20].

2.4 Elements of Ramona mercer's theory: mother-newborn-father support

In the circumstance of hospitalization of the newborn in neonatal care units, the educational intervention that the health professional needs to demonstrate is based on scientific evidence provided by the care models. Ramona Mercer's model would help in part to develop the process of acquiring nutritional knowledge in the newborn by its eager mother.

Nurses have recognized the importance of the process of becoming a mother (BAM) since studies Rubin's, 1967 [21]. This was based on Ramona Mercer's theory that requires extensive psychological, social and physical work toward mother. During this transition, a woman is more vulnerable and faces great challenges. Nurses have a unique opportunity to help women learn, gain confidence, and experience as they come to terms with their identity as mothers [22].

Four stages of the process of becoming a mother have been identified from nursing research reports: (a) commitment, attachment, and preparation during pregnancy to receive the newborn, (b) knowledge and attachment to the newborn (NB), learning the care of the NB and physical restoration during the first weeks after birth, (c) moving and advancing toward the normality of the first 4 months and (d) achievement of a maternal identity around 4 months of age of the infant. The stages are not discrete, they overlap in the maternal, infant, family, and environmental variables [23].

The adoption of the maternal role is a process that follows four stages of role acquisition. These stages have been adapted from Thornton and Nardi's 1975 research [24].

The four stages are: the first stage is anticipation, this stage begins during pregnancy and incorporates the first social and psychological adjustments to pregnancy. The mother generates the expectations of the role, speculates about it, establishes a relationship with the fetus that is in the intrauterine environment and the adoption of the role begins, then comes the formal stage that begins when the newborn is born and is included learning the role and its activation. Role behaviors are accommodated through the formal and agreed expectations of others in the mother's own social system, then the informal stage which begins when the mother develops with her own stamp when performing the role not transmitted by the social system. The mother creates her new role by settling into her lifestyle based on her previous experiences and her future goals, finally, the personal or identity stage of the role appears, where the mother internalizes her own maternal role. The woman feels an effect of harmony, confidence, and aptitude in the way she carries out the role, reaching her maternal role and adapting it to her new reality.

Mercer in 1995, designs a "Maternal Role Adoption" model situated in Bronfenbrenner's in 1979, concentric circles of the microsystem, mesosystem, and macrosystem. The original model proposed by Mercer was modified in 2000, changing the term exosystemic to mesosystem, which groups, influences, and interacts with people in the microsystem. Mesosystem interaction can influence what happens to the developing maternal role and to the child. The mesosystem includes daily care, the school, the workplace, and other entities found in the more immediate community [23].

The limited success of many of the interventions suggests that important areas of BAM have not been addressed, especially the relationship of the father with his newborn daughter or son and the mother, which would mean and determine the process of contention of the binomial, either in the interposition content on the process. For these reasons, the authors propose an expanded model of the complex

Aspect	Description
Author	Ramona T. Mercer
Theory	Becoming a mother (BAM)
Focus area	Obstetric nursing and maternal-infant care
Main goal	Understanding the experience and transition of women toward motherhood.
Key elements	1. Maternal commitment: The mother establishes an emotional commitment to her baby during the pregnancy. 2. Maternal learning: The mother acquires knowledge and skills related to the care and upbringing of the baby. 3. Development of a maternal role: The mother assumes the role of caregiver and establishes a unique relationship with her baby. 4. Maternal adaptation: The mother adjusts physically, emotionally, and socially to her new role.
Importance	It helps health professionals to understand and support the transition to motherhood, promoting quality maternal and childcare.
Applications	1. Prenatal and postnatal education for mothers. 2. Guidance and support in the transition to motherhood. 3. Development of nursing interventions focused on the needs of mothers during pregnancy and postpartum.
Criticisms and developments	Mercer's model has been widely used and accepted in the field of obstetric nursing, but it has also been the subject of debates and revisions to adapt to new realities and approaches in maternal and childcare. After years of research, Mercer has taken this process and simplified it making her theory one of the only theories available for studying and working with families after birth regardless of environment, age, health disparities or socioeconomic class [25].

Designed and made by Mg. Patricia Triviño- Vargas.

Table 1.
Summary of BAM theory by Ramona T. Mercer RN, PhD, FAAN.

elements involved in BAM and the related contextual effects (see **Table 1**). Even if no study can be expected to cover the scope of this model, it provides a structure for selecting key aspects of the transition to motherhood that may be of special significance in specific populations [26]. The mother, infant, and father are shown in the center of cooperating conditions that affect the process of becoming a mother and have the potential to facilitate or inhibit the process. These environment variables and attributes of the mother and infant are important concerns in both nursing interventions and future intervention research construct [26].

The importance of a conceptual base for health professionals in the orientation, guidance and education of mothers or main caregivers. Below is a summary of this important theory of care.

3. Final considerations

Clearly, the assertions and results of the investigations give consequently a positive effect on the knowledge and attitudes of the essential nutrient for infants such as breast milk. Among the findings, the percentage of schoolchildren who believed that breast milk is recommended for up to 2 years of life increased and that all mothers produce adequate milk to feed their child, based on the results of this study, the reference can be established that evidence on breastfeeding is given early before adolescents start life as a couple and include schoolchildren of both sexes in educational programs on breastfeeding because it is known that men will have a vital influence on the woman's decision about the feeding method for her child and the success or failure of lactation. Likewise, these educational intervention programs could be developed using new technologies, through the Internet, App, Social Networks, which could successfully replace traditional methods for the promotion of breastfeeding [27].

Breastfeeding is one of the most effective and cost-effective investments that nations can make for the health of their youngest members and the future health of their economies and societies [3].

In recent studies, political participation, poverty, employment, and income have been associated with breastfeeding practices at the state level and thus may make important contributions to maternal and child health. While peer, professional, and hospital lactation support were associated with state-level breastfeeding rates, only professional support—specifically, the presence of (International Board-Certified Lactation Consultants (IBCLC))—was substantially associated with breastfeeding rates after controlling for women's status. Increasing the number of IBCLCs in each state is an important strategy to make breastfeeding practices a reality in the USA [28].

It should be noted that we must pay attention to variables that can be worked on in such a way that we generate changes in positive and sustainable attitudes over time to enhance the nutrition of infants. These variables or factors that are associated with a longer period of exclusive breastfeeding were: higher maternal education, having a partner, knowledge of breastfeeding, belonging to a lower income level, having a delivery attended by a qualified team, and low birth weight. This study allowed a better understanding of the abandonment of exclusive breastfeeding based on its social determinants, providing evidence to implement more effective interventions for nutrition [29].

Consequently, health education, model theories of nursing, and programs to promote breastfeeding constitute vital support to develop parental skills for mothers and fathers in neonatal units or in any context that requires knowledge support to face the family task regarding nutrition, best for your children. It is a constant challenge for the mother and the consequence for the well-being of the infant.

Author details

Patricia Triviño Vargas
Austral University of Chile, Valdivia, Chile

*Address all correspondence to: patriciatrivino@uach.cl

References

[1] Victora CG et al. Breastfeeding in the 21st century: Epidemiology, mechanisms, and lifelong effect. The Lancet. 2016;**387**(10017):475-490. DOI: 10.1016/S0140-6736(15)01024-7

[2] Innocent Declaration On the Protection, Promotion and Support of Breastfeeding. 1990. Available from: htttp://waba.org.my/v3/wp-content/uploads/2019/04/1990-Innocenti-Declaration.pdf [Accessed: December 10, 2022]

[3] United Nations International Children's Emergency Fund (UNICEF). Nurturing the Health and Wealth of Nations: The Investment Case for Breastfeeding. Global breastfeeding investment case [Internet]. 2017. Available from: https://www.who.int/nutrition/publications/infantfeeding/global-bf-collective-investmentcase.pdf?ua=1

[4] World Health Organization (WHO). Press release. 2017. Available from: https://www.who.int/es/news-room/detail/01-08-2017-babies-and-mothers-worldwide-failed-by-lack-of-investment-in-breastfeeding

[5] World Health Organization. Protecting, Promoting, and Supporting Breast-Feeding: The Special Role of Maternity Services: A Joint WHO/UNICEF Statement. Geneva: World Health Organization; 1989

[6] Balogun O, O'Sullivan E, McFadden A, Ota E, Gavine A, Garner C, et al. Interventions for promoting the initiation of breastfeeding. The Cochrane Database of Systematic Reviews. 2016;**11**(11):CD001688. DOI: 10.1002/14651858.CD001688.pub3

[7] McFadden A, Siebelt L, Marshall J, Gavine A, Girard L, Symon A, et al. Counseling interventions to enable women to initiate and continue breastfeeding: A systematic review and meta-analysis. International Breastfeeding Journal. 2019;**14**:42. DOI: 10.1186/s13006-019-0235-8

[8] Kim S, Park S, Oh J, Kim J, Ahn S. Interventions promoting exclusive breastfeeding up to six months after birth: A systematic review and meta-analysis of randomized controlled trials. International Journal Nursing Studies. 2018;**80**:94-105. DOI: 10.1016/j.ijnurstu.2018.01.004

[9] IRIS PAHO Pan American Health Organization. "Infant and young child feeding: Model chapter for textbooks for students of medicine and other health sciences" [Internet]. 2010. Available from: https://www.paho.org/hq/dmdocuments/2010/IYCF_model_SP_web.pdf

[10] Bernard J, De Agostini M, Forhan A. Breastfeeding duration and cognitive development at 2 and 3 years of age in the EDEN mother-child cohort American Academy of Pediatrics. Grand Rounds. 2013;**29**(6):64. DOI: 10.1016/j.jpeds.2012.11.090

[11] De la Peña G. Evolution of breastfeeding throughout history. From the beginning of humanity to the present [Internet]. 2018. Available from: https://www.revista-portalesmedicos.com/revista-medica/evolucion-la-lactancia-materna-lo-largo-la-historia-desde-inicio-la-humanidad-la-present/

[12] Senior N. Aspects of infant feeding in eighteenth-century France.

Eighteenth-Century Studies. 1983;**16**(4): 367-388. DOI: 10.2307/2738104

[13] Muñoz PF. The implantation of the drops of Milk in Spain (1902-1935): A study from the historical press. Asclepius. 2016;**68**(1):131

[14] Rollins NC, Bhandari N, Hajeebhoy N, Horton S, Lutter CK, Martines JC, et al. Lancet breastfeeding series group. Why invest and what will it take to improve breastfeeding practices? Lancet. 2016;**387**:491-504. DOI: 10.1016/S0140-6736(15)01044-2

[15] American Academy of Pediatrics [Internet]. 2015. Available from: https://www.healthychildren.org/English/ages-stages/baby/breastfeeding/Pages/Where-We-Stand-Breastfeeding.aspx

[16] Atalah E. Current status of breastfeeding in Chile. Medwave. 2006;**6**(05):e3528. DOI: 10.5867/medwave.2006.05.3528

[17] Ilabaca J, Atalah E. Breastfeeding at the southern metropolitan health service. Revista Chilena de Pediatria. 2002;7:127-134. DOI: 10.4067/S0370-41062002000200004

[18] Atalah E, Castillo C, Reyes C. Effectiveness of a national program to promote breastfeeding in Chile 1993-2002. ALAN. 2004;**54**:374-379

[19] Ministry of Health (MINSAL). Technical report. National survey of breastfeeding in primary care (ENALMA) [Internet]. 2013. Available from: https://www.minsal.cl/sites/default/files/INFORME_FINAL_ENALMA_2013.pdf

[20] Martínez P, Martín E, Macarro D, Martínez E, Manrique J. Prenatal education and initiation of breastfeeding: Literature review. University Nursing. 2017;**14**:54-66. DOI: 10.1016/j.reu.2016.11.005

[21] Rubin R. Attainment of the maternal role. Part 1. Processes. Nursing Research. 1967;**16**:237-245

[22] Mercer RT. Nursing support of the process of becoming a mother. Journal of Obstetric, Gynecologic, and Neonatal Nursing. 2006;**35**:649-651. DOI: 10.1111/j.1552-6909.2006.00086. x

[23] Raile M, Marriner A. Models and Theories in Nursing. 8th ed. Barcelona, Spain: Elsevier; 2015. p. 600

[24] Weidman JC, Twale DJ, Stein EL. Socialization of graduate and professional students in higher education: A Perilous Passage? ASHE-ERIC Higher Education Report. Vol. 28, No 3. Jossey-Bass Higher and Adult Education Series; 2001

[25] Noseff J. Theory usage and application paper: Maternal role attainment. International Journal of Childbirth Education. 2014;**29**(3):58-61

[26] Mercer RT, Walker LO. A review of nursing interventions to foster becoming a mother. Journal of Obstetric, Gynecologic, and Neonatal Nursing. 2006;**35**(5):568-582. DOI: 10.1111/j.1552-6909.2006.00080. x

[27] Hernández C, Díaz-Gómez M, Romero M, Díaz M, Rodríguez V, Jiménez A. Effectiveness of an intervention to improve breastfeeding knowledge and attitudes among adolescents. Revista Española de Salud Pública. 2018;**92**:e201806033

[28] Yourkavitch J, Hall SP. Women's status, breastfeeding support, and breastfeeding practices in the United

States. PLoS One. 2022;**17**(9):e0275021. DOI: 10.1371/journal.pone.0275021

[29] Arocha G, Caicedo B, Forero L. Economic, social, and health determinants that influence exclusive breastfeeding in Colombia. Cadernos de Saúde Pública. 2022;**38**(9):e00186621. DOI: 10.1590/0102-311XES186621